WITHDRAWN

Personal, Marital, and Family Myths

Personal, Marital, and Family Myths

Theoretical Formulations and Clinical Strategies

DENNIS A. BAGAROZZI, Ph.D.
STEPHEN A. ANDERSON, Ph.D.

W·W·NORTON & COMPANY · NEW YORK · LONDON

Published simultaneously in Canada by Penguin Books Canada Ltd.,
2801 John Street, Markham, Ontario L3R 1B4.

Printed in the United States of America.

First Edition

Library of Congress Cataloging-in-Publication Data

Bagarozzi, Dennis A.
  Personal, marital, and family myths : theoretical formulations and
  clinical strategies / Dennis A. Bagarozzi, Stephen A. Anderson.
    p. cm.
  "A Norton professional book."
  1. Family psychotherapy. I. Anderson, Stephen A. (Stephen Alan),
1948-   . II. Title.
RC488.5.B27 1989
616.89'156—dc19   88-37213
                                                                    CIP

ISBN 0-393-70065-8

W. W. Norton & Company, Inc., 500 Fifth Avenue, New York, N. Y. 10110
W. W. Norton & Company Ltd., 37 Great Russell Street, London, WC1B 3NU

1 2 3 4 5 6 7 8 9 0

To my loving parents, Joseph H. Bagarozzi and Anna Bagarozzi.

—DAB

To my wife Beth, whose patience, support and perseverence throughout this project reached new heights, and to my children, six-year-old Jacklyn and four-year-old Nathan, who frequently questioned why my one book took so long when each of their many books took only an afternoon to write.

—SAA

Foreword

RECENTLY A FAMILY I was scheduled to see for a first visit "no showed." While waiting for them to arrive, I started doing busywork. I'd wanted to purge my office of some outdated materials in order to make room for some newer additions to my library. As I was separating some of the wheat from the chaff of my hundreds of family therapy titles, it somehow struck me in a way it never had before just how much chaff there was on my bookshelves. Just how many of these books (among the ones I'd read, to be fair) actually offered an innovative perspective? How many had I read and come away certain that I had actually learned something new? How many of them were actually readable?

Thank heavens Dennis Bagarozzi asked me to write this foreword. Because, in order to write it, I had to read *Personal, Marital, and Family Myths*, and in reading it, I have found some of the most creative thinking and writing to appear in this field in years. And some of the most readable: *Myths* is erudite, yet humane; rigorous, yet literary. It is simply a gem. Bagarozzi and Anderson have a rare capacity to bring to bear around a single central theme coherent conceptualization, sound applied empiricism, and compassionate, perceptive clinical reflection.

Had I written this book, I would have called it, "Myths: An Organizing Principle for Integrative Family Therapy." Not really, because a title like that wouldn't help to sell many copies. But that is what the book is really about. It offers, more by example than by exhortation, one of the most persuasive arguments for the wisdom of integrative thinking and practice available to date. There are few writings in family therapy—or anywhere else in psychotherapy—that make it so clear that, once one opens oneself up to the *possibility* of integration, one finds that previously perceived obstacles to integration exist in the mind of the therapist, not in the essential nature of the human clinical phenomena at hand.

Thus, Bagarozzi and Anderson can write fluidly and synergistically about the cognitive, behavioral, psychodynamic, and systemic aspects of myths, not only because they write well, but also because these parameters are inherently fluid and synergistic, inherently complementary and mutually reinforcing. *Myths* provides an organizing framework not only horizontally, i.e., about marital and family relationships in the present, but also vertically, i.e., across time, as it presents a sort of conceptual glue that holds together the multiple levels on which families interact in the present with their personal, marital, and familial experience of change over the life cycle. Thus, not unlike object relations theory, from which (among other theories) the authors derive a good deal of practical wisdom, the style and focus of the therapy based on the centrality of myths in everyday life is pervasively developmental.

Given their integrative biases, the approach to treatment Bagarozzi and Anderson set forth is both structured and open-ended. They provide a perspective on therapy which cannot be easily hooked into only by therapists who rigidly adhere to puristic devotion to single-minded theory-building and clinical practice. But Bagarozzi and Anderson are not merely sophisticated synthesizers; they also compose a lot of their own original music. While, quite frankly, I am not personally inclined to spend nearly as much time in therapy on historical material as these authors, I found their various semistructured interview guidelines for assessing and mapping patients' myth schemata (Family Relations History; Personal Myth Assessment interview; Ideal Child Profile interview) truly fascinating and extraordinarily comprehensive. I am certain that reading just those guidelines (let alone the rest of the book) will have an enduring and enhancing impact on my clinical work. Despite still having overcrowded bookshelves, this is one book that I will be sure to make space for and to place within arm's reach.

Alan S. Gurman, Ph.D.
Professor of Psychiatry
University of Wisconsin
Medical School
Madison, Wisconsin

Contents

Preface

W E THOUGHT IT MIGHT be interesting to readers if we prefaced our explorations into the exciting world of personal, marital, and family mythologies by sharing some of our own memorable experiences with these phenomena. Dennis begins:

I grew up in the bosom of a large, extended Italian-American family system. During my childhood, religious holidays such as Christmas and Easter were always filled with great joy, excitement, and anticipation. Typically, relatives from throughout New York's five boroughs and surrounding states would travel to Manhattan to pay their respects to my maternal grandmother, Christina. The events that I describe below stand out in my mind as very significant, not only because of their symbolic and emotional content, but also because of the fascination and interest in family processes and dynamics that they engendered in me.

I remember this incident as clearly as if it happened yesterday. I could not have been more than 12 years old that bitter cold and snowy Christmas night when these events took place. The women—my aunts, female cousins, and my mother—had all gathered with my grandmother in her kitchen. The men folk had segregated themselves from the females and were relaxing in the living room after their traditional Christmas dinner at my grandmother's. Suddenly, a hush came over the women. An aunt who had been estranged from my grandmother for some time entered the room. Behind her came her eight-year-old daughter, whom she led by the hand. They stopped and stood before my grandmother. With tears in her eyes, she asked grandmother for a special favor. Speaking in the Neapolitan dialect we all understood, my aunt called her daughter to her and presented her to my grandmother. The child had been ill, suffering from a fever of undetermined origin. My aunt was afraid that a spell had been cast upon the child—that a "fattucchiera" or "sorceress" had given her "malocchio," the "evil eye."

It was then that I heard an old Italian woman who was visiting my grandmother refer to her as a "malucchiara," a woman who has the power to take away or remove evil spells. Timidly, the child approached my grandmother, who welcomed her with outstretched arms and a smile that engulfed the whole gathering. She placed her left hand on the child's forehead, stroked it lightly with her thumb, and began to chant softly. The child's eyes began to close and so did my grandmother's. You could see the tenseness leave the girl's body as my grandmother continued to chant. Gradually, the chant became a prayer. The prayer then merged into another chant. The women stood motionless. Suddenly, my grandmother began to yawn and sigh, a sure sign that my young cousin had indeed been a victim of "malocchio." Grandmother's yawning became intense and the child became weak. A stool was brought for my cousin, but no one touched her. Grandmother then turned to one of her daughters and asked her for a sharp object, a knife or a pair of scissors. A knife was brought to her immediately. She took the knife in her right hand, its point directed away from the child and down toward the floor. Slowly she began to circle the child's head with the knife. As she moved the knife in a clockwise direction, the circles became larger and larger and her yawning and sighing intensified. Suddenly, she stopped her chanting, made a large counterclockwise circle with the knife and flung it to the floor—piercing the evil eye. The child swooned and appeared to faint. She was quickly ministered to by her mother and some other women who rushed in with a glass of water.

Grandmother said that someone who was jealous of the child's beauty had wished her evil. Hearing these words, my young cousin (who was not the prettiest of little girls) beamed. Her fever had broken and she no longer had a headache. Her mother, my aunt, was welcomed back into the fold by the other women. The family rift had been healed and my not-too-pretty cousin felt much better, both physically and psychologically.

Steve's recollection is quite different from Dennis':

I was about 16 years old. I had just left my somewhat rural, somewhat suburban home and headed for my favorite spot, a quiet rocky area in the woods about half a mile away. That afternoon I had had a typical falling out with my father on one of the rare occasions when he was home. My mother had attempted to solace me in her protective way while carrying on her own heated exchanges with him. The encounter was familiar and painful. I felt very confused, lonely, and empty as I sat on the rocks. I felt I had nowhere to turn.

It was many years later when I understood why that event had remained so vivid in my memory. I had internalized my family's intergenerational legacy of the strong, silent, independent male facing life on his own, the hero who braves all trials and yet continues the search to understand the emptiness and transcend the pain. My father and his father before him had chosen alcohol as their solution. I chose martial arts, psychology and the study of myths to unravel my own life and to connect with a sense of wonder and mystery greater than myself.

1

Foundations and Theoretical Underpinnings

ANTONIO FERREIRA (1963) first coined the term "family myth." He defined family myths as a series of well integrated beliefs shared by all family members. He postulated that these beliefs prescribe the complementary role relationships that all participants are required to play vis-à-vis other family members. For Ferreira, the family's myth was thought to be the focal point around which all family processes revolved. He described how these beliefs and roles went unchallenged by family members in spite of the reality distortions required in order to keep the myth intact. The family myth was conceptualized as the way the family appears to its members (insiders), not the way the family is viewed by others (outsiders). Myths were thought to offer a rationale for familial behavior while concealing their true motives, i.e., their homeostatic and defensive functions (Ferreira, 1966). Family myths also were seen as providing ritual formulas for action at certain defined crisis points in the family's development. The regularity with which these ritualized patterns appeared in families led Ferreira to speculate about their importance as overt manifestations of covert family rules used to maintain the family's status quo.

Our views of family myths (Anderson & Bagarozzi, 1983; Bagarozzi and Anderson, 1982) differ significantly from those originally postulated by Ferreira. For example, we do not believe that family myths remain static, that their sole purpose is to maintain a homeostatic balance, that myths are consciously shared by all family members, and that there exists only one family myth serving as a focal point around which the family process revolves. In our research and clinical work with well families and severely distressed family systems, we have come across a few instances where Ferreira's observations seem to have been borne out. However, we found these to be the exceptions rather than the rule.

In our work and in our discussions with other clinicians (in the United States and abroad) who share our fascination with family myths, we confirmed what we had suspected when we first began our investigations: Families have a variety of myths which continually change and evolve with the passage of time and the unfolding of the family life cycle. Furthermore, these myths exist at various levels of individual (personal) consciousness and group (family) awareness. Indeed, some myths are persistent and serve a homeostatic function, but this does not make them dysfunctional. Negative feedback is essential for the maintenance and stability of any system. On the other hand, some myths promote change, growth, and development. These can be seen as positive feedback loops which enable the system to remain viable. It is our contention that family myths are universal and not necessarily pathological. Their functionality can be determined only by assessing the degree to which they contribute to or curtail the growth and development of each family member and the family system as a whole.

Family myths are comprised of a number of interrelated components and processes. These include:

1. The personal myths of each spouse. Frequently personal myths include a number of intergenerational themes.
2. Conjugal myths which begin to take shape during the dating-courtship-engagement process.
3. Family group myths which emerge from the meshing and integration of all family members' personal myths, the conjugal myths of the spouses, parents' expectations for their children, and the shared experiences of all family members as a family group.

The development of personal, conjugal, and family myths will be dealt with in later chapters. General formulations and definitions of myths are discussed below.

DEFINITIONS OF MYTHS

Our primitive ancestors, during the dawn of consciousness, made little distinction between an objective, law-governed, external universe and their own internal world of subjective experiences. Boundaries between conscious and unconscious experiences were blurred, indistinct, porous and fluid. Awareness of the self as a separate entity with an independent existence apart from one's primary group was achieved only by a select few—the heroes of myth and legend (Neumann, 1954a, 1954b). During these primeval times, probably the closest the average person came to such awareness was to distinguish what was sacred from what was profane or secular. However, this distinction was largely fluid and unpredictable, except when it was crystallized by some definite symbol, rite, ritual, story, or some priestly authority (Wheelwright, 1962). Whenever an aspect of life and existence was seen as problematic or fraught with anxiety or danger, and hence found to be extraordinary, it entered the realm of the sacred, mystical, magical and mysterious (Perry, 1966).

In order to make some sense of and bring order to this confluence of experiences, stories or myths were created. For our ancestors, these mythological explanations were truth. Each story, each myth gave meaning and purpose to specific aspects of everyday life and existence. In addition to prescribing behavior, myths also proscribed action. To go against the wisdom of the myth was to tamper with a preordained order. To stray from this predetermined path was to step beyond the bounds of one's "Moira." For the ancient Greeks, such behavior constituted the unpardonable sin of "hubris," excessive pride. Such action could lead only to personal and familial catastrophe (e.g., the stories of Oedipus and Orestes). Myths were regarded as demonstrations of an inner meaning and order of the cosmos and in human existence (Watts, 1954). They were attempts to explain a perception or experience and, at the same time, to justify that very perception.

Magical rituals evolved in conjunction with these myths. Their meaning and purpose varied with the needs of the individual or group. Some rituals were devised to insure that cosmic harmony and order were maintained. Others were meant to bring about desired changes or to influence the course of natural events (Frazer, 1942). Essentially, rituals can be seen as being either predominantly homeostatic or morpho-genetic.

Very much like our primitive forebears, we are born into and raised by a family group from which we must separate and individuate. As we attempt to master each successive developmental task, to disentangle thoughts from feelings, to develop a true self (as opposed to a false or pseudo self), to free oneself from the enmeshed confines of an undifferentiated family ego mass (Bowen, 1978), to achieve self-realization (Jung, 1940), and to actualize our inherent potentials (Maslow, 1954, 1962; Rogers, 1951, 1961), we create our own personal mythology, complete with attendant rituals, rites, and taboos. Our individual struggles with differ-

entiation and self realization can be conceptualized as a personal recapit-
ulation of our primitive ancestors' struggles to free themselves from the
confines of the participation mystique and to separate the self from an all
encompassing, preconscious existence in the primal group (Neumann,
1954a, 1954b).

Knox (1964) identified four characteristics of myths. Although he discusses these basic characteristics in terms of their importance to groups
and communities, we have found them to be central to the formation of
personal, conjugal and family myths as well. For example:

1. Myths are stories, imaginative narratives, that deal with cosmically
significant acts of gods or superhuman beings, i.e., heroes. A cosmically
significant act or event is an act of decisive importance for the world,
especially for the world of humans, whose response to it may have taken
place in prehistoric or historic epochs. However, it recounts particular
actions taking place at particular times.

Personal identification with a particular hero or character in a myth/
story plays an essential part in the development of one's personal mythology. For example, the late Reverend Martin Luther King Junior was
named after the German theologian who led the Protestant Reformation.
The reformation King spearheaded, although social and political, drew
strength from his identification with other religious revolutionaries (e.g.,
Christ, Moses and Gandhi). Shortly before his assassination, King's personal identification with Moses became evident in the famous speech in
which he metaphorically stated that he had "been to the mountain top"
and had seen "the promised land." In his identification with Jesus
Christ, King knew his fate. He was driven by forces larger than himself,
compelled to live his life to its inevitable conclusion. Such is the power of
one's personal mythology.

Time after time, in clinical practice, we have seen a person overcome
by the power of his/her personal mythology. Such a man/woman seems
possessed, driven, compelled to behave in a particular fashion. As if in a
dream or surrealistic passion play, the person goes through various ritualistic behavior patterns in an attempt to relive and resolve some conflict
or to master a particular life task.

2. Myths always have their source in the common life and experiences of
a particular human community. They will bear the mark of that community's culture and persist over generations as part of its tradition.

This second characteristic proposed by Knox (1964) addresses the communal and intergenerational nature of myths. In some instances, an
individual's or family's mythology may be inextricably tied to a common

group, ethnic, racial, or religious identification and experience. For example, it would be extremely difficult, if not impossible, to separate one's Jewishness or one's blackness from the self-concepts, personal themes, and conjugal/family mythologies that Jews and black Americans develop and pass down to succeeding generations.

3. The community will prize the story/myth because it suggests and answers something distinctive and important in human existence and particularly in the community's existence.

One needs only to turn to the beliefs and doctrines of any religious group or community to find numerous examples of this third characteristic. However, this characteristic may be less evident in the structure of personal, conjugal and family myths.

In our work with individuals, couples and families, the "suggested answer" to a particular problem usually appears in the form of a person's, couple's or family's agreed-upon belief system. However, this agreement may not be consciously acknowledged or recognized. More will be said about this process later in this volume.

4. Because of the relation in which the story stands to the actual existence of the community, it will become an inseparable and indispensable part of the community's life and, for those sharing in that life, an irreplaceable symbol.

Myths, whether personal, familial, cultural or universal, persist and are passed down from generation to generation because the message they carry is thought to be critical for the survival of the individual, the group to which he/she belongs, or the species. In some instances, belief in a particular myth and the performance of certain rituals associated with the myth are thought to be necessary for the survival of an entire people (e.g., the ancient Mayans practiced human sacrifice daily in order to insure that the sun would rise). One way to conceptualize myths, therefore, is to consider them as supernatural explanations which legitimize, justify and preserve personal values, behaviors, norms and mores of a given individual, family, group, community and society. Myths serve the additional function of externalizing and objectifying those shared phenomena which are problematic and incomprehensible. In doing this, myths also foster group identity and cohesion.

It is impossible to separate an individual's personal myths from those of his/her family, community and culture. In our work, we focus our attention on understanding one's personal myths in terms of how they affect relationships with significant others in the context of marital/family systems. Individuals, couples and families are seen as actively selecting and adopting, as their own, those cultural myths whose various components, symbols, rituals, etc., have meaning and importance for each family member and the marital/family system as a whole. These cultural myths are modified and reworked by the individual in ways that fit into his/her personal mythology. In this way, they are used to maintain one's self-concept and preserve one's personal integrity. Similarly, cultural myths are used to stabilize the organizational structure of marital/family systems and maintain predictable patterns of interaction between and among family members. In a true systemic fashion, this process also works to reinforce and stabilize the cultural myths themselves. Modification of personal, conjugal, family and cultural myths can come about gradually, according to the step function (Ashby, 1954; Watzlawick, Beavin, & Jackson, 1967), or abruptly through second order changes (Watzlawick, Weakland, & Fisch, 1974) or discontinuous leaps (Hoffman, 1981).

THEORETICAL UNDERPINNINGS

Our orientation to individual behavior and systems functioning relies heavily upon developmental theories and principles. For example, we accept that:

1. Development progresses in an orderly and predictable fashion. Although the rates of development may differ from individual to individual and from system to system, the progression remains orderly and predictable.
2. Individuals and systems pass through a series of hierarchically ordered and invariantly sequenced stages.
3. Each stage contains a series of developmental tasks that must be resolved completely if the individual, couple, family, etc., is to proceed successfully to the next higher level of development. Each stage can be conceptualized as constituting a critical period.
4. Developmental tasks present themselves in four interrelated domains: biological and maturational, psychological, learning and cultural. Developmental tasks that are not successfully mastered persist as issues to be resolved and affect the successful resolution of all successive developmental tasks encountered throughout the life of the individual or system.
5. Development does not occur in a vacuum. It is the product of the dynamic interaction of the system with its environment.

6. Development consists of the simultaneous and compatible processes of differentiation and integration.
7. Each developing system utilizes morphogenetic processes as well as homeostatic processes in its progression toward maturity and greater complexity.

In their classic work, *Systems of Psychotherapy: A Comparative Study*, Ford and Urban (1963) put forth some basic assumptions about the practice and evaluation of psychotherapy. Later, these authors elaborated on their formulations in Bergin and Garfield's (1971) *Handbook of Psychotherapy and Behavior Change: An Empirical Analysis*. Essentially, these clinical researchers postulate that:

1. The practice of psychotherapy must be rooted in a more general theory of human behavior and human development.
2. Theoretical statements are needed to account for how unwanted behavior or undesirable behavior patterns develop.
3. Theoretical statements are needed to explain how and why such unwanted and undesirable behavior patterns are maintained.
4. A theory of therapy (which is internally consistent with this theory of human behavior and deviance) should specifically identify reliable procedures designed to correct those interactional or developmental processes that have gone awry.
5. Increased understanding and effectiveness of theories of psychotherapy rest upon the systematic and rigorous application of the scientific method of inquiry and evaluation.

We sincerely believe that the practice of marital and family therapy should be guided by the five principles outlined above. Therefore, it is essential that any theory of marital/family behavior and development rest upon, and be consistent with, a theory of individual development, relationship formation, and marital/family development across the marital/family life cycle. The theories of individual development that have most influenced our conceptualizations of cognitive functioning and the nature and content of developmental tasks that become the central foci of various themes later interwoven into one's personal mythology are based upon the seminal works of Erikson (1950, 1968) and Flavell (1963, 1985), Freud (1913, 1927, 1963a, 1963b), Kohlberg (1963, 1964, 1966, 1969), Piaget (1926, 1928, 1929, 1930, 1932, 1952, 1954) and Sullivan (1953, 1954). Unresolved developmental tasks also manifest themselves as drives, needs, and motives. When viewed as such, personal myths and their interwoven themes can be conceptualized according to the theories of Maslow (1954, 1962) and Murray (1938). However, in our work with severely disturbed personality disorders, such as narcissistic characters and borderline personalities, we have found it most helpful to use theories of personality formation that have been developed specifically for understanding and treating such individuals (e.g., Grotstein, 1981; Gunderson & Singer, 1975; Jacobson, 1964; Kaplan, 1980; Kernberg, 1967, 1968, 1970, 1974a, 1974b, 1975, 1978, 1980; Klein, 1932, 1975; Kohut, 1965, 1966, 1968, 1969, 1971, 1977; Mahler, 1963, 1965; Mahler & Kaplan, 1977; Mahler & Lapierre, 1965; Mahler & McDevitt, 1968; Mahler, Pine, & Bergman, 1970; Masterson, 1972, 1975, 1981, 1985; Masterson & Costello, 1980; Stone, 1980; Winnicott, 1965; Zetzel, 1970). Our theoretical orientation concerning the nature of systems development and systems functioning draws heavily upon the works of Buckley (1967, 1968), Lewis (1972), Miller (1971a, 1971b), Speer (1970), and von Bertalanffy (1968).

The logical links between individual dynamics and systems dynamics must be shown in order for any theory of marital/family behavior and therapy to be given serious consideration. For us, the logical link between individual dynamics and marital/spousal dynamics is seen in the meshing of personal themes and myths between prospective mates. The processes by which personal myths develop and evolve into conjugal and family myths are described in subsequent chapters. In the following chapter, we offer some additional formulations regarding the major characteristics and structures of myths.

2

Myths: Major Characteristics
and Structures

K NOX (1964) PROPOSED that myths are irreplaceable symbols. However, to
say that myths are symbols is to simplify their true structure. For
us, it is more accurate to say that the symbol is only one component of
the myth and that myths are composed of a complex of symbols, rituals,
themes and stories, each standing in intricate and frequently contradictory and paradoxical relationships to each other. In addition to symbols,
myths make use of analogies and metaphors to put forth their meanings.
A brief discussion of these concepts is offered below.

SYMBOLS AND MYTHS

In order to fully comprehend the true nature of symbols and the fascinating processes associated with their formation and development, it is
essential for the reader to have some basic understanding of primary
process thinking (Freud, 1963b). Essentially, primary process thinking
takes place unconsciously and is not governed by the laws of logic. The
type of thinking associated with primary process was thought to be the
original way in which the primitive psychic apparatus functioned. Freud
and his colleagues believed that the id functioned according to primary
processes throughout life and that the ego did so during the first years of
life when its organization was immature and still much like that of the
id.

In primary process thinking, representations by allusion or analogy are
frequent and any part of an object, person, memory, or idea may be used in
place of the whole. Conversely, any whole object, person, memory, or idea
may be substituted for its parts. In addition, several different thoughts,
ideas, objects, concepts, etc., may be represented by a single thought,

idea, object, concept, etc. Verbal representation is rare, and visual or other sense impressions often appear in place of the spoken word. Indeed, an entire paragraph may be condensed into one visual representation.

In primary process thinking there is no time. It is always the present. There is no such thing as a logical sequence of events. Before and after do not exist. Present, past and future stand together side by side. Thoughts, ideas, or concepts are not subject to mutual contradictions; good and evil, black and white, right and wrong, back and front, male and female, yes and no, up and down, all exist together in harmony without the slightest bit of conflict, confusion or contradiction. Finally, primary processes substitute psychic reality for external reality. Whatever occurs psychically is real. There is no distinction between what is fantasized and what actually takes place.

The predominant mode of expression in primary process thinking is the symbol. Symbols are relatively stable and repeatable elements of perceptual experiences that stand for some larger meaning or set of meanings which cannot be given or fully communicated through perceptual experiences (Wheelwright, 1962). Symbols cannot be entirely or explicitly stated, since their essential quality draws life from a multiplicity of associations, subtly and for the most part unconsciously interrelated. The symbol and things associated with it are joined in the past, so that there are accumulated potential meaning and significance available for elaboration when the symbol is explored. Symbols may be personal or shared by a couple, family, community or society. Symbols may also develop ancestral significance by being shared over generations within a particular family or group. Finally, symbols may be archetypal, in that they have significance for all or a major portion of humankind throughout history (Jung, 1951, 1953, 1954, 1956, 1959, 1960, 1961, 1973). The relationship of symbols to myth is well established (Bettelheim, 1976; Campbell, 1949; Graves, 1955a, 1955b; Jung & Kerenyi, 1950). A clear statement about the relationship of symbols and myths is offered by Church (1975):

> It is not the literal contents of the myth but its central symbols that in fact form the content of revelation. The specific contents of myths and actual historical circumstances of the tradition change from age to age through time, only the symbols remain. (p. 51)

The above definition of symbol is illustrated in the case of a 35-year-old, single-parent mother of four who was divorced a year earlier. The mother was currently an undergraduate in the physical sciences and had recently expressed hopes of becoming a medical doctor rather than following her earlier plan of becoming a nurse. Since her divorce, she had worked on weekends in a hospital and also managed an apartment complex. Recently the family house had been sold and the mother and her children were living in cramped quarters with a friend. They were hoping to build a new house, but complications (financing, construction help from relatives, expense, etc.) had arisen and the mother was unsure whether to commit to the building project, to buy an already constructed older home, or to remain with her friend in their current living arrangement.

The presenting problem was the oldest, 13-year-old son's uncooperativeness and misbehavior. He was perceived by his mother as attempting to fill his father's role in the family, reminding the family of the father who had moved out of state, and protecting his father's good name in his absence. The result was a power struggle between mother and son reminiscent of the previous marital relationship. Additionally, the youngest daughter, 9 years old, suffered from asthma which was worse on weekends when mother worked. This daughter was extremely sensitive to her mother's absence and strongly reacted to her increased unavailability.

The therapist in the case, a supervisee of the second author, had focused on a number of issues, including appreciating the many changes the family had experienced in a short period of time, helping family members to verbalize their feelings about the recent divorce, restructuring the interactions surrounding the son's fighting and disobedience, helping mother resolve her conflict between her parental responsibilities and her own personal goals, and focusing on mother's indecision about how their current housing dilemma should be remedied. The symbol chosen to understand the many issues and conflicts facing this mother and her children was their "home." The loss of the original family dwelling was viewed as a metaphor for the loss of the original family role structure and the husband/father. The current chaotic, overcrowded living arrangement was seen as representing the family members' turmoil and unresolved feelings about the divorce and the father's/husband's absence. The son's misbehavior was viewed as a constant reminder that neither the housing situation nor the divorce was yet resolved. The "complications" which had arisen regarding the construction of a new home were seen as a reflection of the complications that mother and children were having in their attempts to move on to a new lifestyle. Mother's indecision regarding whether to commit to building a completely new house, to buying an already constructed home, or to remaining at her friend's home was seen as paralleling her indecision about committing to the many years of schooling necessary to become a medical doctor, opting for a more easily obtainable nursing degree, or remaining a dedicated parent and homemaker in the security of what was most familiar. Thus, the "home" symbol was affectively charged, contained multiple associations operating simultaneously at multiple levels of awareness and organized valuable information into a theme depicting the family members' perceived reality, current role relationships, and shared identity.

SYMBOLIC BEHAVIOR AND ANALOGY

In order to gain a fuller understanding of how myths evolve, we think of the behaviors exhibited by individuals and the behavioral patterns shared between and among family members as being symbolic and having analogical qualities. To understand analogical behavior is to see behavior as having an "as if" quality. For example, a wife responds to her husband "as if" he were a Roman soldier coming home from battle, or a father treats his daughter "as if" she were a princess. Such roles become part of a family myth when the "as if" quality disappears and the labeled family member actually becomes the "Roman soldier" or the "princess" and is treated accordingly by all other family members.

METAPHOR AND MYTHS

Many statements and gestures have to do with communicating what is happening in our actual, sensual, moral, ethical or emotional experiences. These experiences are subjective, having a reality only in terms of their relevance for an individual at a particular point in time and in a particular context. If we move beyond simply communicating the existence of subjective experiences, we will frequently, if not always, use literal descriptions in a nonstandard way. When we talk about abstract concepts, we tend to use language drawn from some concrete domain. Employing literal, digital language in a different context or in a nonstandard manner is characteristic of metaphorical communication. For the purpose of this discussion, metaphors will be considered phrases or word structures that analogically assert something about the reality of a relationship between and/or among two or more individuals or family members.

In family therapy, the presenting problem is often viewed as a metaphor for disturbed interaction patterns elsewhere in the family system (Haley, 1976). For instance, a child's misbehavior is often construed as a metaphor for a disturbed marital relationship. Our view extends beyond an emphasis on symptoms by seeing metaphor as a communicational vehicle representing multiple aspects of a person's or family members' interpersonal experiences. For example, a Hispanic woman from a close-knit, patriarchal, old world family married a man whom her father and brothers disliked. After her divorce from this man, the woman turned to her father and brothers for emotional support and guidance in raising her two adolescent sons. She described her periodic visits to her family of origin as "appearing before the Knights of the Round Table." The "Round Table" was a metaphor which brought home the power and authority of this woman's family of origin.

The multiplicity of images or pictures which can be used to describe the quality of one's experience is the essential difference between symbols and metaphors. Symbols are more stable and enduring than metaphors and can be conceptualized as extensions of metaphorical activity.

RITUALS AND MYTHS

Historically, rituals were behavioral dramas which enacted a myth or a portion of a myth. They were socially shared experiences common to a community or larger territory. Fontenrose (1966) discusses a number of relations between myths and rituals:

> A ritual drama may clearly enact the events of a myth, or a myth may account for nearly every act in a rite, each ritual act in order; other myths, however account for rites in a less systematic way; still others tell only how the rites were introduced. Moreover, once ritual and myth become associated, one affects the other. (p. 50)

As each affect the other, both may suggest additions to or revisions in the main text. Perry (1966) has suggested that myth was the outcome of primitive man's attempt to account for his universe and that ritual was then the expression of this. According to Perry (1966), ritual also was intended to preserve the social group and was the basic source of communal action. Myth and ritual were seen as being intimately related vehicles for the symbolic expression of man's perceptions of his reality in both a spoken and acted form.

Ritual also can be seen as a person's attempt at maintaining a personal homeostatic balance. For example, compulsive behaviors of neurotic or psychotic persons can be seen as rituals that have idiosyncratic meaning for the individuals who perform them. Indeed, the manifest picture of the compulsive ceremonials of psychiatric patients and religious rituals (due to the similarities of the underlying unconscious conflicts believed to be present) led Freud (1963a) to call compulsive neurosis a "private religious system" (p. 25). Personal rituals, therefore, can be seen as overt manifestations of specific aspects of one's personal mythology.

Behavioral sequences in marital and family systems that are repetitive and cyclic have a ritualistic and stabilizing quality to them. Empirical support for the stabilizing function of these redundant patterns has recently been offered (Rogers & Bagarozzi, 1983). A ritual commonly focused upon in therapy is the behavioral sequence within which the presenting symptomatic behavior is embedded. For instance, father's style of disciplining the identified patient may provoke mother's criticism. This criticism only serves to evoke father's sense of frustration and anger and leads to a symmetrical escalation between mother and father. The parental struggle over discipline is then deflected by the identified patient's misbehavior. Here the cycle begins again. While the understanding of such symptom-oriented rituals is essential in therapy, our attention to ritualized behaviors extends beyond the "symptomatic cycle" (Hoffman, 1981) to include a broader spectrum of ritualized behaviors. Family celebrations, family traditions, patterned family interactions (Wolin & Bennett, 1984), and rites of passage (Kobak & Waters, 1984) all behaviorally portray portions of individual and family mythologies.

Having concluded our discussion about the nature, character and functions of myths, we are ready to proceed with our explorations into the development and evolution of personal, conjugal, and family mythologies.

3

Personal Mythologies:
Theoretical Formulations
and Assessment Guidelines

PERSONAL MYTHS SERVE the function of explaining and guiding human behavior in a manner analogous to the role played by cultural and religious myths in all societies. They give meaning to the past, establish continuity, define the present and provide direction for the future (Feinstein, 1979). Personal myths allow us to organize our experiences (biological, personal, familial, social, and cultural) in a way that gives them some psychological meaning and significance (Bagarozzi & Anderson, 1982). The family of origin is where one's personal mythology has its genesis. Personal mythologies are complexes of symbolic and affectively laden themes comprised of three basic structural components: the self, the self-in-relation-to-other-selves, and the internalized ideals of significant others.

The *self*, as we conceptualize it, is a superordinate personal structural system having cognitive and affective components operating at both conscious and unconscious levels of awareness. The self's primary function is to organize one's experiences (both internal and external) into some coherent whole. The self attempts to bring order and meaning to one's life and one's existence. Although the self strives for wholeness and completeness, traumatic experiences during critical periods of individual development often retard, impede or prevent full integration and actualization. In extreme cases, the self may become fragmented or disintegrate entirely. One's personal behavior and the behaviors of others are perceived, experienced, interpreted, and responded to according to

15

how these experiences are cognitively organized and viewed by the self. The assumption that human thoughts, behaviors and affects are mediated by personal cognitive structures and processes is a central tenet of cognitive psychology (e.g., Forgus & Shulman, 1979; Kelly, 1955; Kohlberg, 1966, 1969; Piaget, 1977), cognitive behavioral psychotherapy (e.g., Beck, 1987; Beck, Rush, Shaw & Emery, 1979; Ellis, 1962, 1973, 1987; Ellis & Grieger, 1977; Mahoney, 1974; Meichenbaum, 1977), and analytic psychology (Jung, 1940).

Interpersonal styles evolve as one confronts and attempts to master the various developmental tasks and interpersonal conflicts with significant others that occur during each stage of the life cycle. The more difficulty one has in one's efforts to master a particular developmental task, the more this unresolved task will persist as a motive throughout one's life. *Such unresolved conflicts with significant others continue to resurface as major themes in one's personal mythology.*

It is our contention that persons attempt to rework unresolved conflicts with significant others symbolically through the selection of personally meaningful fairy tales, folk stories, nursery rhymes, novels, short stories, motion pictures, television programs, etc. These later become woven into the themes of one's personal mythology. These stories are retained as important because they are thought to suggest solutions to one's personal conflicts. Frequently, parts of a fairy tale, short story, etc., are remembered in place of actual childhood events. When this occurs, the fairy tale or story becomes a screen memory for significant (sometimes traumatic) events. In such instances, the fairy tale or story can be compared to the manifest content of a dream and can be treated as such in therapy (i.e., as a symbolically disguised wish or attempt to solve an important relationship conflict or developmental task that is pressing for expression and successful resolution).

As we develop in our families of origin, significant persons with whom we come in contact become associated symbolically with specific characters in these fairy tales, stories, etc., through the processes of projection and transference. We also identify with characters in these stories through modeling, introjection, projective identification, and object splitting. It is important to understand that *significant others and the relationships between and among these persons also take the form of, and are represented to the self as, cognitive structures.* For example, when one thinks about (consciously or unconsciously) one's parents, siblings, grandparents, etc., their relationships and one's relationships with them, what one actually remembers is a reconstruction of events and experiences with idealized versions of these persons. Truth or accuracy has little to do with how these persons and one's relationships with them are perceived, recalled, and stored cognitively. Similarly, these reconstructed relationships between and among significant others also become the schematic models for conjugal and familial role expectations and relationship themes.

One important internalized ideal image, which is central to understanding the development of conjugal myths and their evolution into family myths, is the self-in-relationship with one's *ideal spouse*. The *ideal spouse* becomes the central figure in those personal themes having to do with intimate heterosexual relationships. Closely interwoven with themes concerning the *ideal spouse* are those having to do with the *ideal marriage* and, later on, one's *ideal children* (i.e., the expectations and role assignments one has for each child that is brought into the family). These are discussed below.

The Ideal Spouse

As a result of one's experiences with significant members of the opposite sex and of repeated exposure to familial models and other significant male-female, husband-wife relationships, one develops a cognitive representation of one's *ideal spouse*. This ideal has both conscious and unconscious components and becomes the standard against which all prospective mates are judged and evaluated. The *ideal spouse* usually contains certain characteristics of one's parents and significant others, as well as aspects of the self that have been projected.

The degree to which one's ideal is composed of unconscious archetypal elements (e.g., animus/anima, good mother/bad mother, good father/bad father, shadow) is a matter of speculation and personal choice. However, we accept the proposition that archetypes do exist (and play some role in the development of one's ideals), in the same way that we accept Piaget's belief in universal and enduring genetically transmitted cognitive structures that condition and limit what an individual is capable of perceiving, understanding, and learning (Flavell, 1963, 1985).

The notion that individuals seek out, develop intimate relationships with, and subsequently marry persons whom they perceive to be similar to an internal ideal has been proposed by Bagarozzi (1982a, 1986) and Bagarozzi and Giddings (1982, 1983b) and is referred to as the *cognitive matching hypothesis*. This hypothesis draws its empirical support from sociological studies, which have shown that the greater the congruence between what one expects from one's spouse (in terms of physical attractiveness, personality characteristics, sex-role behavior, etc.) and that spouse's actual behavior, the greater the person's satisfaction with the partner and their marriage (Burgess & Locke, 1945; Lewis & Spanier, 1979; Sabatelli, 1984). Indirect empirical support for the *cognitive matching hypothesis* can be found in a number of studies (Frank, Anderson, & Rubinstein, 1980; Goode, 1962; Hawkins & Johnsen, 1969; Luckey, 1960a, 1960b; Schulman, 1974; Tharp, 1963).[1]

The Ideal Marriage/Family

The idea that spouses come to the altar with a preconceived set of beliefs and expectations of achieving some idealized version of marriage and family life is not new. It was first described by the noted anthropologist, Ray Birdwhistell (1970). One's *ideal marriage/family* is not as well defined and crystallized as one's *ideal spouse*; nevertheless, it persists as a goal to be achieved. Like images of the *ideal spouse*, one's conceptions about one's *ideal marriage/family* have both conscious and unconscious components. Here again, these ideals are derived from one's exposure to family models and other important intimate male-female relationships and family environments that serve as prototypes.

The Ideal Child/Children

Each spouse brings to the marriage his/her internal representation of the ideal son and the ideal daughter and the role each child is expected to play in the family vis-à-vis each parent and his/her siblings. The *ideal child*, like all ideals, is a composite structure containing conscious and unconscious elements as well as portions of the self that have been projected and with which one is identified. However, it is our contention that projective identification and splitting of the self may play a more significant role in the formation of the *ideal child/children* than they do in the development of the *ideal spouse*. Again, let us mention that analytic psychologists would consider the ideal child/adolescent to have archetypal roots also (Jung & Kerenyi, 1950).

The term "ideal," as we use it, does not connote perfection. It simply represents an enduring, fairly stable, internal, cognitive representational image of

---

[1]Popular music abounds with contemporary examples of individuals relentlessly seeking the "ideal" woman/man. It does not matter whether the music is mainstream pop, acid rock, heavy metal, punk, country and western, soul, jazz, rap, new wave, reggae, etc.— the "theme" is the same. The quintessence of the "theme" can be seen in the lyrics of "Mystery Woman" (Allman & Toler, 1980).

one's desired mate, children, etc., that becomes the standard against which all prospective mates and children are measured, compared and judged. Behaviors, values, beliefs and the personality characteristics of one's spouse-to-be and one's children are assessed in terms of their goodness of fit with these ideals.

For most people, these ideals possess predominantly positive qualities and desirable traits. Negative attributes, when consciously recognized and acknowledged, are minimized so long as they do not pose a serious threat to the integrity of these internal structures. However, in some cases, the *ideal spouse* or *ideal child* may come to represent a standard of perfection. For example, persons who have had traumatic experiences with severely rejecting, punishing, abusing, inadequate or ineffectual models may construct a *perfect ideal* (i.e., the "good object") as a survival defense against this traumatizing or *negative ideal* (i.e., the "bad object"). When this happens, the *negative ideal* is repressed, banished to the unconscious where it resides as a central character in an unresolved conflictual theme or myth. Much more will be said about this phenomenon in later chapters.

The family of origin and the relationship dynamics that occur therein can be considered to constitute a rough blueprint for the development of central themes in one's personal mythology. A more complete blueprint would also include extrafamilial, subcultural, ethnic, social, and cultural themes.

The development of personal themes depicting the self, self-other relationships, and idealized others is illustrated in the case of a young woman who was raised by strict authoritarian parents. Her early childhood years and grade school experiences with peers had been painful and unrewarding. She had developed a central theme in her personal mythology which, if translated concretely, might be expressed as: "I am a fragile person. Therefore, I must avoid taking risks at any cost, and I should not expect much from others. By making myself invisible, I can avoid rejection and the embarrassment of failure that inevitably occur when I take any kind of risk. I also must protect myself from the disappointment that always results when I expect too much from others."

Based upon her early childhood experiences, this woman developed a fairly rigid world view, as well as a fixed set of beliefs and cognitions concerning herself and people in general. She also developed a particular interactional style, "becoming invisible," which characterized much of her interpersonal life. This personal theme organized the woman's memories of her previous experiences, dictated her present behavior, and prescribed a formula for her future behavior. Once a particular theme becomes crystallized, it takes on the qualities of a belief system that is extremely difficult to alter. At times, such a belief system might reach delusional proportions. Eventually, this young woman's personal theme was aggressively challenged when she was introduced to a young man who became very interested in her and who admiringly persisted in his attempts to date her. This new dimension in her life activated a latent "prince charming" theme and attendant image. She viewed her new suitor as the perfect gentleman, considerate, supportive, and genuine. She envisioned herself as having been swept off her feet and freed from her previous, emotionally constraining lifestyle.

Environmental experiences and other persons often serve as stimulus cues which activate a particular personal theme. In other instances, a person may seek out situations and/or other individuals who unconsciously collude to enact complementary role patterns and thematic dramas. This process allows the person to enter into (seemingly) new and different relationships which, nevertheless, have familiar patterns and predictable behavioral outcomes. Frequently, this repetitive, almost ritualistic, process involves elements of transference and projective identification and is an attempt to rework and correct unresolved past conflicts.

In this section, we have defined the components of personal myths as cognitive structures, which form symbolic and affectively laden themes. By defining the self, self-other relationships, and one's idealize images of significant others as cognitive structures, we can use the empirical findings from cognitive psychology for a more scientific description and further elaboration of personal myths. The following review of empirical studies is selective and is not intended to be comprehensive. Rather, the goal is to summarize some major research findings in the area of cognitive psychology, brain hemispheric functioning, and cognitive behavioral therapy in order to further elaborate our definition of personal mythology and to establish a rationale for using an understanding of mythological systems in therapy.

BRAIN HEMISPHERIC FUNCTIONING AND MYTH FORMATION

Recent research into brain functioning has emphasized two hemispheres, each with a separate set of functions and each capable of perceiving external reality from a different frame of reference. The left hemisphere, frequently referred to as the verbal or major hemisphere, functions to translate perceptions into logical thought, which then are communicated to the outside world through language. It is competent in areas such as speaking, logical thinking, reasoning, reading, writing, counting, and essentially, all forms of digital communication.

The right hemisphere, in contrast, is highly specialized in the holistic grasping of complex relationships, patterns and configurations. The right hemisphere possesses those cognitive abilities necessary for the construction of logical classes and, therefore, the formation of concepts—two abilities without which perception of reality would be chaotic and unintelligible (Watzlawick, 1978). The language of the right hemisphere, however, is archaic, underdeveloped, and characterized by primary process thinking. Its conceptions and representations to the person are ambiguous and ill-defined. It tends to draw illogical conclusions because it has the tendency to confuse the literal with the figurative, the concrete with the symbolic, the sign with what is signified. Its primary mode of representation is symbolic, using analogies, metaphors, puns, etc., to convey meaning. Even though it is considered to be the more primitive hemisphere (or maybe because of it), the right hemisphere is capable of spontaneously grasping the whole, the gestalt, or the total "world image," rather than the component parts of perceptual experiences (Dimond, 1972; Eccles, 1973). For analytic psychologists, the right hemisphere would be the most likely location for genetically inherited cognitive structures, such as archetypes.

Research on brain functioning suggests that we are capable of experiencing the world in very different ways and that these two modes of cognition, while interrelated, may be relatively independent of one another (Watzlawick, 1978). This further suggests that what are typically considered the unconscious elements of myths are not totally out of conscious awareness but are simply processed through alternative cognitive structures and pathways. These "unconscious" myth elements may be beyond the logical, digital awareness of the left hemisphere yet nevertheless responsive to analogic forms of communication (e.g., symbolic representations, nonverbal behaviors, rituals, metaphors, analogies).

Thus, given the role of the right hemisphere in perceiving and organizing holistic images and patterns, it is probable that it is from this source that personal mythologies (and by implication conjugal and family myths) originate, are maintained, and are transformed over time. It is from this source that mythologies would derive much of their power to organize perception and influence behavior. This formulation, while admittedly itself only a heuristic myth, also offers an explanation as to why individuals, couples and families are typically more aware of particular beliefs, values and attitudes and less aware of symbolic images, recollections, themes, etc., until these are brought to light and unraveled in therapy. Through the therapeutic process, symbolic mythological material may be accessed from the right hemisphere and brought into left hemisphere "awareness." Alternatively, mythological material may be accessed directly from the right hemisphere through analogical and symbolic forms of communication. This material can be used to organize a person's or system's behavior while bypassing the left hemisphere's logical awareness.

The ritualized prescription is one example of how this process may be used in therapy. Here the therapist prescribes a symbolic task or ritual sequence of behaviors which edits or rearranges key portions of a personal, marital, or family theme. Another example is the metaphorical discussion used to hint at or suggest alternative solutions to the client's, couple's, or family problems. When such strategies are employed, symbolically meaningful material is chosen to highlight or underscore aspects of the client's or family's presenting problem, without ever making the connections explicit (Anderson & Bagarozzi, 1983). Our assumption is that the individual, couple, or family members will use this material to find more satisfying and functional ways of resolving the particular problems that brought them into therapy.

Bettelheim (1976) postulates that fairy tales (i.e., metaphorical discussions) offer hope and suggest solutions to universal existential problems and developmental crises by using a language that children understand intuitively. While we do not agree with Bettelheim's strict psychoanalytic interpretation of fairy tales, we do believe that the solution or resolution of many existential problems (personal, interpersonal, and transpersonal) are suggested in fairy tales, cultural myths, and religion. These solutions, however, are not clearly spelled out; rather, they are suggested through metaphors. This permits the person or persons hearing the stories to devise their own unique solutions to their current life circumstances. The vagueness of fairy tales (in terms of time and place, the paucity of specific details, and the simplicity of the plot) permits one to "fill in the details" for oneself. It is this "filling in" of details by the right hemisphere that the therapist hopes to activate by assigning ritualized prescriptions, telling anecdotes, or elaborating symbols and metaphors.

INTERNAL DIALOGUE, COGNITIVE SCHEMA, AND MYTH FORMATION

The field of cognitive behavior therapy has provided ample evidence of the role of the internal dialogue (the process of speaking and listening to oneself) as a mediator among cognitions, behaviors, and emotions (Beck, 1987; Beck et al., 1979; Ellis & Grieger, 1977; Meichenbaum, 1977).

In addition, considerable attention has been given to the meaning system or structure that gives rise to a particular set of internal statements and associated images. For instance, Meichenbaum (1977) has emphasized that, in order to understand why people change their behavior, it is necessary to consider not only the functions of their inner speech but also how such inner speech "fits" into the individual's cognitive schema. He postulates the existence of cognitive structures that organize those aspects of thinking responsible for monitoring, directing, routing, and selecting thought patterns. These structures are believed to serve as an "executive processor which holds the blueprints of thinking and which determines when to interrupt, change or continue cognitive thought" (p. 213). These structures are "believed to be the source of scripts from which all dialogues borrow" (p. 213).

Beck et al. (1979) have approached the same problem from a slightly different angle. They have proposed that individuals selectively attend to specific stimuli, combine these stimuli into set patterns, conceptualize situations, events or persons according to these patterns and *then* respond to what is perceived. These patterns, or cognitive schema, are considered to have stable structural characteristics that are capable of differentiating, coding, and categorizing stimuli. It is these structures that lend form and meaning to one's phenomenal field, the self, and one's world. They also are credited with lending continuity to one's past, present, and future.

Beck et al. (1979) also postulate that, as these schema develop, they can become activated by a wider range of stimuli that are less logically related to them. In some instances, this process may get out of hand, and the person actually loses control of his/her thought patterns. When this happens, the individual may be unable to call up other, more appropriate schematic patterns (Beck et al., 1979). These more generalized schemata have been found to constitute the dominant stream of negative thoughts, ideas, and self-statements of depressed patients (Beck et al., 1979) and the self-defeating beliefs and attitudes of anxious, phobic, and under assertive individuals (Ellis & Grieger, 1977). It is interesting to note the uncanny similarity between Beck's and Meichenbaum's descriptions of cognitive structures and those of contemporary analytic psychologist's conceptions of archetypes (Stevens, 1982).

Meichenbaum and Beck do not explain how cognitive structures and patterns develop, nor do they explain how specific thoughts, feelings and behaviors become associated. It is our contention that such internal dialogues and self-statements are actually complex response chains that have become associated with specific structural configurations. Frequently, these structural configurations and attendant feelings became associated during specific critical periods of individual development (e.g., infancy, childhood, adolescence), when the person was struggling to resolve specific developmental crises (e.g., trust, autonomy, separation-individuation, competition, identity formation).

Identification, introjection, projection, splitting, etc., play an important role in the development of a person's unique response chain. Our clinical work with individuals, couples, and family members has repeatedly shown that, upon close examination of such response chains (i.e., internal dialogues and self-statements), one finds them to be strikingly similar to statements made about the person or statements made directly to the person by significant others during critical periods of development. As we have stated earlier, unresolved developmental conflicts become the major source of themes in one's personal mythology. It should not be surprising to find that there are specific affects, behaviors, and cognitions (in the form of internal dialogues, self-statements, belief systems, expectations, or attributions) associated with a particular structure, theme or complex of themes. Psychoanalysts have known for decades that words, sentences or phrases which are heard in one's dreams are frequently those that have actually been heard or spoken by the dreamer at some important moment in his/her waking life.

According to cognitive behavioral models of therapy, change comes about as the result of an interplay among three processes: (1) the person's behaviors and the responses they elicit in the environment (i.e., whether behaviors are reinforced or punished); (2) the person's internal dialogue and self-statements which precede, accompany and follow a particular behavioral sequence; and (3) the cognitive structures which give rise to a particular internal dialogue, group of self-statements, beliefs or behaviors. Empirical studies have shown that a change in any one of these three responses will evoke changes in the other two (Beck et al., 1979; Ellis & Grieger, 1977; Meichenbaum, 1977).

At first glance, it appears that one's internal dialogues and self-statements are products of the left hemisphere. However, this may not be altogether accurate. For example, Feinstein (1979) has discussed how internal dialogues often take the direction of deliberate, conscious self statements that, once learned, become automatic and later occur outside of the person's immediate awareness. Meichenbaum (1977) uses the example of learning how to drive an automobile to illustrate how logical and conscious self-instructions become subvocal and less conscious as the behavioral sequences become patterned and automatic. It is likely that as self statements, internal dialogues, and response chains become generalized and habitual, allowing for an economy of effort, they are transferred from the domain of the digital left hemisphere to the right hemisphere, where they can be stored more economically in symbolic, analogic, metaphoric and holistic forms.

This explanation may hold true also for logical chains and sequences (e.g., as in learning to drive an automobile) learned as an adult. However, it is extremely important to keep in mind that personal themes, as well as the response chains that have become associated with them, were organized primarily in one's childhood during preoperational periods of cognitive functioning (Flavell, 1963, 1985; Inhelder & Piaget, 1958; Piaget, 1969). Thus, they were not organized and stored in accordance with the logical, concrete, or formal-operational thought patterns and cognitive structures of adults. Certain interpersonal experiences, situations and environmental circumstances can serve as stimulus cues which evoke a certain theme and set in motion a cognitive-behavioral-affective response chain that one learned as a young child.

THE NATURE OF INTERNAL STRUCTURES

We should remember that personal myths and their associated internal structures (self, self-in-relation-to-others, ideal images and themes) are not static or rigid. Myths evolve and change over time. Structural changes can evolve gradually or come about abruptly (through discontinuous reorganization). Structures change and evolve through the processes of assimilation and accommodation. When new input is dissonant with one's personal myths, disequilibrium results. These new data may be assimilated to fit the current myth or the myth may accommodate itself to the new data. New structures emerge whenever existing structures become outdated or whenever environmental inputs exceed the structure's "accommodation capacity" (Piaget, 1977), so that higher order structures are needed to replace them (Feinstein, 1979).

New, superordinate structures, in the form of self reorganizations, modified relationship themes, or revised ideal images, are necessary whenever conflicting aspects of the self are experienced, whenever two or more themes appear to be in direct opposition, and whenever old ideal images no longer serve their purpose. This dilemma comes about because cognitive structures within a single system may organize data in conflicting ways. For example, a woman's self definition as a "loving wife" who behaves in ways that she believes will produce a "successful marriage" may conflict with another self-definition as a "devoted daughter" who is unable to deny any requests from parents, siblings, and extended family members (no matter how inappropriate these requests may be). In such a situation, the conflicting self-definitions, the attendant themes, the affects, and the self-in-relationship are in conflict. This conflict may be experienced unconsciously as tension, anxiety, depression, or some psychosomatic symptom. Or this woman may become consciously aware of her dilemma whenever she perceives herself to be in a situation that she believes requires her to choose between her husband and her family of origin.

The resolution of this conflict can be brought about in a number of ways:

1. A redefinition and restructuring of the self that allow this woman to function in both situations without internal conflict.
2. The creation of a different, superordinate theme that permits these two conflicting subthemes to become compatible.
3. Some combination of 1 and 2.

We assume that the presence of anxiety, depression, tension, or any psychiatric symptom is an indication that a successful resolution has not been found. How such symptoms maintain an internal homeostatic balance and serve to maintain a systemic balance (i.e., a marital and/or family balance) will be discussed in detail in the following chapters.

As we said earlier, new personal themes, myths, or self definitions are often needed to help individuals resolve developmental crises. For example, a 16-year-old client's emerging sexual urges came into direct conflict with her ideal self-definition as a woman who would remain a virgin until she was married. A persistent theme for this girl had been one of purification, premarital abstinence, and self-denial. In order to resolve this dilemma, the client modified her self-concept to fit with a revised theme permitting sexual intercourse with someone whom she "really loved."

The emergence of a new theme or myth or the transformation of any of its associated structures to a higher, more encompassing level of organization may be preceded by an ambivalent (conscious or unconscious) personal struggle, which may include debilitating stress and/or symptom development. For example, a 33-year-old borderline male, whose developmental struggles having to do with separation-individuation manifested themselves in themes of engulfment and abandonment, became "alcoholic" during that part of his individual treatment when he began to experience fears of rejection, abandonment, and annihilation. Old myths and their accompanying themes are powerful, and the habitual behavioral patterns associated with them often become highly resistant to extinction. In such cases, these may take on an existence of their own, become autonomous, and continue to operate in spite of one's conscious attempts to relinquish them.

The transformation of a personal theme is illustrated in the case of the woman referred to earlier who believed that she must always remain "invisible" to others. This personal style enabled her to avoid overwhelming social anxiety until a young man activated a "prince charming" theme and an antithetical theme of freedom from an emotionally constraining lifestyle. These conflicting themes resulted in an ambivalent struggle, in which she had to weigh the safety of her earlier "invisibility" against the promise of a "totally fulfilling" emotional relationship. In this case, the woman was able to accommodate to her new experiences and in therapy work toward an integration of the two conflicting themes. The result was a redefinition of self as a woman who could be selective in making herself "visible" to others, who could take calculated risks in some interpersonal situations, and who could develop a more realistic set of expectations for her intimate relationships. The theme of "calculated risk" then replaced the dysfunctional theme of "invisibility."

For us, all psychotherapy (whether it be focused on the individual, a couple, a family system, or a group) deals with helping the client or clients develop new and more functional themes, myths, and self-definitions. Regardless of the therapist's theoretical orientation, the therapeutic process is the same, i.e., the client or clients adopt the new myth of psychotherapy, which enables them to: (a) redefine themselves; (b) reinterpret their relationships with significant others; and (c) develop new and more rewarding behavior patterns that allow for increased mastery, control, personal efficacy, and self development.

As we have discussed so far in this chapter, personal myths are made up of symbolic and affectively laden themes depicting the self, the self-in-relation-to-significant-others, and idealized images of significant others. These themes represent incomplete developmental tasks and unresolved personal, as well as interpersonal, conflicts that arose during critical periods of development. These conflicts continue to press for resolution throughout the course of development and manifest themselves as secondary drives, motives, needs, etc. In this next section, we will outline our approaches to assessing these personal themes.

PERSONAL MYTHOLOGY: ASSESSMENT GUIDELINES

In order to gain insight into the content of the major themes concerning the self-in-relationship, we developed the *Family Relationships History*. This semi structured interview consists of 41 open ended questions. These are presented below for discussion:

1. What is your first memory about your family of origin?
Early recollections were used by Adler (1968), who believed that the memories presented by clients were important for understanding an individual's lifestyle, the core constructs that made up one's personality, the person's characteristic ways of perceiving the world, and the typical manner in which a person can be expected to respond to his/her environment. Some clinicians have gone so far as to say that from one's earliest recollections it is possible to formulate a person's self-concept (Forgus & Shulman, 1979). Our understanding of one's earliest recollection concerning one's family of origin is much more modest. We see the person's first memory as representing the theme or themes with which he/she is most concerned at the present time. We do not assume that the client will always remember the same event or series of events. Indeed, in our clinical experience, we have found that clients' first memories do change over time. As therapy progresses and conflicts are resolved, one would expect the client's first memory to change.

2. What circumstances, do you think, played an important part in your parents' decision to marry?

3. How do you think your father's parents reacted to your parents' decision to marry?

4. How do you think your mother's parents reacted to your parents' decision to marry?

Questions 2 through 4 provide valuable background information about the beginnings of the person's family of origin, as well as shedding some light upon the possible motives and circumstances surrounding the individual's parents' decision to marry. These questions also allow one to speculate about the atmosphere and affective tone of the person's family of origin at this critical first stage of the family life cycle (Bagarozzi, 1986, 1987; Bagarozzi & Bagarozzi, 1982; Bagarozzi, Bagarozzi, Anderson, & Pollane, 1984; Bagarozzi & Rauen, 1981). The degree to which the individual's parents had successfully mastered the critical tasks of separating, individuating and achieving personal authority vis-à-vis their own families of origin (Bray, Williamson, & Malone, 1984; Williamson, 1981, 1982a, 1982b) can be assessed informally, to some degree. For example, one can learn if: (a) one or both parents married to get out of an intolerable home life; (b) the parents married with parental consent and support or, like Romeo and Juliet, against parental wishes; (c) the parents married because of pregnancy, etc.

The relevance of the above questions is illustrated in the case of a middle-aged woman. The circumstances leading up to this woman's parents' marriage included a five- or six-month dating period during which the father made numerous proposals of marriage. Each of these proposals was met by the mother's declining and expressing ambivalence and uncertainty about the strength of her feelings for the would-be husband. It appears that there was another man for whom she also had some feelings. However, this suitor had joined the armed services and had been away for some time. The pattern of proposals by the prospective husband followed by refusals by the prospective wife continued until the man had an industrial accident which severed the fingers from his left hand. When, in this pained state, the man desperately proposed again, the woman accepted.

The maternal grandparents disapproved of the marriage, with the grandmother, in particular, expressing dislike for the man and the circumstances under which the proposal had been accepted. Her feeling was that the man was not "good enough" for her daughter and that he would never amount to much of anything. The paternal grandparents were never really consulted about the wedding, because the grandmother was confined to a state psychiatric hospital and the grandfather was a chronic alcoholic.

The circumstances surrounding the beginning of this middle-aged woman's family of origin provided evidence of several themes which continued throughout most of her childhood years. The conflictual triangle between her mother, father and maternal grandmother resulted in intense loyalty conflicts. She eventually chose to side with her mother and grandmother against her father, who had developed an alcohol problem like his father before him. This pattern continued into the woman's early dating years as ambivalence about establishing relationships with the opposite sex. A second early theme involved her father's professed love for his wife along with his enduring uncertainty about whether she had married him out of love or pity. This theme continued for this woman as skepticism about the degree to which others really cared about her and whether their expressions of caring could be believed.

5. *What circumstances, beliefs, values, etc., do you think played a part in your parents' decision to have the number of children they had?*

6. *What circumstances, beliefs, values, etc. do you think played a part in your parents' decision to have you?*

7. *How do you think your parents reacted to finding out that your mother was pregnant with you?*

We said previously that the family of origin is where one's personal mythology takes shape. The circumstances surrounding the child's conception play an important part in the way the newborn is welcomed into the family and how he/she is treated by parents, grandparents, siblings, and extended family members. Consider the following questions concerning conception: (a) Were the parents married at the time of conception? (b) If pregnancy occurred after marriage, was the pregnancy planned? (c) Was the child wanted? (d) Did the parents struggle with such issues as abortion, adoption, single parenthood, etc., if the child was born out of wedlock? (e) Was the child conceived to replace a loved one that was lost by one or both parents? (f) Was the child intended to be a replacement for a deceased sibling? (g) Was conception an attempt, by one or both parents, to salvage a failing marriage?

The reasons for having a child are varied and complex. They color the parents' perceptions and expectations and also affect how they will treat their child. For instance, conceiving a child to replace a loved one may place expectations on that child to develop similar personality traits or to behave in ways similar to those of the person he/she was meant to replace. Conceiving a child to save a marriage may place pressure on him/her to mediate a couple's conflicts at the expense of his/her own developmental needs. On the other hand, a child who is wanted and planned for may become a symbol of the couple's love and affection and caring and may become the focus of increased nurturance and caretaking.

The power of the circumstances surrounding one's birth to influence one's personal mythology and subsequent behavior is illustrated in the case of an 18-year-old boy. This boy was born out of wedlock when his mother was 16 years old. He never knew his father. All this boy knew about his father was that his reaction to hearing that his girlfriend was pregnant was to leave her. Several years later, while the boy and his mother were living with her parents, the boy's mother again became pregnant out of wedlock. The boy's younger sister, born from this second relationship, also never knew her father because he, too, soon departed following the girl's birth. The boy's early childhood years were difficult. His mother had become bitter toward men following these experiences and directed much of her anger toward him.

When this boy was 16, the girlfriend he was dating became pregnant.

His girlfriend, who was living with her parents and trying to complete high school, already had a one-year-old daughter. This boy was determined not to abandon his child to the same fate he had experienced. He vowed to marry the mother and to raise his child. He quit high school, found an apartment, got a job, and attended night school to complete his education.

Once the child is born, however, other factors play a part in parental perceptions, expectations, and reactions. How the parents, siblings, and extended family members perceive and experience the child will profoundly affect his/her developing self-concept and self-esteem. Questions 8 through 13 are used to gain some understanding of parental and sibling effects upon the developing self.

8. What do you think your mother's reactions were after seeing you for the first time?

9. What do you think your father's reactions were after seeing you for the first time?

10. What do you think your siblings' reactions were to knowing that your mother was pregnant with you?

11. What do you think your siblings' reactions were to seeing you for the first time?

Janine Roberts (1989) offers an excellent illustration of how parental and sibling reactions to the birth of a child play a significant role in the development and evolution of family and personal myths. Roberts describes the family's "myth of displacement of the firstborn son" as an explanation and justification for the oldest son's acting-out behavior. The parents believed that their son had never been able to get over the birth of his younger brother. The mother's experience was that her son had "never forgiven (her) for the fact that she had had a second son." The explanation that the oldest son had somehow been hurt by his brother's birth seemed to make the parents more lenient with his behavior and inconsistent about setting limits. The result, for the two sons, was a good/bad split object dichotomy, with the older boy internalizing a self-image of "bad boy" and the younger internalizing a self-image of "good boy."

12. How do you think your mother felt about your gender (sex)?

13. How do you think your father felt about your gender (sex)?

Questions 12 and 13 are included in this section on parental and sibling reactions to a newborn child because of the consistent empirical support for a relationship between parents' gender and sex-role expectations and the child's self-concept and behavior (Chodorow, 1978; Pleck, 1984). Clinically, it is not uncommon for some clients to report such experiences as, "after having three girls, my parents really wanted a boy, but they got me instead," or, "My father always wanted a son. I guess that's why he treated me so much like a boy." Historically, most cultures have shown a preference for sons, who represent the continuation of the family name (McGoldrick & Gerson, 1985). Research indicates that, while this preference for sons is diminishing, there is still a greater likelihood that families with only female children will continue to try for another, while families with only sons will stop with fewer children (Broverman, Vogel & Broverman, 1972; McGoldrick & Gerson, 1985).

In addition to gender, the ages of the parents when the child is conceived and born, the parents' previous experiences with children and childrearing, the number of children already in the family, the stage of the family life cycle, the nature of the developmental tasks associated with that particular stage of the family life cycle, the family's socioeconomic status at the time of the child's birth, the family's religious beliefs, its ethnic and racial background, the family's regional and geographical location, and the parents' political beliefs all play an important part in determining how the child is perceived and treated and, in turn, how the child interprets his/her place and role in the family. Each parent and sibling will form an opinion, develop an impression, and entertain certain hopes, fears, expectations, and aspirations for the newborn child. Essentially, each family member constructs, consciously and unconsciously, an ideal of each new child. As soon as the child is born, each family member begins to treat him/her "as if" this ideal were, in fact, a reality. More will be said about this process in Chapter 10. For the time being, however, we will simply list questions 14 through 18 which pertain to familial expectations for the child's behavior.

14. *Who named you and why do you think you were given your particular name?*

Frequently, one can learn a great deal about parental expectations for a child and the role for which that child is being prepared by the name he/she is given. For example, the first author once treated a South African family. The members' names, when translated into English, revealed much about the role each person was expected to play in the family drama. The firstborn child, a female, was named "Princess" by her father. Both parents were pleased with her and treated her "as if" she were royalty. The parents' response to the birth of their second child, also female, was very different. They had hoped for a boy and mother was depressed when she found out that this child was also female. This second child was named, by her maternal uncle, for the time of day she was born. The English translation of her name is "Night" or "Obscure

One." Their third child, the long awaited male, was given a distinctly African name which, roughly translated, meant "Unique." He was named after his mother's favorite sibling, an older brother with whom she had a very close relationship. From birth, this male child stood out as different.

This family came in for therapy with their son, who was 11 years old at the time, as the presenting problem. The parents were very concerned about the boy. He had no friends at school or in his neighborhood and refused to ride the school bus, because other children teased him and made fun of him. He was obese and sloppy in his personal appearance, changed his clothes infrequently, and did not bathe regularly. These behaviors as well as others at home, became a constant source of friction between him and his oldest sister, the "Princess," who had lost her favored place in the family with the birth of this male child. The power she once had as "big sister" with parent-like responsibility for her two younger siblings began to dwindle as these children grew older and challenged her authority.

By the time this family presented itself for treatment, familial roles had become rigidly fixed and highly stylized. The son was seen as truly "Unique" by his family, school, and community. The oldest sister's role as "Princess" had changed into one of critical, wicked sister and parental child. The middle child, the second daughter, progressively withdrew from the family. By the age of 17, she had completed high school, gotten a full-time job, and traveled abroad. She spent most of her time away from home, with friends whom her parents did not know. She still lived with her parents, but rarely spoke to them or to her older sister. She came and went without notice. No one knew much about her personal life. Family members made sure not to infringe upon her privacy. As she grew more distant, she became an enigma to her family, removed from them, "Obscure" and silent like the "Night."

Nicknames and pet names given to family members also can be thought of as labels which prescribe and proscribe behaviors and familial roles. However, the reader should not assume that all such names carry with them specific directions and role assignments, or that a person, once labeled and scripted, is forever locked into a predetermined role or life motif. We, as humans, are proactive as well as reactive to our environments and others' attempts to influence our behavior. We, in turn, respond to these influence attempts in our own unique ways. We also attempt to influence others and shape our environment so that it conforms to our personal needs, motives, and desires. Through this process of give and take, assimilation and accommodation, mutual influence and familial exchange, the self evolves. However, in order to understand the familial forces impinging on individuals, we ask the following questions regarding parental expectations and prescribed roles.

15. *What do you think your mother's hopes, desires, and expectations were for you as you were growing up? How were these communicated to you?*

16. *What do you think your father's hopes, desires, and expectations were for you as you were growing up? How were these communicated to you?*

17. *What role were you expected to play in your family?*

18. *What role did you actually play in your family?*

We believe that human development is goal-directed. This goal is to achieve a dynamic state of maturity, self-realization and self-actualization, with all aspects of the self integrated into one harmonious whole. Although this dynamic union is rarely achieved by most individuals, the drive to fulfill one's potential propels the person forward and carries him/her through each successive stage of development. If one's quest for selfhood is to be realized, he/she must reconcile those aspects of the self that are in conflict and those aspects of the self which act as internal censors to prohibit full expression of one's true nature. It does not matter whether these internal censoring agents are called conditions of worth (Rogers, 1951, 1961) or referred to as the superego (Freud, 1927)—some harmonious integration must be achieved among all conflicting components if full maturity is to be attained. In order to gain some understanding of the person's internal censoring agent and its effect upon the developing self and the ideal self, we use the following questions:

19. *What did you have to do in order to be loved by your mother?*

20. *What did you have to do in order to be loved by your father?*

21. *What did you have to do in order to be loved by your siblings?*

22. *What topics of conversation, behaviors, thoughts, feelings, etc., were forbidden expression in your family?*

23. *What secrets existed in your family that could not be talked about openly?*

24. *What secrets were there in your family that had to be kept from outsiders?*

25. *What secrets about yourself could you not share with your parents and siblings?*

Although the list of potential secrets in any given family is innumerable, there are some universal toxic issues around which secrets may cluster. These include money, sex, substance abuse, death, suicide, religion, unwanted pregnancies, incest, and extramarital affairs. Pincus and Dare (1978), echoing Freud (1913), emphasized how incestuous sexual fantasies are an important part of the secret life of every family. They noted, "Intense family bonds of love and caring spring from passionate feelings which must invariably carry the possibility of forbidden wishes for physical closeness" (p. 81).

A case of a daughter sexually abused by her father illustrates the importance of questions related to what children must sometimes do to feel loved and what secrets must be kept within the family. In families with father-daughter incest, one often finds either a tyrannical and dominating or a shy, ineffectual father whose ambivalence toward his wife leads him to his daughter for emotional and sexual gratification. Also typically present is a strained marital relationship and a passive, uninvolved wife unable or unwilling to meet the husband's emotional and sexual needs and also unable or unwilling to protect her daughter from her husband (Finkelhor, 1978, 1984; Shaw & Bagarozzi, 1986; Vander Mey, & Neff, 1984).

In one such setting, the daughter came to associate being loved and not being abandoned with submitting to her father's sexual demands. These feelings were further reinforced when the daughter finally confided in her mother and her mother's response was disbelief and inaction. Though feeling terribly abandoned and angry, the daughter came to see her role as caretaker and replacement spouse for her father. She became "the little mother" who was responsible for the needs of other family members. This role and the associated one of abused, depersonalized plaything became the prototype for her future relationships with men.

The next four questions deal directly with the predominant conscious beliefs and rules the individual believes have had the greatest influence upon the self. These questions also help capture clients' fears, as well as their unfulfilled wishes and imagined solutions to their own self-integration. These questions often take on additional significance when they are contrasted with the individual's responses to the *Personal Myths Assessment* questions discussed later. Then, both conscious as well as unconscious elements of one's core conflicts and associated symbolic themes become evident.

26. What important values, beliefs, and rules in your family do you think played an important part in shaping who you are?

27. How do you think these values, beliefs, and rules for behavior helped you to become the person you are today?

28. How do you think these values, beliefs, and rules for behavior can help you to become the person you would like to be?

29. How do you think these values, beliefs, and rules for behavior prevent you from being the person you would like to be?

Family clinicians have identified two salient dimensions of family structure and process—adaptability and cohesion. Adaptability refers to the degree of flexibility families exercise in their efforts to change their power arrangements, relationship rules, and individual roles. Cohesion refers to the way closeness and distance/separateness are regulated among family members and the degree of emotional bonding that characterizes the family system as a whole (Anderson, 1986; Beavers & Voeller, 1983; Epstein, Bishop, & Levin, 1978; Olson, Russell, & Sprenkle, 1983). A number of reliable and valid instruments, such as FACES III (Olson, Portner, & Lavee, 1985) and the Family Environment Scale (Moos & Moos, 1981), have been developed to help clinicians gain insiders' perspectives of these two dimensions. These instruments also allow one to type families so that they can be assigned to one of a number of functional/dysfunctional categories depending upon their derived scores on adaptability and cohesion. *In our work with personal, marital, and family mythologies, we are not interested in constructing family typologies or in assigning families to specific diagnostic groups or categories. We are primarily concerned with each person's phenomenological experiences and perceptions of these two dimensions as they occurred in one's family of origin.* To this end, we developed this final series of open-ended questions:

30. *What were the unwritten rules in your family of origin?*

31. *What phrase, motto, or saying best describes how your family functioned as a unit?*

32. *How would you characterize and describe your parents' relationship?*

33. *Who was the person you liked most while you were growing up? Why?*

34. *Who was the person you liked least while you were growing up? Why?*

35. *Who was the person you feared most while you were growing up? Why?*

36. *Who was the person you were closest to while you were growing up? Why?*

37. *Who was the person in your family with the most power? What form did this power take? How was this power used?*

38. *What person owned you emotionally? What was the nature of this emotional relationship?*

39. *How did this emotional relationship change over the years?*

40. *In what way did this emotional relationship remain the same over the years?*

41. *If you had the power to go back in time, or even now in the present, what changes would you make in your family's life circumstances, its members, and their relationships to each other?*

Once we have collected information about an individual's early recollections of his/her family and parents' marriage, the circumstances surrounding the individual's birth, parental expectations and prescribed roles for the individual, family secrets, values and beliefs, and family adaptability and cohesion, we are ready to proceed to an assessment of unconscious, symbolic, and affective personal themes. We have already said that unresolved tasks from previous stages of individual development persist throughout life as conflicts which take the form of interpersonal themes. We developed the *Family Relationships History* interview as one way of determining the content of these themes and of identifying those family members who played central roles in the development and maintenance of core conflicts. We also proposed that individuals select specific fairy tales, folk stories, nursery rhymes, novels, movies, etc., as important and meaningful to them, because they suggest a solution to these central conflicts. Once the *Family Relationships History* interview is completed, we use the *Personal Myth Assessment Interview* as a projective technique to further our understanding of central conflicts, themes, and relationship dynamics. The questions which make up this interview are given below.

1. What is your favorite fairy tale, book, short story, play, movie, television show, etc., and why do you like this particular story? Please give a brief summary of the story, in your own words.

It has been our clinical experience to find that the story chosen usually contains the core conflicts, themes, and role relationships with which the person is struggling. Frequently, the story selected is one that was learned in childhood.

It is important to allow the person to tell the story in his/her own words, as he/she remembers it. Each person's version of the same story will be different, and each person will edit and add certain material to suit his/her own unconscious needs. Therefore, the therapist should refrain from interfering with the person's recounting of his/her particular story. If a person omits certain facts, characters, or material that are considered to be important by the therapist, such omissions are just as meaningful (if not more so) than the material, facts, and characters that are included. Any such omissions should be noted, as should any significant addition or gross distortion. However, the therapist should make no attempt to correct the person's version of the story, to help him/her recall specific facts, details, materials, or characters that have been omitted, or to edit the material in any way during the client's initial telling of the story. *It is the person's version of the story that is significant.* This narration should be treated as the person's projections. Truth or accuracy is not at issue here. The story, as told by the person, also can be treated as the manifest content of a dream.

2. Who is your favorite character in the story and why do you like this character so much?

It has been our experience to find that the favorite character chosen by the person may change over time depending upon external circumstances or in response to some personal reorganization that has taken place. The therapist should not assume that the character designated as "most liked" is the person with whom one is actually identified. This character may represent only one aspect of the self, not necessarily the primary figure with whom one identifies. To find the identity of the character who serves as the central figure for conscious modeling and identification, question 13 is used. Frequently, the person's favorite character and the character he/she would like to be are one and the same. However, this is not always the case.

3. How is this character treated by others in the story?

Question 3 is useful in underscoring salient relationship conflicts and interpersonal themes.

4. What important things does this character do in the story?

This question helps one learn more about the person's drives and motives and highlights those developmental tasks which have not been successfully mastered and with which the person may still be struggling.

5. What important things happen to this character throughout the story?

Significant, sometimes traumatic events are often described in response to this question. Frequently, what happens to this character occurs repeatedly (e.g., in fairy tales, significant and symbolic events often take place three times in succession). Here again, meaningful material, unresolved conflicts, interpersonal themes, and incompleted developmental tasks come to the fore in response to this question.

6. What happens to this character at the end of the story? How does the story end?

In many instances, the end of a story offers a solution to the character's central problem or provides a resolution to an interpersonal conflict between various characters. In fairy tales, this solution is often brought about miraculously through the intervention of supernatural beings, magical characters, charmed animals, etc. In other instances, the means by which problems are solved and conflicts are brought to a happy resolution are not clearly detailed or outlined in the story. Such vagueness is deliberate and can be used therapeutically. Much more will be said about how vagueness is used in treatment in later chapters.

7. What character in the story do you dislike the most? Why do you dislike him/her?

It is our contention that each character identified in one's favorite story symbolically represents not only significant persons in one's life (or at least an aspect or certain aspects of these individuals) but also significant aspects of the self. For example, a hero might represent a person's ego ideal; a harsh and demanding character may represent one's superego or conditions of worth; characters of the opposite sex may stand for undiscovered "male" or "female" (animus and anima) qualities or components of the self; animals or monsters and fantastic figures may represent instincts, drives, motives, etc., that the person has not been able to accept and integrate into his/her self-concept; villains and malevolent figures may symbolize those denied, repressed and projected Shadow parts and split aspects of the self that are totally unacceptable to conscious awareness.

Splitting of the self and splitting of introjected objects is a central defense mechanism used by individuals having borderline, schizoid, and narcissistic personality disorders. Therefore, in working with such persons, couples and family members, it is essential to remember that characters, in the stories, frequently represent split or part objects. Finally, it is not unusual to find that various characters may stand for the same individual (self or other) at different times in one's life or at different stages of personal development.

Questions 8, 9, 10, and 11 correspond to questions 3, 4, 5, and 6. They are used to gain additional depth, breadth, and insight into central conflicts, motives, or themes and to unearth additional conflicts, motives, or themes that might be important.

8. How is this character treated by others in the story?

9. What important things does this character do in the story?

10. What important things happen to this character in the story?

11. What happens to this character at the end of the story?

12. How does the character you dislike treat your favorite character and what is the nature of their relationship?

Question 12 usually crystallizes the major dynamic of a central conflict. However, we would like to stress that one should not assume that the narrator's primary identification always rests with either (or both) of these two main characters, because the conflict described may actually represent one that the person observed between or among significant others. The narrator, in such cases, might have been involved only peripherally or as a passive spectator. Nevertheless, the impact of this conflict was traumatic for him/her and has been internalized. Under

such circumstances, the fairy tale, story, etc., related by the person becomes important because it offers the narrator some means of mastering
the traumatic event through its retelling. The following example will
serve to illustrate this point.

The first author once treated a family consisting of two sisters (aged 12
and 14) who had been adopted by their maternal uncle and his wife after
the girls' father was convicted of stabbing their mother to death during a
domestic argument. The maternal uncle and his spouse had had only
one child, a boy aged 16. The identified patient was the youngest daughter. Her presenting problems included stealing from her adoptive mother, lying and shoplifting.

The young girl chose the film *Aliens* as her favorite story. The character
with whom she identified (her answer to question 13) was the female
child who is instrumental in helping the heroine elude the Aliens. Later
in the film, the child is captured and imprisoned by the "Mother Alien."
The child is then rescued by the heroine after a brutally violent battle in
which the "Mother Alien" is destroyed.

The significance of this film seemed obvious at first. However, the
Family Relationships History interview revealed some important information about the events that had taken place on the night of the murder
which had never before been permitted open expression. First, although
both parents were inadequate, the girls' father had actually been the
more nurturant of the two. Since he did not have a steady job, he spent
most of his time at home taking care of his two daughters while their
mother worked. Second, the mother was heavily involved with drugs
and alcohol and often stole and shoplifted to get money to support her
habit. Third, on the night of the murder, both parents had been drinking
and arguing over money and drugs. In the heat of this violent argument,
the father threatened to kill his wife and brandished a butcher knife. In
response to this threat, the wife fled their mobile home. The husband
put down the knife and pursued her into the woods. While both parents
were gone, the identified patient crept out from under her bed (where
she and her sister had been hiding throughout the course of the argument). She took the knife and hid it under her bed in order to protect her
mother. When their father returned, he searched for the knife, found it,
and left the mobile home. Shortly thereafter he stabbed his wife to
death. At the time of the murder, the identified patient was four and a
half years old.

13. *If you could be any character in the story, who would you be and why?*

This question is important because it underscores the person's conscious identification and brings to light some of the beliefs, expectations,

attributes, values and attitudes that the person consciously holds concerning his/her role in finding a possible solution to the presenting problem. Frequently, the person has tried to solve the presenting problem by employing behavioral solutions used by the character with whom he/she identifies. The person may continue to use these methods in spite of their being inappropriate to the circumstances at hand. Strategies for helping individuals use such identifications in a more creative and productive fashion are offered later in Chapter 4.

14. *If you could change any part of this story, what changes would you make and why?*

This question corresponds to question 41 in the *Family Relationships History*. Both questions allow the therapist to see the person's desired outcome from his/her own unique perspective.

When we examine the person's responses to these 14 questions and compare them to his/her discussions of the *Family Relationships History*, the parallels between the two become strikingly obvious. It is not uncommon for an individual to develop significant insights about current relationship dynamics simply by participating in these interviews. In the next chapter, we present a case history which demonstrates how personal mythologies are used in individual psychotherapy.

4

Personal Mythologies in
Individual Psychotherapy

I N THIS CHAPTER, we present a case study illustrating how personal mythologies are explored in individual psychotherapy. For heuristic purposes, the ideal course of treatment is presented in outline form. We do
not intend to offer the reader an in-depth explanation or analysis of the
psychotherapeutic process. Stages of treatment are outlined in an orderly, sequential, and linear fashion simply for purposes of clarification and
demonstration. The actual course of treatment is not rigidly structured;
rather, therapy is a fluid and dynamic developmental process. The therapist and the client constitute a developing dyadic system which functions as do all living systems. It is goal directed and uses both positive
and negative feedback to achieve its ends. It is a system of mutual influence (Bagarozzi, 1983c) whose hierarchical structure changes as therapy
progresses, with the client taking increasingly more responsibility for:
identifying themes; understanding the true nature of their underlying
conflicts; devising new strategies for dealing with these conflicts; recognizing when he/she has been using faulty or inappropriate solutions;
becoming aware of transferential patterns that get in the way of relating
to others as real people and altering one's behavior accordingly; modifying one's internal ideals; correcting irrational beliefs, unrealistic expectations (for self and others), and faulty perceptions; setting realistic and
achievable goals; and devising effective strategies and plans for achieving these goals as therapy draws to an end.

In practice, themes are identified and dealt with as they emerge. Ideal-
ly, one would expect to help the client resolve the underlying conflicts
around one theme before going on to the next one. However, in clinical
work this is rarely the case. In many instances, one theme may be laid
aside temporarily while the client turns his/her attention to another the-

42

matic issue that has been activated by some external, real life circumstance. In other instances, two or more themes may emerge together to form a *problem complex* which must be dealt with as a gestalt. Rarely, if ever, do all themes and their underlying conflicts get resolved. However, resolution of the central themes that one brings into therapy is the desired outcome of a successful treatment. In the following case example, we focus on just a few of the central themes and conflicts that made up this client's extremely complex personal mythology.

MR. G.

Mr. and Mrs. G. initially contacted the first author for marital therapy; the presenting problem was Mrs. G.'s lack of sexual desire. This symptom was global and not specific to Mr. G. Mrs. G.'s decreased sexual responsiveness began three years earlier, immediately following the birth of the couple's third and final child. When the couple presented for therapy, Mr. and Mrs. G. were having sexual intercourse on the average of once every three to four months.

After a series of conjoint and individual diagnostic interviews, it became evident that there had always existed a desire discrepancy between Mr. and Mrs. G. However, this discrepancy had gone undetected by previous therapists. As is sometimes the case with adult women who were incest victims or who had been sexually molested as children, Mrs. G. was orgasmic and highly sexually active with her husband during their courtship and prior to the birth of their first child. However, her sexual behavior during this period of time was not a valid predictor of her post pregnancy level of desire. Frequently, the woman's true level of desire only surfaces when she feels herself to be secure in the marriage. When Mrs. G.'s true level of desire surfaced, a gross discrepancy between her and Mr. G.'s level of desire became apparent (Bagarozzi, 1987; Shaw & Bagarozzi, 1986).

Relatively short-term sex therapy helped Mr. and Mrs. G. recognize what had taken place throughout the course of their relationship, and the frequency of the couple's sexual intercourse gradually increased to an average of once or twice a month. However, Mr. G. still was not satisfied with this frequency. He felt disappointed, angry, and sad about the turn of events. He expressed his belief that he had been manipulated by his spouse, deceived by her and tricked into marrying her under "false pretenses." At this time, his feelings of mistrust for all women surfaced, and he and his wife agreed that it was time for Mr. G. to enter individual treatment to deal with these feelings and related problems.

Work with Mr. G. was chosen over couples' therapy or individual therapy with Mrs. G. because in treating incest survivors, it is important not to push them prematurely into disclosure and intensive therapy— especially if the therapist is male. This only reenacts the violation, invasion, and intrusion experienced previously by the woman. The approach is to allow the woman to move at her own pace. She is in control, not the man.

CLIENT PREPARATIONS

In all our work with individuals, couples, and families, we begin with some type of induction procedure to prepare and orient the client for what to expect throughout the course of treatment. Research has shown that pre therapy preparation enhances the probability that clients will not terminate prematurely; in addition, they will be more likely to profit from psychotherapy than clients who have not been so prepared. This is especially true for disadvantaged clients and persons from lower socioeconomic strata (Lorion, 1978; Sattler, 1978).

Mr. G. was from a lower-middle-class, rural family. Even though he was intelligent, and education and achievement were valued in his family (his brothers had all been helped to attend college), Mr. G. had not been encouraged to reach the same level of achievement as his siblings and held a "blue collar" position. Therefore, pre-therapy preparation was considered to be a crucial prerequisite to his treatment.

Major Ingredients: Goal Setting and Outlining the Treatment Process

Pre-therapy preparation begins with asking the client what he/she hopes to accomplish and achieve at the end of successful therapy. Short-term and long-term goals are specifically identified. The therapist's responsibility, at this juncture, is to help the client assess and evaluate whether his/her goals are realistic and whether the therapist will be able to help him or her achieve these goals or whether referral to another therapist is warranted. If it is determined that our clinical approach is appropriate for treating the client and that the client's goals are realistic and achievable, we discuss with the client our theoretical and philosophical views concerning the nature of how human developmental crises come about, how unresolved developmental conflicts and crises evolve into central life themes, and how these conflicts continue to press for resolution throughout the course of a person's life. Next we outline the treatment process for the client. We explain that the beginning phase of treatment is devoted to helping him/her identify major life themes and that the second phase is concerned with helping the client: (a) understand the central dynamics of these conflicts; (b) identify the significant others who are centrally involved in each of these conflicts; (c) recognize the role played by each participant (including the client); and (d) identify the attempted interpersonal solutions that the client has used (and is presently using) which only serve to perpetuate the conflicts. The third phase of treatment is explained as the learning phase of therapy. Here the client learns new, more adaptive interpersonal and cognitive strategies that can help him/her resolve and work through past conflicts. The final phase of therapy is described as a self-evaluation and redecision phase. Here the client evaluates the extent to which long-term and short-term goals have been achieved, whether further psychotherapeutic work is necessary, or whether termination is appropriate.

Engendering Hope and Creating Positive Expectancies for Successful Outcome

An important part of any induction process consists of engendering realistic hope for change and creating positive expectancies for successful problem resolution and mastery of the unresolved conflicts that brought the client into therapy. Toward these ends, we emphasize the importance of completing homework assignments, which are an integral part of treatment. We stress that homework assignments will be given when appropriate and that such assignments are designed to increase mastery, self-sufficiency and self-efficacy (Bandura, 1977), so that the client will not remain dependent upon the therapist for help in resolving conflicts once formal treatment has been terminated. In addition, we state our view that we expect the client to take more and more responsibility for critical self-observation, objectivity, insight, and goal-setting and for devising homework assignments and strategies for achieving these goals as treatment progresses.

We assure the client that we have no predetermined timetable and that each client is expected to progress at his/her own rate of speed and development. We also explain that we do not expect him/her to resolve a specific number of developmental conflicts in order for therapy to be brought to a successful conclusion. We underscore our position that cognitive insight into one's motives and conflicts and the subjective experiencing of one's own emotions are not therapeutic ends in and of themselves and that problem resolution and behavior change are of primary importance. However, we also add that self realization and self actualization of one's inherent potentials are considered to be legitimate goals that one might wish to pursue once the presenting problems have been resolved. We explain that such a contract can be renegotiated with the therapist during the self-evaluation and redecision phase of treatment.

Unconscious Processes and Transference Considerations

We conclude our induction procedures with a brief discussion and explanation concerning the nature of unconscious cognitive processes, the role played by these processes in the development and maintenance of interpersonal difficulties, and the way people use these processes in their attempts to solve problems. We also explain how unconscious attempts to resolve central conflicts can be seen in the form of defense mechanisms, dreams, and transference phenomena that occur regularly in the client's everyday life. We explain the importance of the client's sharing any feelings, thoughts, questions, concerns, etc., about the therapist, so that any transferential elements can be identified, explored, understood, and worked through to successful resolution.

Clients must develop the ability to stand back, to role-take, to decenter, and to reverse perspectives if therapy is to be effective and if they are to cultivate more satisfying interpersonal relationships outside the therapist's office. Therefore, each client is told that the ability to observe oneself and to assess one's actions objectively will be called upon continually by the therapist throughout the course of therapy, so that transferential distortions in the form of misperceptions, irrational beliefs, or faulty attributions can be reduced. The desired outcome of such a procedure is clients' relating and interacting with intimate others in more satisfying and realistic ways, free from transferential distortions, projections, etc.

ESTABLISHING TRUST

Psychotherapy begins with the initial contact between therapist and client. It does not matter whether this initial encounter takes place via a telephone conversation or in a face-to-face interview in the therapist's office. The client must feel, on some intuitive level, that the therapist is a person he/she will be able to trust, that the therapist will not do anything intentionally to hurt or exploit the client and that the therapist possesses the knowledge, skill and expertise necessary to help him/her resolve whatever the difficulties or conflicts were that brought him/her into therapy.

Initially, during the beginning phase of treatment, the therapist uses client-centered interviewing techniques to establish rapport: reflecting content and underlying affects as the client talks about his/her difficulties; responding with accurate, empathic understanding; accepting the client unconditionally and demonstrating genuine concern and warmth for the client. As the client becomes more secure and comfortable in the therapeutic relationships, the therapist can impose more structure in the sessions by introducing questions taken from the Family Relationships History. As treatment progresses, the therapist begins to paraphrase what the client says in ways which begin to highlight central themes in the client's personal mythology. After several months of therapy with Mr. G. he disclosed his deep mistrust and fear of all people, not just women. His first memory about his family of origin is quite telling. He recounts:

> I am lying in my crib. I guess I must have been about a year and half years old. I see these gigantic figures standing all around my room. They are yelling and screaming and demanding things from each other and from me. I feel scared and helpless.

Mr. G. was the youngest of four children. There were two brothers, 14 and 11 years older than he, and a sister, nine years his senior. She was a parental child charged with the responsibility of raising Mr. G. He believed that he was conceived in error by parents who were both in their early forties when he was born. He always felt unloved and unwanted as a child. He described his family atmosphere as hostile and tense and recalled feeling alienated and estranged from other family members. He characterized his role in the family as "scapegoat," "slave," and "whipping boy." He lived in constant fear and apprehension, carefully watching his parents and siblings for the slightest cue or sign that signaled that an attack was imminent or that he was about to be shamed, ridiculed, or berated.

The key themes that emerged during the early phases of treatment had to do with trust: suspiciousness of people's motives, concerns about being exploited by others, and his constant vigilance. These were accompanied by feelings of impending doom, anxiety, and dread.

The following dream serves to illustrate Mr. G.'s perception of his family environment:

It is night, and I am a young child in my parents' house. I am in my room, and it is very dark. I am very scared, because I know that there is a monster in the room who is waiting to get me. I am petrified, afraid to look behind me, because the monster might get me.

I look across the room to the other side, and I see some light coming out from under the door. I know that if I can just get across the room and out the door I can use the telephone in the hall to call for help, but I am too frightened to move. I hear the monster coming.

The fear became so intense that Mr. G. woke up in a cold sweat. His associations to the dream symbols revealed that the monster was "sexless" or of "both sexes." He recalled using the hall telephone frequently to call his grandfather when he was a child. His grandfather was one of the few people Mr. G. loved and trusted.

Obviously, the degree of trust that the client is able to develop will depend upon the extent to which basic trust had been established in the client's childhood. The less trusting the client's primary relationships were in critical, formative years, the more time it will take for the client to begin to trust the therapist.

At the same time that Mr. G. reported this dream, his suspiciousness of the therapist began to increase. Any changes in the therapist's body posture, body position, or body orientation were interpreted, by Mr. G., as the therapist's boredom or impatience with him. Minute alterations in facial expressions, changes in respiration rates or eye movements prompted Mr. G. to question the therapist's true motives and his sincerity. He wondered what such changes "really meant." Was the therapist angry? Was the therapist afraid of him? Was the therapist tired of listening to Mr. G.'s complaints? Was the therapist disappointed in Mr. G.? If the therapist was a few minutes late to the therapy session, was this the therapist's way of making Mr. G. suffer? If the therapist had to cancel or reschedule Mr. G.'s appointment, was this a sign of "rejection" or "abandonment" by the therapist?

During this part of Mr. G.'s treatment, the therapeutic atmosphere was extremely tense. Throughout this period, the therapist responded warmly and empathically, reflecting Mr. G.'s fears, suspicions and concerns. All Mr. G.'s questions and inquiries about the therapist, his motives, his feelings about Mr. G., his likes and his dislikes were answered openly, honestly, and candidly. After about one year of treatment, Mr. G. revealed that he was beginning to trust the therapist "a little." He then disclosed that, even though his everyday life experiences with people and the therapist caused him to question his long held belief that the world was not a "safe place" and that everyone would eventually "exploit" him, he still could not trust his experiences and still felt "unsafe," "isolated," and "strange."

However, the most significant change occurred in his relationship with his wife. He began to wonder whether many of his sexual demands of Mrs. G. were not, in fact, veiled requests for love, approval, physical contact, reassurance, and acceptance from a "parental substitute." With this insight came a more sympathetic attitude toward his wife. He became less demanding, less hostile, and less angry with her, and he began to accept the differences in their sexual desire levels as "real differences" and not as Mrs. G.'s willful attempt to "deny," "punish," and "demean" him. He began to attribute malevolent intentions to his wife less and less as therapy progressed. She, in turn, became less fearful and more affectionate with her husband, and the frequency of their sexual relations increased to an average of once a week.

As we said earlier, the time needed to build a trusting relationship with a client differs depending upon the degree to which the client experienced basic trust in infancy and was able to make up deficits in basic trust during his/her childhood and adolescence (Sullivan, 1953). The more traumatized the client during these critical periods, the more difficult it will be for him/her to establish trusting relationships in later life. For some individuals, true trust may never develop, because they have been so traumatized that the damage done is irreparable. Nevertheless, such individuals can learn to adopt a personal mythology which permits them to trust a few, select people with whom they can interact in highly circumscribed areas of their lives without too much fear that they will be betrayed and exploited.

Mr. G. was fortunate in that he had had some genuinely loving, trusting and satisfying relationships with extended family members (e.g., a maternal grandfather and a female cousin).

The Dynamics of Trust in the Therapeutic Relationship

As therapy progresses, issues of trust continue to surface. One should not assume that trust, once established, is forever securely maintained. As therapy continues and the relationship between the therapist and the client deepens, the client becomes increasingly vulnerable, because he continues to disclose more about himself and his conflicts and insecurities than does the therapist. This state of affairs produces an asymmetrical relationship. *Each new theme that emerges or each attendant conflict that one unearths becomes another area where trust is tested as the client plays out each new conflict with the therapist via the transference.*

We accept the psychodynamic concept of transference and work with transference phenomena when treating individuals. However, in our work with most couples and family systems transferences to the therapist are not dealt with in therapy, although we make use of positive transferences to the therapist to motivate and influence family members to carry out enactments and complete homework assignments or ritual prescriptions. However, the first author has found that in the treatment of certain client populations (e.g., borderline and narcissistic couples and family constellations) direct and immediate interpretation of negative transference phenomena is critical if therapy is to succeed. More will be said about this in later chapters.

Analysis and evaluation of transference distortions are a central thrust of our work with individuals. This practice is in keeping with Beck's (1987) cognitive behavioral approach. He states, "Transference reactions also are valuable and can be used to demonstrate the distortions embedded in the patient's cognitive reactions to the therapist" (p. 157). In discussing the use of procedures from both psychoanalysis and behavior therapy in his cognitive therapy approach, Beck also noted that, "other therapies seem to encompass features similar to those already expressed. Perhaps a common feature of relationship therapies is the *corrective emotional experience*" (p. 159, *italics ours*).

By being open, honest, and direct with Mr. G., the therapist was able to offer him a "corrective emotional experience" (Alexander & French, 1946; Beck, 1987). This experience paved the way for the modification of Mr. G.'s perceptions, attributions, interpretations of events, and the cognitive schema that were responsible for organizing his experiences in ways that were consistent with significant themes in his personal mythology. *We believe that each significant theme will surface in therapy as a transference issue between the client and the therapist. Each time this occurs, the trust that has been developed between the client and the therapist is tested.* When the therapist responds appropriately and not out of his/her own countertransference, the client benefits from this corrective emotional experience and trust is deepened. However, whenever the therapist's response is countertransferential, a homeostatic deadlock is created which blocks further therapeutic progress and inhibits the development of trust in the relationship.

IDENTIFYING CENTRAL THEMES

The Family Relationships History and the Personal Myth Assessment Guidelines are two semi-structured interview formats that we have developed to gather information about the central symbolic and affective themes regarding the self, the self-in-relationship to significant others and the internalized ideals in one's personal mythology. In our work with couples and families, we have been able to isolate four *indicators* which also are helpful in identifying salient conjugal and family themes. These are:

1. Recurrent topics of concern.
2. Redundant interaction patterns.
3. Repeated surfacing of specific, affect-laden conflicts.
4. The couple's/family's predominant affective tone.

When we work with couples and families, we pay very close attention to the content of topics that continue to concern family members, the redundant interaction patterns that are symptomatic of marital/family homeostasis and the repeated resurfacing of specific affect-laden conflicts. However, in our work with individuals we do not have the opportunity to observe these behaviors directly. Therefore, we ask a number of questions that deal specifically with interpersonal transactions and the contexts in which they occur. For example, we ask the client to attend to his/her thoughts, feelings, perceptions, interpretations of events, attribution of intentions, and the internal dialogues that precede, accompany, and follow the specific *indicator* (i.e., the topic of concern, repetitive interpersonal patterns and affect laden conflicts). We also ask the client to identify what it was that he/she had hoped to accomplish by behaving in a particular manner. This enables us to identify the specific behavioral contribution that the client makes which (paradoxically) maintains the interpersonal problem.

Another modification that must be made in work with individuals involves focusing on the tone of the affective relationship that exists between the client and the therapist. In our work with couples and families, we also pay close attention to how being with a particular couple or family makes us feel. We use this experience in therapy and comment about our feelings in order to spotlight and underscore the central affective tone of the couple or family that accompanies a particular theme. In work with individuals, the affect tone of the client/therapist relationship is targeted as a surface expression of some significant theme.

IDENTIFYING SOURCES OF CONFLICTS, TRACING THEIR ORIGINS,
AND RECOGNIZING TRANSFERENCE DISTORTIONS

This phase of individual psychotherapy recurs throughout the course
of treatment as each conflict or theme comes to the fore. It consists of
helping the client reach back into his/her past to find the origins of a
particular conflict and to identify how he/she has continually attempted
to resolve this conflict through past and present interpersonal relationships. However, insightful understanding in and of itself is not sufficient
to bring about change in the attendant repetitive patterns that persist,
because the client is unable to give up the accompanying fantasy (which
is usually not consciously available) that he/she will be able to find
someone who will right past wrongs, make up for deficiencies that were
lacking in one's parents and siblings, protect the client from injustices,
love the client as his/her parent should have, reestablish or establish (for
the first time) a nurturant mother-child relationship, etc.

The realization that one must give up such fantasies and expectations
comes hard to the client. Although the client may verbalize conscious
and rational acceptance of this state of affairs, he/she is usually unable to
relinquish these hopes and expectations in the unconscious and affective
realms of experience. A therapeutic milestone is reached when the client
begins to recognize that he/she has been unconsciously relating to the
therapist as the person who is expected to correct past wrongs and
inequities. *This realization marks a turning point in therapy.* At this juncture, the client usually becomes disappointed with the therapist and
disillusioned with therapy. His/her expectations for a "quick" or "magical cure" are exposed as unrealistic, and the therapist becomes the target
of his/her anger and disappointment. It is at this point in treatment that
many clients leave therapy in hopes of finding someone (another therapist, another spouse, another lover, etc.) who will correct past wrongs
and inequities. It is our contention that many divorces are precipitated
by such dynamics. More will be said about this in the following
chapters.

It is not unusual for symptoms to erupt or intensify during this phase
of treatment. During this very crucial period, the therapist has nothing
to rely upon except the strength of the bond of trust that has been
developing between him/her and the client throughout the course of
treatment. The therapist must have faith that he/she will be able to
address the rational, objective, reality-focused aspects of the client's ego,
so that the client will be able to: (a) identify and recognize how these
unrealistic and irrational beliefs and expectations have prevented him/

her from cultivating more satisfying and reality-based interpersonal relationships; (b) appreciate how transference, projection, projective identification and object splitting have distorted his/her ability to appreciate the true identities, motives, or intentions of persons with whom he/she has become intimately involved; (c) objectively evaluate which aspects of the therapeutic relationship have likewise become distorted; and (d) understand his/her own part in constructing an interpersonal environment designed to perpetuate such distortions and the defensive purpose such environments serve.

In addition to helping the client identify his/her transferential distortions, their childhood origins and the defensive functions they serve, we actively explore with the client any possible therapist contributions that help to maintain these fantasies, beliefs, expectations, or distortions. We also investigate with him/her how we, as therapists, might be unconsciously colluding with the client in ways that prevent change.

Here is a dream reported by Mr. G., when he reached this stage of treatment:

> I am standing in the kitchen of my house where I live with my wife and children. My wife is standing to my right and my parents are to my left. I feel myself becoming angry, and I turn to my wife. I then begin to scream something at her. Suddenly, I realize it is not my wife with whom I am angry, but my parents. I stop yelling at my wife and ask her to wait in the living room. I turn to confront my parents, but they are gone. I let out my frustrations by punching the refrigerator several times.

Mr. G.'s interpretation of this dream reveals his awareness of his plight. He realizes that he has turned to his wife for fulfillment of his unmet needs for nurturance, love, and support. He knows intellectually that she cannot do this and he turns to confront his parents. They disappear, for in real life both of them are deceased. He vents his frustrations on the refrigerator, which he believes represents the therapist and the therapeutic relationship. The refrigerator contains food, but it is cold. It does not offer the kind of nurturance he has been seeking ever since childhood. He realizes that the warmth, tenderness and unconditional love that he wanted so desperately from his parents cannot be gotten from his wife or the therapist. This therapy session ended with Mr. G. saying, "Well, at least I can go to the refrigerator, take what food there is and cook it myself."

Each time the client reaches such an insight into a core conflict, the therapist helps the client explore how this theme is related to other significant themes that make up his/her personal mythology.

OUTLINING THE CLIENT'S PERSONAL MYTHOLOGY

Once significant themes have been identified, material gathered from the Personal Myth Assessment Guidelines is used to construct an overall gestalt picture of the client's personal mythology. The conduct of the therapeutic interview will vary with the client and the nature of the therapeutic relationship. For example, one or two clinical sessions may be scheduled to deal specifically with the 14 questions included in the Personal Myth Assessment Guidelines. When this procedure is followed, the therapist can either audiotape the client's responses to each question or take written notes as the client responds. Another technique is to give the client a copy of the Personal Myth Assessment Guidelines to complete as a homework assignment. When the assignment is completed, the client and the therapist can use as much time as they need to explore each question in depth.

The central themes, their underlying conflicts, their origins, and the interpersonal contexts in which these conflicts arose in Mr. G.'s present life circumstances are outlined below:

1. *Mistrust of all people and their motives, intentions, etc.* As we have already shown, Mr. G.'s childhood experiences made it extremely difficult for him to trust others. His suspiciousness was pervasive and entered into all interpersonal relationships. This conflict had its genesis in the early mother-son relationship. Later, as Mr. G. grew older, he found that he could not turn to his father for nurturance, support and protection. Separation-individuation was seriously hampered as a result. His older siblings were seen as constant threats who did not support his attempts at independence.

In his everyday dealings with employers, coworkers, and his wife, Mr. G. was constantly on the look out for deceit and malevolence. He frequently attributed evil motives to others' behaviors. The simple act of walking down a crowded street sometimes precipitated what Mr. G. referred to as his "paranoia" and his "fear of attacks." Feelings of suspiciousness, resentment, and dislike for his siblings caused him to sever relationships with them and most extended family members. Suspiciousness of his wife took the form of seeing her as being exploitive and selfish and as controlling him by making her sexual responses contingent upon his compliance with her wishes.

2. *Feelings of estrangement and difference.* Closely associated with the theme of mistrust was the theme of his "differentness" and his belief that he

did not "belong" to his family of origin. As is frequently the case, this theme seems to have developed as a rationalization to defend Mr. G. against feelings of rejection by parents and siblings. What better way to explain such harsh treatment from nuclear family members than to develop a belief system which places one's origin in doubt. For example, on numerous occasions Mr. G. voiced his belief that he might have been adopted or that he really might not be the natural child of his parents. Perhaps he was the child of some distant relative, a child abandoned by his natural parents and found by strangers.

As Mr. G. was growing up, he nurtured his "differentness." Fear of people caused him to avoid any close or intimate relationships. He learned early in life that, if he behaved "differently" or dressed "differently" from other people his own age, they would be less likely to approach him. His "differentness" gradually became a source of pride. It served two important purposes: It singled him out as "special" and kept him at a safe distance from people. As an adult, Mr. G. would use his "differentness" selectively to distance himself from others whom he perceived were getting "too close" emotionally or to reduce the mounting anxiety and self-consciousness that he sometimes experienced in crowds, social gatherings, and public events. At such times, he might make inappropriate comments about the proceedings, jokingly insult other participants, ask highly personal questions of people he had just met, or stand up and conspicuously walk around the room during a public lecture.

3. *Illness as a way to secure nurturance.* Mr. G. was frequently rewarded with attention and comfort whenever he became ill as a child. Illness usually caused his mother to dote upon him. As he grew older, he learned that he could receive attention from his mother for "psychological" as well as physical illness. This "psychological" illness took the form of depressions, moodiness, and pouting whenever things did not go his way. "Psychological" illness played a significant role in Mr. G.'s relationship with his wife. Their dating and courtship began when Mr. G. was in his early twenties and Mrs. G. was still a teenager. Their coming together was precipitated by Mr. G.'s breakup with a former girlfriend. It appears that the major dynamics of their premarital relationship had to do with mutual support, concern, and pity. Each seemed to identify with the other's pain and feelings of rejection by parental figures. This dynamic persisted in the form of a marital theme. Physical and emotional illness continued to be the only channel through which

love, caring, concern and regard for the other were communicated. More will be said about this type of communication between spouses in the next chapter.

4. *Ambivalence concerning interpersonal closeness and distance.* This issue is believed to be the core dynamic in Mr. G.'s personal mythology. Although it can be said that all individuals who form intimate associations must struggle with and negotiate mutually agreed upon levels of separateness and connectedness (Hess & Handel, 1959), some persons are unable to achieve a successful balance between the two. Masterson (1981, 1985) has demonstrated how such difficulties in adult life stem from unresolved conflicts associated with the critical period of separation-individuation which occurs at one and a half to three years of age. Incomplete separation from a maternal figure is believed to have profound influences upon the development of the self, its integrity, its continuity, and the self-in-relationship with others throughout the life cycle. Such incompleteness in the self is later manifested in the person's inability to disengage from enmeshed family relationships (Minuchin, 1974) and to separate from an undifferentiated family ego mass (Bowen, 1978).

Individuals who have not successfully resolved the developmental tasks associated with separation-individuation are extremely ambivalent about interpersonal intimacy. They desperately crave human contact and closeness, but experiences in their families of origin have left them cautious about any type of interpersonal intimacy. The fears that one associates with intimacy in adult life are derived, to a large degree, from what transpired during this critical period. This is especially true for persons who did not have the opportunity to have a corrective interpersonal experience with a "chum" during preadolescence (Sullivan, 1953). For some, whose ego boundaries have become damaged as a result of their attempts to gain independence, interpersonal closeness may carry with it the threat of absorption and dissolution of the self. For others, attempts at separation-individuation may have been met with threats of rejection and abandonment. Such persons may learn that only total dependence and submission are acceptable. As a result, interpersonal closeness becomes associated with the loss of personal control. To escape these perceived consequences, individuals usually find it necessary to withdraw (physically and/or emotionally) from intimacy. This withdrawal is a transferential attempt to achieve separation-individuation. However, the more one withdraws, the more one begins to feel isolated and abandoned. Depression inevitably results. When the depression associated with abandonment becomes intolerable, the person is again drawn to the object of his/her dependence (or some other individual) and the approach-avoidance cycle begins again.

Shortly after he entered individual treatment, Mr. G. began to grapple with the issue of whether or not to divorce his wife because of her sexual unresponsiveness. During this period of indecision, Mr. G. was asked by his employer to attend a series of job-related retraining seminars that were being offered in a distant southwestern state. This trip represented the first time that Mr. G. had been separated from his wife in the 12 years of their marriage. The first two days of his eight-day trip produced feelings of relief and freedom. By the third evening, however, he had become anxious and depressed. Leaving his hotel room only made matters worse. Walking along the city streets and being in the midst of strangers caused him to become more frightened and depressed. Telephone conversations with his wife were the only thing that made him feel secure. For the remainder of his stay, he left his hotel room only to attend training seminars and to take his meals. He telephoned his wife each evening in order to reassure himself that she had not abandoned him.

In our earlier work concerning the ordering and structures of the various themes that make up personal, conjugal, and family myths (Anderson & Bagarozzi, 1983; Bagarozzi & Anderson, 1982), we thought that themes might be organized in some type of logical or hierarchical manner. However, our clinical experiences did not support this assumption (Anderson & Bagarozzi, 1989; Bagarozzi & Anderson, 1989). Because themes and myths are products of the unconscious, they are organized according to primary process thinking. Therefore, to say that personal, conjugal and family myths are logically sequenced or hierarchically arranged is incorrect. As therapists we may construct our own order and arrange our clients' themes in ways that are meaningful for us, so that we can develop and carry out a specific treatment plan or intervention strategy. However, we should not forget that the order we impose is nothing more than a myth itself, a convenient method used to organize and make sense out of the wealth of clinical data collected throughout the course of therapy.

We contend that a person's world view is a reflection of that individual's personal mythology. This world view contains material concerning the self and the self-in-relationship with others and can be reduced, for our purposes, to a finite number of axiomatic statements about the individual. Our summary of Mr. G.'s personal mythology is as follows:

The world is a dangerous place where people cannot be trusted. People in general, and women in particular, are uncaring, self-centered, and exploitive. They are only interested in what they can get from you and what you can do for them. I have a number of basic needs and urges, such as a desire for closeness and sex. These needs are bad, and I am bad for wanting to satisfy them. This makes me different from most people. If I let these needs be known, I will be punished, rejected, and abandoned. However, my different-ness is also a strength. Whenever I feel threatened by other people, I can show my differentness and this keeps them at a safe distance. There is one way that I can get some of my needs and desires met. When I become sick or ill, the people upon whom I am dependent will take care of me for a little while. However, I dare not remain ill for any long period of time, because they will become impatient with me and I will be abandoned by them.

Life is a constant struggle to get these needs satisfied. For this reason, I am constantly drawn toward others, especially women, but my fears of rejection, punishment, and abandonment make it impossible to trust them, so I must distance myself. The more I distance myself, however, the more fearful I become. I go back and forth between these two extremes. Sometimes I think I might be able to get my needs met by other men. This thought frightens me because it may mean that I am a homosexual. Therefore, I keep my distance from most men.

THE PSYCHOTHERAPEUTIC PROCESS AND THE DYNAMICS OF CHANGE

We make no claim to have identified all of the components, ingredi-ents, factors, and conditions responsible for bringing about the cogni-tive, behavioral, and affective changes that occur throughout the course of therapy. However, we would like to outline what we believe to be some of the central processes and dynamics that operate to produce desired therapeutic outcomes.

Cognitions

The modification of cognitive structures takes place gradually through-out the course of therapy. The cognitive structures that are the primary targets of our therapeutic efforts include the self, those cognitive ideals that represent significant others in one's personal mythology, and the major themes involving the self-in-relationship with these significant others.

Changes in the self come about as a direct result of the client/therapist relationship. The supportive, empathic, nonjudgmental atmosphere created by the therapist allows the client to experience all aspects of his/her being, to express all his/her thoughts, feelings, and beliefs, and to integrate those aspects of the self that have been repressed, split off from conscious awareness, denied and projected onto others, or otherwise defended against. As therapy proceeds and the client begins to feel less constrained by conditions of worth or an overly harsh superego, he/she develops a personal value system, sets self-generated goals and develops plans and strategies to achieve these goals. In this therapeutic milieu, the client's true self can begin to emerge and become actualized. As therapy progresses and transference distortions are reduced, the client begins to experience the therapist as a real person and not as a totally good object or perfect parent, sibling, etc. As this transformation is taking place, the client begins to introject and identify with the therapist and to incorporate the therapist's nonjudgmental attitudes, objectivity, and openness to exploring and understanding the dynamics of his/her conflicts with significant others. *This new stance, on the part of the client, makes it possible for him/her to accept interventions made by the therapist that will significantly alter cognitive structures.*

The techniques used to bring about modifications in the client's cognitive structures range from those that are subtle, indirect and perceptually focused to those that are straightforward, direct and behaviorally focused.

*Perceptually Focused Strategies for Editing Portions
of One's Personal Mythology*

1. *Psychodynamic interpretation* was used throughout Mr. G.'s treatment, because Mr. G. was an avid reader of popular, self-help books and many of his beliefs, values, and interpretations of his own and others' behavior were colored by psychoanalytic theory. By aligning with Mr. G.'s psychodynamic viewpoint, the therapist was able to interpret critical experiences with significant others in ways that were acceptable to Mr. G. and yet changed the nature of Mr. G.'s cognitive representations of these people.

Information gathered from Mr. G.'s Family Relationships History interviews was used extensively. For example, the lack of "basic trust" between Mr. G. and his mother was a primary source of his anger toward women, fear of others, and mistrust of people in general. He obsessed about how his mother had neglected him, how she paid little or no attention to his needs as he was growing up, how she showed favoritism toward his older siblings, and how she devoted more time and energy to her own mother and her mother's family than to her husband and her children. Essentially, Mr. G.'s cognitive ideal of his mother was that of an unloving, controlling, and critical woman who cared more about herself and her own needs than those of her husband or children.

Making certain not to discount, disqualify, or deny any of Mr. G.'s experiences and feelings, the therapist offered a number of psychodynamically oriented interpretations as alternative explanations for his mother's actions. Based upon information supplied by Mr. G., the therapist remarked that his mother seemed to have had a number of unresolved conflicts that prevented her from giving him the nurturance, care, and support needed for the development of "basic trust." Mr. G. had stated on a number of occasions that his mother was "overanxious," suffered from "periodic depressions," and was a "compulsive house cleaner." The therapist used these observations to suggest that Mr. G.'s mother seemed to show her nurturance and concern for him in a way characteristic of "people with obsessive-compulsive character traits," i.e., they tend to "overcontrol their children." The therapist added that "frequently the children of such parents interpret their behavior as restricting, especially when they are just beginning to assert their independence." Staying within the framework of "character traits," the therapist explained that "because of the overly harsh superego of persons with obsessive-compulsive character traits, they tend to use criticism as a disciplinary technique with their children." However, the intention is not to ridicule the child but to teach him/her certain "values" and to "build character." In short, this technique was used to build a child's "unconscious conscience or superego."

Favoritism toward his older siblings was interpreted within the framework of "sibling rivalry." Since his siblings were older, they had developed much more skill in monopolizing mother's time. While it seemed that she was favoring his siblings, she was probably responding to the children who "made the most noise," because the "squeaky wheel always gets the grease."

Mother's overinvolvement with her family of origin was attributed to a number of personality factors and unresolved psychodynamic conflicts. For example, her involvement with her family of origin, especially her mother, was interpreted as her having "her own difficulties" with "basic trust," "dependence," and "separation-individuation." Mr. G.'s grandfather, his mother's father, had died when she was an adolescent. The therapist used this information to explain Mr. G.'s mother's "periodic depressions." The "unresolved grief and mourning" for her father were viewed as another factor contributing to her "unavailability" to her children and her husband.

These psychodynamically based interpretations were accepted as plausible alternative explanations by Mr. G. Gradually, his cognitive ideal of his mother began to change, as did the affects associated with this internal representation. Rather than seeing his mother as a harsh, uncaring, controlling and critical parent, he began to picture her and refer to her as a "tired and overworked woman with her own problems." The affects associated with this revised ideal were pity and sadness rather than anger and resentment. During this period of cognitive reorganization, Mr. G. decided to pay a visit to his mother's grave, something he had not done since her burial some ten years earlier.

2. *Positive reframing of themes.* Positive reframing is a technique used by strategic therapists in their clinical work. Watzlawick, Weakland, and Fisch (1974) use reframing as a technique designed to "change the conceptual and/or emotional setting or viewpoint in relation to which a situation is experienced and to place it in another frame which fits the 'facts' of the same concrete situation equally well or even better, and thereby changes its entire meaning" (p. 95). What is changed through reframing is the meaning attributed to the situation, and therefore its consequences. However, the concrete facts remain unchanged.

Psychoanalytic interpretation can be viewed as a reframing technique. While psychoanalytic interpretations do not necessarily attribute positive intentions to others, they do offer a different explanation for the same set of concrete data. In our approach, alterations in the client's perceptions of situations, contexts, and events are not our central focus. Our primary concern is the modification of the client's *cognitive ideals and the reconstruction of entire relationship themes.*

For example, Mr. G. described his father as being physically and emotionally removed from the family. He spent very little time with his son and was unresponsive to any of his son's requests for guidance and direction. On those occasions when he did heed his son's requests for help or assistance, his response was to instruct Mr. G. to "figure it out for yourself" or "go to the library and find the answer in one of those books."

A positive reframing of this father/son relationship was accomplished by the therapist's use of the country and western song popularized by singer Johnny Cash, "A Boy Named Sue." The song tells the story of a young man's search for his father, who deserted his mother when the boy was still an infant. Before leaving, however, the boy's father named him "Sue." The son finally tracks down his father, after years of searching, and challenges him to a gun duel. Enraged over the humiliation he has had to suffer because of his name, the young cowboy is bent on revenge. However, instead of trying to outdraw his son, the father points out that his son has grown up to be a self-sufficient man, even though he did not have a father throughout his formative years. He knew that with the name "Sue" his son would have to learn how to fight and survive in his absence. Therefore, it was out of love, caring, and concern that the boy was given a girl's name.

Mr. G., a lover of country and western music, responded positively to the comparison of his father to the father in the song. The therapist pointed out how Mr. G.'s father had not had any formal education and really could not answer many of Mr. G.'s questions about math or science. The best Mr. G.'s father could do, with his limited resources, was to urge Mr. G. to "do it on your own." The therapist added that Mr. G.'s father was a proud man who could not admit that he did not know the answers to questions asked by his son and did not want his son to think poorly of him. Therefore, rather than to admit his ignorance, he was silent, while encouraging his son to get an education.

In addition to altering cognitive structures and person-in-relationship themes, these strategies also facilitate the development of empathy and the reduction of egocentrism.

3. *Reattribution of responsibility.* In reattribution of responsibility, the reason for a person's behavior or for the occurrence of a specific act is attributed to something, someone, or some factor beyond the actor's control. This technique is used to reduce the client's perceptions and attributions of malice to other family members and significant others.

Labeling the differences between Mr. and Mrs. G.'s desire for sexual intercourse as individual differences resulting in a "desire discrepancy" that was physiologically based and beyond either spouse's control is an example of how reattribution of responsibility was used to reduce conflict and resentment in this relationship. It also played a large part in altering Mr. G.'s cognitive representation of his wife. The shift occurred when his internal ideal took the form of a "woman with different sexual needs," rather than a "hostile bitch who uses sex to punish and control."

4. *Analogies* are used in individual therapy to crystallize specific relationship dynamics central to a client's personal mythology. Once a relationship theme has been identified and symbolized via an analogy, a different, more functional analogy can be suggested by the therapist. Such an analogy provides the client with a flexible alternative that he/she can adopt and modify. It allows for maximum elaboration and works at both conscious and unconscious levels of awareness.

For example, Mr. G.'s childhood relationship with his mother was characterized as resembling a "moth who is drawn to a flame." The "moth to flame" analogy was also used to describe the dynamics of Mr. G.'s relationship with his wife. In order to present Mr. G. with an alternative relationship dynamic, the therapist remarked, in passing, that he wondered if there was anything that Mr. G. could do to make it possible for him and his wife to live more like "two peas in a pod." This analogy inferred two separate, autonomous individuals living in harmony within the security of a marital system with distinct boundaries setting it apart from other systems and protecting it from unwanted intrusions from external sources.

Several days after the "two peas in a pod" alternative was mentioned, the therapist received a call from Mrs. G. She indicated that she and her husband had been discussing their relationship and had decided to try again to work together, as a couple, to bring about more "harmony" to their marriage.

5. *Telling Metaphorical Stories.* As we have already described in some detail (Anderson & Bagarozzi, 1983; Bagarozzi & Anderson, 1982), metaphorical stories are used to suggest alternative themes, to modify cognitive representations, and to offer possible solutions to unresolved conflicts. The use of metaphors in psychotherapy has been popularized by Haley (1973, 1980, 1985) and other followers of Milton Erickson (e.g., Lankton & Lankton, 1983; Rosen, 1982; Rossi, 1980; Zeig, 1980). The construction and use of therapeutic metaphors seem limited only by the therapist's imagination.

Clinicians who use metaphors, as part of their work, usually develop their own unique methods of presentation. Space and time constraints make it impossible for us to review various methods of presentation; however, we will outline one method used often by the first author. In this approach, the clients, couple, or family members are never directly told a specific metaphorical story. Instead, the therapist introduces them to a family of animal characters (his pets and various forms of wildlife that live on the therapist's property) in what appears to be an innocuous or accidental fashion. Throughout the treatment process, the therapist mentions these characters, makes reference to their unique "personality traits," and recounts stories about their relationships with one another, with him, and with the members of his family.

For example, shortly after Mr. G. began individual treatment, the therapist arrived late for an appointment. He apologized for his lateness and then gave Mr. G. this explanation for his tardiness: "Our youngest dog, Baby Tyrone, ran away from home, and I had to find him before I could leave for the office." The therapist continued: "He was abandoned by his mother when he was a puppy, and sometimes he does this just to see if someone will come after him. It is almost as if he is testing us to see if we really care about him. He never goes too far from our house. He stays within a safe distance, but refuses to come when he is called. He really fears the outside world, but wants to have some freedom. If I call him and offer some food or a dog biscuit or something to eat, he will eventually come to me. He gets a lot of attention for his naughty behavior."

This metaphorical vignette actually was a description of the newly formed therapeutic relationship, of Mr. G.'s ambivalence about beginning therapy and becoming involved with the therapist, and of his unvoiced concerns about whether the therapist "really cared" for him and his well-being. The symbolic messages implied in this brief story are that the therapist does have some understanding of Mr. G. and his conflicts, that the therapist can be patient, that he will not abandon Mr. G. and that therapy does offer Mr. G. some form of nurturance and security. It also acknowledges that some of Mr. G.'s inappropriate behavior is an attention getting, yet distancing device.

The second author's use of metaphors often involves listening intently to the content offered by clients during therapy sessions and emphasizing, elaborating and exaggerating it beyond the client's original productions. Such elaborations are used to highlight central affective and conflictual themes on a symbolic level and to add missing elements to the current script. For example, a father once described his son as having a "Dr. Jekyll/Mr. Hyde" personality. At times, the son could be responsible, sensitive, and successful in school (he had been tested and found to have a high I.Q.). However, at other times, he was a "monster." He would belligerently disobey any request, pound walls, and verbally threaten his parents. He was presently failing in school.

The original story of Dr. Jekyll and Mr. Hyde was reviewed with special attention given to the intellectual, bold, and pioneering scientific mind of Dr. Jekyll, the potion that Dr. Jekyll created and then drank, the absence of an antidote to reverse the repeated "conversions" of Dr. Jekyll into the "monster" Mr. Hyde, and the inevitable outcome of this script—the death of Dr. Jekyll along with the monster. The metaphor positively highlighted the boy's yet-to-be-developed creative potential, while dramatically exaggerating the irreversible and lethal consequences of his destructive behavior. The context of these metaphorical elaborations was an initial interview, before the father's commitment to the therapy was established. The issue of death, initially addressed in this metaphor, later emerged as a central, unresolved theme in the therapy.

· Prolonging individuals' or families' attention to the metaphor or symbol to the exclusion of their ordinary mental constructions (e.g., presenting problems, ongoing conflicts, other daily "hassles") or ways of viewing the world appears to have a *centering effect* similar to that provided by meditation or deep relaxation. As the emphasis on the metaphor or symbol is maintained, clients are able to slow down and to narrow their focus to the detailed, finite, and overlooked elements of their experience. In so doing, they are able to develop an expanded awareness of themselves and their relations to significant others.

6. *Role taking* is the ability to: (a) view the world through the eyes of another, (b) perceive what another person perceives from that person's unique vantage point, and (c) reverse perspectives so that one can see himself/herself as others see him/her. This cognitive ability is critical for the development and maintenance of a mature interpersonal relationship. Role taking begins to develop during middle childhood (at about the age of seven) and should be fairly well established by the beginning of adolescence (approximately by age 12), according to Flavell (1985). This ability to decenter is frequently impaired in clients. Many can see the world and others only from their own egocentric standpoint. In order for clients' cognitive representations of others to become modified, a certain amount of training in perspective reversal and decentering is necessary.

Once trust has been established between the client and the therapist, one method that can be employed to foster perspective reversal is for the therapist to ask the client to envision himself or herself in the role of a significant figure in his/her family of origin. The client is then asked to imagine what life must have been like for that person, what experiences might have caused this person to behave as he/she did toward the client, and how the client thinks this person perceived him/her at various significant points in the client's development.

When using this technique, proper timing is essential. The therapist must be certain that a solid foundation of trust has been established and that the client will not experience this intervention as the therapist's siding with or defending the other person's actions. The therapist must be sure not to communicate, verbally or nonverbally, that the client's perceptions of the person and the events that have taken place are inaccurate, distorted, or fabricated. The therapist must also be sure not to discount the client's feelings or to disqualify what the client has said. The central thrust of this intervention should always be to enable the client to decenter, so that some modification can take place in the client's internal representation of key figures. Extreme caution should be exercised in using this technique with clients who are victims of incest, with persons who have been physically assaulted as children, with clients who are extremely hostile and suspicious, and with individuals who exhibit paranoid ideation.

The major differences between this intervention and positive reframing and psychoanalytic interpretation are that the client is asked to come up with alternative explanations for others' behavior and to adopt a different perspective from the one he/she has always held to be true. This technique was used judiciously with Mr. G. to bring about some modifications in his cognitive ideals of both parents.

Behavioral Strategies for Editing Portions
of One's Personal Mythology

When parents and significant others are still alive and available to the client, yet unavailable to the therapeutic system, homework assignments, behavioral tasks, or structured enactments, which are designed to bring about cognitive dissonance between the client's internal representations of these figures and actual experiences, are prescribed. Clients usually are afraid to encounter parents, siblings, grandparents, and other significant persons because the internal representations of these individuals have not undergone revision since they were formed during infancy and childhood. Encountering one's parents as an adult and discussing important issues with them in a way that produces a different outcome will necessitate a reorganization of one's cognitive representations of these figures. Encouraging the client to enact specific assignments by explaining that he/she may not encounter the parent of his/her "childhood" usually helps reduce the anxiety and uncertainty that develop the first time such an assignment is introduced. It is important that the homework assignment, task, or prescription be designed in a way that requires the client to behave toward the target figures in a manner different from his/her customary way.

1. *Role playing* is often used in conjunction with role taking in order to help clients decenter, reverse perspectives, and increase empathy. However, our primary purpose in using this technique is to foster changes in the client's self-concept and his/her posture in relation to significant others, as well as to enhance the client's sense of self-efficacy, esteem, mastery, control, and confidence through the successful completion of specific, conflict-based, tasks.

Modifications in the self and in one's self-concept as a direct result of enacting a specific role or role complex is a central component of George Kelly's fixed role therapy (Kelly, 1955). According to this cognitive theory of personality formation and behavior change, individuals are what they represent themselves to be. In fixed role therapy, clients are encouraged to behave differently and to represent themselves to others in new and different ways. As a result, clients modify their personal construct system (i.e., self-concepts and self-representations) and their interpersonal behaviors. These modifications are then reinforced through changes in the responses clients receive from significant others.

In our approach, clients are asked to select or to create a role model (based upon characters described in their Family Relationships History and their Personal Myth Assessment interview) whom they would like to emulate. With the help of the therapist, clients then construct a series of person-in-relationship roles, outlining specific behaviors they would like to exhibit with selected individuals. Next, clients identify a specific interpersonal context and role play the new character role with the therapist, who responds to the client as would the target individual in that particular context. When clients can enact these roles satisfactorily and comfortably, they can begin to play out these new character roles with selected target persons in predetermined contexts. The contexts initially chosen are those that offer the highest probability of successful role performance.

The integration of a new role into the client's behavioral repertoire and the development of the accompanying changes in the client's self-concept are facilitated by the creation of *internal dialogues* tailored to meet the client's unique needs. After internal dialogues have been developed, they are recorded on 3" × 5" index cards so that clients can refer to them as needed. Once the dialogues have been committed to memory, they are recited aloud. Gradually, subvocal recitation replaces vocal performance. Finally, the client pairs these subvocal recitations with specific character/role performances in real life settings.

2. *Ritual prescription* is used to edit certain elements of one's personal mythology at the unconscious levels of awareness. The ritual is designed by the therapist and assigned to the client as part of his/her role enactment or as a component of an internal dialogue. The ritual is always constructed in a way that addresses unresolved conflicts underlying personal themes. In this way the client may be able to arrive at solutions to interpersonal conflicts in a less affectively charged or anxiety-producing manner. Once behavioral changes have been brought about and modifications in the self become evident, insight may occur. However, insight is

not the goal here. Ritual prescriptions are meant to help the client *unconsciously* work through key conflicts that form the basis for themes in the client's personal mythology.

In accordance with systems formulations of human behavior, alterations in any one of the client's personal themes will have an effect upon other themes associated with it. However, how these associated themes will be affected cannot be predicted. Additionally, changes in the client's personal themes can be expected to result in behavioral changes, which will be reinforced by significant others in the client's interpersonal context who respond to the client in new and different ways.

EDITING CENTRAL THEMES IN MR. G.'S PERSONAL MYTHOLOGY

Earlier we outlined four basic themes that were part of Mr. G.'s personal mythology. These were:

1. Mistrust of all people and their motives, intentions, etc.
2. Feelings of estrangement and difference.
3. Illness as a way to secure nurturance.
4. Ambivalence concerning interpersonal closeness and distance.

Here we demonstrate how information gathered from Mr. G.'s Personal Myth Assessment Interview was used to edit the fourth theme in his overall personal mythology, ambivalence concerning interpersonal closeness and distance.

Sometimes we come across clients who cannot recall a favorite fairy tale, short story, play, or motion picture, but readily identify a television show or series as having special significance. Mr. G. was one such person. He chose the television series *ALF* as having special significance for him. For readers not familiar with this situation comedy, a brief synopsis of the plot and central characters is offered.

ALF is the name given to an extraterrestrial voyager from the planet Melmac whose spaceship accidentally crashlands in the garage of a typical, everyday American family. Fearing that this alien will be subjected to scientific experimentation by NASA, the family agrees to hide and protect him from the authorities. He then becomes an adopted member of the family, so to speak, who is confined to the house and the garage where his spaceship is stored. The family names this furry, diminutive, midget-giraffe-like muppet ALF, an acronym for "Alien Life Form."

Mr. G.'s description of the family dynamics in this sit-com are as follows: The family that adopts ALF consists of a mother, a father, and their two children: an adolescent daughter and her prepubescent brother. ALF's relationship with the father is characterized by Mr. G. as "antagonistic" and "conflicted." The relationship with the family's mother is seen as "less antagonistic" yet still fraught with "periodic conflict." However, ALF's relationship with the mother figure is more "complex" and "ambivalent" than his relationship with the father figure. She is seen as more "understanding" and "comforting" than her husband, although she too becomes exasperated with ALF's antics.

Mr. G. depicts ALF as a "peculiar mixture" of a "self-centered, unsocialized child" and "adult with impaired reasoning abilities" who seems unable to distinguish between the "literal" or "concrete" and the "symbolic" meaning of words and communication. For this reason, he is continually "getting himself into trouble." ALF is not "bad" or "malicious," and his intentions are not designed to "hurt" anyone, but he often makes a "mess of things that others have to clean up." ALF's relationship with the two children in the family simulates a sibling relationship, with the two human children playing the roles of older brother and sister.

One interesting theme that resurfaces from time to time is ALF's bungling attempts to help the "parents." However, his efforts always seem to produce disastrous results for the entire family.

Mr. G. discussed, at length, his identification with ALF. The themes of being "alien," "different," "apart from," and "distant" from those with whom one lives and upon whom one is dependent for survival were readily recognized by Mr. G. as similar to the feelings he experienced throughout his childhood and adolescence.

As the similarities between Mr. G. and ALF were reviewed, Mr. G. came to the realization that many of the same "childhood feelings" were still with him. Mr. G. also began to recognize that ALF's earthly parents seemed to possess many of the same undesirable traits and characteristics that he found so distasteful in his own parents and siblings. However, his most startling discovery was that he perceived his wife to possess many of these same negative traits. That is, Mrs. G. was perceived as having the same negative qualities as significant family members with whom he still had unresolved conflicts.

On the other hand, many of the positive qualities, traits, characteristics, and resources that he had hoped to find in a nurturant maternal/paternal surrogate were also attributed to Mrs. G. However, he perceived his wife as deliberately and intentionally withholding these resources (e.g., sex, affection, love, attention, emotional support) from him to punish him or offering them to him contingently, only if he complied with her wishes and desires. As was the case in his family of origin, Mr. G. perceived himself to be totally dependent upon another person for psychological and emotional sustenance and trapped in a relationship from which there was no escape.

The Socialization and Maturation of ALF

Once the therapist and the client have identified a particular theme in the client's personal mythology that requires editing or revision, the client is helped to revise the role that he/she has characteristically played. Treatment goals are outlined in terms of specific behavioral, cognitive, and affective changes that are to take place. For example, Mr. G.'s identification with ALF produced both positive and negative consequences for him. He could use his ALF-like sense of humor and mischief to achieve closeness and intimacy, to put himself and others at ease, and to make new acquaintances. However, this same sense of humor could be used hostilely to distance himself from others whenever the threats associated with interpersonal closeness became too menacing. With his wife, extended periods of closeness and excessive amounts of intimacy awakened fears of ego disintegration, of loss of control, and of being dominated and overpowered by a larger-than-life negative maternal figure. In his relationships with male friends and acquaintances, prolonged closeness or intimacy produced feelings of intense competition and rivalry, fears of mutilation, destruction, and homosexual submission. Unfortunately, Mr. G.'s use of this different, ALF-like hostile humor eventually produced irreversible negative consequences. His friends had disappeared, and his relationship with Mrs. G. had deteriorated.

Within this broad theme of ambivalence concerning interpersonal closeness and distance, three subgoals were identified by Mr. G. These were:

1. To learn socially acceptable and appropriate ways to structure comfortable and nonthreatening levels of interpersonal closeness and separateness with his spouse and with male companions.
2. To learn how to identify, distinguish, and discriminate the true nature of his personal needs.
3. To recognize the appropriate persons who would be able to satisfy his actual needs once these needs were accurately identified.

For Mr. G. a number of needs were undifferentiated and consolidated into one mode of expression. For example, needs for physical closeness, emotional support, acceptance, nurturance, approval, etc., were all expressed through genital sexual activity. Therefore, most, if not all, of Mr. G.'s approach behavior toward his wife took a sexual form. His desire to become friends with members of the same sex was also interpreted as his desire for sexual intimacy. The inability to distinguish the true nature of his needs sometimes resulted in outbreaks of intense anxiety accompanied by obsessive fears of being "homosexual."

Here, we limit our discussion to the first and second subgoals. The outline in Table 1 illustrates how these subgoals fit into Mr. G.'s personal mythology. These particular sub-goals were selected as primary targets of our intervention in order to help Mr. G. acquire the interpersonal skills necessary to develop a more satisfying relationship with Mrs. G., so that she would be willing to reenter marital therapy.

1. *Developing a self-instructed performance model.* The first step was to help Mr. G. identify which of ALF's socially acceptable character traits he possessed and would like to retain as part of his behavioral repertoire. Next, Mr. G. was asked to select those socially acceptable character traits that ALF exhibited that he did not possess but wanted to acquire. Finally, Mr. G. was asked to identify the unacceptable character traits that he and ALF shared in common. These would become the targets for extinction and/or modification.

To complete the performance model, Mr. G. was directed to identify any additional persons, characters, or figures from all sources available to him (e.g., the ALF sit-com, other television shows, movies, books, short stories, fairy tales, popular songs or actual persons from his own life experiences) who possessed traits that he wanted to incorporate into his new character. Once these traits were identified and the behaviors associated with them were specified, they were grouped into a number of *role constellations*. These were designed to be enacted with specific individuals (e.g., spouse, siblings, employer) or classes of persons (e.g., male friends, female friends, neighbors, acquaintances). Depending upon Mr. G.'s relationship with a particular person and his needs at the time, he could activate the appropriate role constellation (and the accompanying cognitive-behavioral response chain associated with that role constellation) to achieve the degree of interpersonal closeness or separateness that was comfortable to him.

2. *Discriminating personal needs and differentiating appropriate responses.* In order to help Mr. G. determine which behavioral responses within a

TABLE 1 Schematic outline of Mr. G's personal mythology

Theme 1: Mistrust of all people and their motives.

Subgoals: (a)
　　　　　(b)
　　　　　(c)
　　　　　(etc.)

Theme 2: Feelings of estrangement and difference.

Subgoals: (a)
　　　　　(b)
　　　　　(c)
　　　　　(etc.)

Theme 3: Illness as a way to secure nurturance.

Subgoals: (a)
　　　　　(b)
　　　　　(c)
　　　　　(etc.)

Theme 4: Ambivalence concerning interpersonal closeness and distance.

Subgoals: (a) To learn socially acceptable and appropriate ways to structure comfortable and nonthreatening levels of interpersonal closeness and separateness with his spouse and with male companions.
　　　　　(b) To learn to clarify, distinguish, and discriminate the true nature of his personal needs.
　　　　　(c) To learn to recognize the most appropriate persons who would be able to satisfy his actual needs once these were accurately identified.

---

given role constellation were the most appropriate, discrimination training was necessary, because Mr. G. was unable to distinguish precisely what needs were pressing for fulfillment and motivating his behavior.

We began training by introducing Mr. G. to Murray's (1938) concept of basic needs and providing him with a list of 20 needs and their definitions. Next Mr. G. was asked to keep a behavioral diary, which was to include the following: (a) a list of all interpersonal situations and contexts where he experienced any strong emotion or affect that felt like a pressing need; (b) the individuals, circumstances and events that produced these feelings; (c) his actual behavioral responses in each situation; (d) any accompanying thoughts and internal dialogues; (e) the consequences and outcomes of his actions; and (f) his thoughts and feelings immediately following each sequence of events. Finally, Mr. G. was asked to identify what need he thought was motivating his actions and whether or not the behavior he exhibited actually helped him satisfy this particular need.

After several weeks of self-observation, Mr. G. was able to discriminate his needs more accurately. Specific role constellations were then revised so that Mr. G. could enact them with more precision, thus enabling him to satisfy his needs more appropriately.

3. *Restructuring and revising cognitive-behavioral response chains and internal dialogues through the use of ritual prescription.* Role constellations are made up of a series of interrelated sub-roles. Each sub-role consists of one or more cognitive-behavioral response chains and internal dialogues. These are designed to replace the client's outmoded, dysfunctional, and inappropriate cognitive-behavioral response chains. We have found it very useful to conceptualize cognitive-behavioral response chains as personal rituals that require editing. For example, Mr. G.'s new role constellation (centered around the ALF character) was named "Alfred the Mature Adult" by Mr. G. "Alfred the Mature Adult" was made up of several interconnected sub-roles: "Alfred the Patient Listener," "Alfred the Sensitive and Understanding Husband/Lover," "Alfred the Direct but Tactful," and "Alfred the Fun Loving Adult."

Cognitive-behavioral response chains and internal dialogues are automatically activated by specific stimuli, environmental cues and interpersonal contexts. These stimuli may be external to the person or internally generated, unconditioned or conditioned, consciously perceived or unconsciously experienced. Regardless of their origins, they activate a predictable sequence of thoughts (which are frequently accompanied by specific emotions) leading to a specific class of behavioral outcomes. For example, whenever Mr. G. perceived his wife to be "angry," the following cognitive-behavioral response chain would ensue:

"She *is angry.*"
"I wonder what *I have done to upset her?*"
"I wish *she* would say something *to me.*"
"Her *silence* is *driving me crazy.*"

"She is doing this to punish me."
"She is using silence to control me."
"I'll show her, she *won't control me."*

The above cognitive sequence usually resulted in Mr. G.'s exhibiting angry, hostile, and distancing behavior (e.g., insulting Mrs. G., retreating to another room in their home, going for a drive by himself, drinking "a few beers" in the privacy of his workshop).

Cognitive restructuring in the sub-role of "Alfred the Direct but Tactful" incorporated a ritual prescription that paradoxically led to increased interpersonal closeness and intimacy (responses incompatible with distancing):

1. Mr. G. was asked to identify the specific behaviors, facial expressions, body postures, nonverbal communications, etc., exhibited by his wife that he perceived to be indications of her anger.

Then he was asked to:

2. Identify what feelings he experienced whenever he perceived Mrs. G. to be angry.
3. Institute a "stop think" procedure that would prevent the dysfunctional cognitive-behavioral response chain from becoming activated.
4. Devise a different cognitive response chain that could be used in place of the dysfunctional one.
5. Record the new cognitive response chain on 3" × 5" index cards.
6. Practice reciting this new response chain aloud until it was completely memorized. Then practice the chain subvocally. Finally, "think" the response chain in a variety of settings and interpersonal contexts.
7. Introduce a different, more personally satisfying and socially appropriate behavioral outcome at the conclusion of the new cognitive response chain and internal dialogue.
8. Role play the new cognitive-behavioral response chain with the therapist until complete mastery was achieved.
9. Identify and list, in ascending order of the anxiety experienced, at least three persons (e.g., coworkers, acquaintances, friends, relatives) with whom Mr. G. could begin in vivo, practice trial runs before attempting to approach his wife.
10. Enact the cognitive-behavioral sequence with Mrs. G.

The new cognitive-behavioral response chain (outlined below) was instituted immediately after the "stop think" procedure was introduced. The "stop think" procedure served as a discriminative stimulus that automatically set in motion the new internal dialogue. The dialogue was incompatible with the old, dysfunctional cognitive-behavioral response chain and prevented its activation.

The new associative chain instituted by Mr. G. was:

"My wife (co-worker, acquaintance, friend, relative, etc.) *appears* to be angry."

"This makes me feel _____ (anxious, uneasy, angry, frightened, etc.) *because she reminds me of my mother who never expressed anger directly.*"

"Since I *don't really know* what she is *feeling* or *thinking*, I must *ask her directly* to find out."

"I will approach her *tactfully* in order to find out *whether she is angry* and *with whom* she is angry."

At this juncture in the response chain, Mr. G. approaches the target figure and says:

"You seem to be *upset*. Is there something troubling you that you would like to talk about?"

When developing a new cognitive-behavioral sequence for a particular sub role, it is extremely important that the new sequences (a) address the underlying conflict theme (ambivalence concerning interpersonal closeness and distance); (b) call attention to distortions in perception based upon transference phenomena, projective identification, etc. (the connections Mr. G. had begun to make between his negative projections onto his wife and his unresolved conflicts with his mother); and (c) provide a behavioral alternative that can be used to edit this particular portion of the client's personal mythology (replacing the distancing response with approaching behaviors).

OUTCOME

Once the "Alfred the Mature Adult" role constellation was firmly in place, Mr. G. was able to approach his wife differently. She, in turn, became more responsive in a variety of ways. Not only did she consent to having sexual intercourse more frequently, but she also agreed to resume marital therapy.

Individual treatment with Mr. G. was temporarily discontinued during the time he and his wife were in marital therapy. It is obvious that much more individual work could have been done with Mr. G. If individual treatment were to continue, the next step would have been to identify subgoals for another of the significant themes selected for editing earlier. This same process would continue until all four themes were successfully edited either independently or as a result of interactive changes in several themes simultaneously.

The reader must keep in mind that the presenting problem in the above case was a marital one. Individual treatment, therefore, was employed in order to prepare Mr. G. for the marital work that was to follow. In the best of all psychotherapeutic worlds, the therapist would have the opportunity to edit all major themes in the client's personal mythology. However, this is rarely the case. Such an undertaking takes a considerable amount of time, more time than most clients are willing to devote to the psychotherapeutic process. It has been our experience that individual clients usually terminate after the successful editing of one or two central themes. Many of these clients return to resume their work on remaining themes after a period of time (sometimes several or more years). Others return with their spouses and children to work on marital and family themes.

Therapists who desire complete closure for all themes will find themselves thoroughly frustrated in their work with individuals, couples and family systems. We ask those therapists who want their clinical outcomes neatly packaged and complete at the end of treatment to consider the wisdom of the oriental rug makers. These weavers deliberately leave a small segment of their handwoven carpets unfinished as a reminder, to themselves and others, that only Allah can create something that is complete and perfect.

5

Couples' Mythologies:
Theoretical Formulations and
Assessment Guidelines

A S WE SAID EARLIER, *the logical link between individual dynamics and marital/spousal dynamics is seen in the meshing of personal themes and myths between spouses*. This meshing of two distinct personal mythologies forms the basis of the couple's conjugal mythology. This process begins during the mate selection and courtship stages of relationship development. By the time the couple formally marries, the blueprints for the couple's conjugal mythology have, to a large degree, already been drawn.

Conjugal myth-making begins with mate selection. We assume that individuals actively seek out and attempt to marry persons whom they believe will behave in accordance with their internal cognitive *ideals*. As we noted earlier, the term *ideal* does not connote perfection or only positive attributes; rather, it is a comparative standard by which significant others are measured, compared and judged. For instance, an individual's negative experiences with her own parents during childhood may result in a personal mythology including the cognition, "my parents taught me a lot about how not to relate to my own husband." Wamboldt and Wolin (1989) have referred to this type of internalized standard as a "disengage and repudiate" posture with regard to one's family of origin.

The cognitive matching process is both conscious and unconscious. Family sociologists Lewis and Spanier (1979) have summarized the wealth of research findings related to conscious mate selection. These researchers reviewed a large number of empirical studies which suggest that mate selection is an active process wherein both parties seek potential mates to match their cognitive ideals. In the initial stages of relationship formation, physical attraction and similarity on a number of salient dimensions are important (e.g., race, ethnic background, religion, socio-economic status, intelligence, age, values). As the relationship progresses, however, more subtle and less tangible factors become crucial in determining whether the relationship will progress or dissolve. These factors include the fulfillment of complementary needs, a satisfactory role fit between the persons, and a congruence between the role expectations for one's future spouse and the actual role performances and behavior of the spouse-to-be. Lewis and Spanier propose that the greater the congruence between one's expectations and the actual behaviors of one's mate, the higher the quality of the marriage. Although these family sociologists do not address the unconscious dynamics of mate selection, they are keenly aware that individuals continually evaluate the behaviors of their intended spouses according to some internal comparative standard of which they may not be fully aware.

MATE SELECTION AND THE DEVELOPMENT OF CONJUGAL MYTHOLOGIES

Experiences with significant members of the opposite sex and repeated exposure to familial models and other important male/female relationships contribute significantly to the development of conscious and unconscious cognitive representations of one's *ideal spouse* and one's *ideal marriage*. In addition, it is assumed that persons become seriously involved only with others whom they believe match (Bagarozzi, 1982a, 1986; Bagarozzi & Giddings, 1983b) and will most likely behave in accordance with these internalized ideals. In our research, we have identified seven factors which persons take into conscious consideration in their attempts to match prospective spouses with their cognitive ideals (Anderson, Bagarozzi, & Giddings, 1986): (1) emotional gratification and support, (2) sex-role orientation and physical attraction, (3) satisfaction, (4) parent-sibling identification, (5) emotional maturity, (6) intelligence, and (7) sociological homogamy.

The ideal spouse and the ideal marriage, as well as their relation to the self, become central themes when one is preparing for marriage and actively seeking a mate. Prospective spouses are chosen because they are perceived as being able to "fit" well within the individual's personal mythology.

Major Components of the Matching Process

When one's prospective spouse's behavior is perceived to be in accordance with one's ideal, personal and dyadic equilibria are simultaneously maintained. However, when one's prospective spouse's behavior deviates too drastically from the ideal, disequilibrium results. At such times, the person will behave in ways designed to restore congruence between the spouse-to-be and his/her ideal.

A variety of strategies, both cognitive and behavioral, can be used by a person to deal with such discrepancies:

1. The first option open to a person who perceives a gross mismatch is to terminate the relationship with the unsuitable candidate and begin a new quest for another person who more closely approximates the ideal spouse.
2. A second possibility is for the ideal to undergo modification by accommodating to external realities. When this occurs, discrepancies are reduced and the ideal becomes more closely aligned with the perceived spouse-to-be.
3. A third option is for a person to attempt to bring about changes in his/her prospective spouse so that the spouse becomes more like his/her ideal.

In order to explain how this third option operates, we will describe a process called *mutual shaping toward the ideal* (Bagarozzi & Giddings, 1983b). In mutual shaping toward the ideal, both partners selectively reinforce those behaviors, characteristics, traits, and roles of their mates-to-be which are consistent with their ideals. However, behaviors, characteristics, and traits that are not perceived to be consistent with the ideal, that cannot easily be assimilated into the ideal, or that cannot be accommodated to (because this would require an unacceptable change in the essential character of the ideal) are ignored, denied, or in some other way defended against by the individual. Because discrepant behaviors are ignored, they are not reinforced and tend to fall into extinction. However, behaviors which are periodically reinforced become highly resistant to extinction. Any behaviors or characteristics that (a) are resistant to extinction, (b) cannot be assimilated into the ideal, (c) cannot be accommodated to because such accommodation would drastically alter the ideal, and (d) cannot be defended against because this would require gross reality distortions will create problems later on in the relationship.

In such cases, it is not uncommon for an individual to resort to using punishment (sometimes physical punishment) to modify undesirable traits and characteristics of a prospective spouse. However, punishments tend to be reciprocated (Patterson & Hops, 1972), and the excessive use of coercion of any type may lead to termination of the relationship if more attractive and less punishing alternatives are perceived (Bagarozzi & Wodarski, 1977). When punishment is used to modify a mate's behavior, it provides only a temporary solution to the problem, because when the threat of punishment is removed the undesirable behavior or trait will tend to resurface in a more exaggerated form. Most therapists have seen cases where the threat of punishment (in the form of abandonment by one's spouse-to-be) temporarily puts an end to an undesirable behavior or trait (e.g., the threatened individual refrains from drinking, taking drugs, gambling, dating other persons). However, the problem behavior resurfaces after marriage.

In sum, mutual shaping toward the ideal consists of four related processes:

1. Reward for those behaviors, traits and characteristics which are congruent with one's ideal spouse.
2. Extinction of undesirable behaviors, traits and characteristics which are not consistent with the ideal.
3. Punishment of unacceptable behaviors, traits and characteristics which cannot be assimilated into the ideal or accommodated to by the person.
4. The use of intrapsychic mechanisms (repression, denial, projection etc.) to avoid dealing with behaviors, traits, and characteristics which cannot be assimilated into the ideal or accommodated to by this structure.

Personal and Interpersonal Homeostasis: The Delicate Balance

The active quest for and ultimate selection of a mate who closely resembles one's ideal involve cybernetic goal seeking and mapping. This behavior serves a homeostatic function, because the closer the match between one's actual spouse and one's ideal, the less one is required to modify one's cognitive structures. Similar matching along behavioral and interactional dimensions of the relationship also occurs. For example, interpersonal and personal homeostasis is maintained, to a large degree, if one is able to find a spouse whose interactional style and rules for conjugal relationships do not require major changes or revisions in one's characteristic way of relating (i.e., in his/her interpersonal style). However, perfect matching rarely occurs and conflicts develop whenever spouses attempt to impose their own relationship rules on the marriage or force their mates to behave in ways which are consistent with their ideals.

Coercive strategies used to force one's mate to conform to an ideal or to behave according to certain relationship rules persist because they receive periodic reinforcement. The redundant interaction patterns that result have a ritualistic quality to them. These become woven into the fabric of the couple's conjugal mythology and give the couple system its unique rule-governed character. When assessing couples' conjugal mythologies, we pay particular attention to both idealized cognitive structures *and* the primary interactional rules. We use a number of perspectives in order to identify the couple's primary relationship rules. This involves exploration of their: (a) rules for interpersonal closeness and separateness; (b) rules for distributive justice and social exchange; (c) rules for marital power sharing, influence, and leadership; and (d) rules for communicating love, value, and worth.

Rules for interpersonal closeness-separateness. Pioneering family therapists recognized the importance of spouses' being able to negotiate and resolve their differences concerning individual needs for interpersonal distance, i.e., "closeness" and "separateness" (Hess & Handel, 1959). Since Hess and Handel first identified this central dynamic of family process, other family clinicians have incorporated it into their theories of family behavior and family therapy. For example, the extremities of "closeness-separateness" have been described as "emotional fusion" and "emotional divorce" (Bowen, 1978), as "enmeshment" and "disengagement" (Minuchin, 1974), and as "binding centripetal force" and "expelling centrifugal force" (Stierlin, 1981). Reiss (1971) labeled these two extremes as "consensus sensitive" and "interpersonal distance sensitive." Olson, Sprenkle, and Russel (1979) used Minuchin's two polar dimensions, "enmeshment" and "disengagement," to describe the extremes of the cohesion dimension in their Circumplex Model of Marital and Family Systems.

In our view of marital interaction, the differences between individuals' rules for "closeness" and "separateness" are conceptualized as behavioral reflections of individual personality differences in the critical area of one's need for interpersonal intimacy. Intimacy itself is not a unitary construct. There are at least *eight* subcomponents, including physical, sexual, emotional, psychological, intellectual, spiritual/aesthetic, social, and recreational intimacy.

It would be erroneous to assume that a person experiences the same level of need in all eight subcomponent areas or that any two people would share the same depth of need in all of these areas of potential interpersonal intimacy. In addition, it would be highly unlikely to find two individuals who attach the same meaning to all areas. For example, sexual intercourse may symbolize deep intimacy, love, and commitment for one person but mean only superficial coupling for his/her partner.

Finally, for some individuals, intimacy of any kind may produce severe anxiety, because interpersonal closeness has become associated with the loss of autonomy, the loss of control over one's life, or the loss of one's individuality, integrity or identity. Such fears are rarely verbalized as such because they are usually unconscious.

Persons who fear intimacy usually develop a number of defensive strategies that allow them to regulate interpersonal closeness and gain the separateness they desire. However, whenever too much distance is felt, these same persons frequently become anxious and depressed because this isolation evokes fears of abandonment and destruction. When this happens, they often initiate attempts to reestablish interpersonal closeness of some kind. The ambivalence associated with interpersonal intimacy for such individuals usually manifests itself behaviorally in the person's "inability to make a commitment."

At the other end of the continuum are those individuals who seem to want an inordinate amount of closeness, who attempt to merge with their partners, who seek to share the deepest intimacies possible in all eight areas, who actually lose themselves in the relationship, who willingly give up their own identities as individuals and become totally identified with their partners. Such persons often experience "separateness" as intolerable, perceive any sign of difference as a threat to personal integrity of the relationship, and become extremely threatened and suspicious whenever their spouse acts, feels, or thinks independently.

Differences between the spouses' rules for interpersonal closeness and separateness (i.e., interpersonal intimacy) constitute the first area where ideal spouse/perceived spouse discrepancies can become a source of conflict and struggle. These differences will generally manifest themselves in an interactional pattern where one spouse assumes the role of "pursuer" and the other the role of "distancer" (Fogarty, 1976; Guerin & Pendagast, 1976). While distressed spouses typically persist in their roles, these roles may at times become reversed, with the distancer becoming the pursuer and the pursuer the distancer. The net effect of these variations, however, is to maintain an unconscious, collusively negotiated level of interpersonal closeness and distance (Ryder, 1987).

Rules for distributive justice and social exchange. Social exchange theorists assume that spouses evaluate the fairness of conjugal exchanges according to the norms of equitable sharing and distributive justice and that prolonged perceptions of inequity between spouses lead to marital dissatisfaction (Bagarozzi & Wodarski, 1977). It is important to note that a dissatisfied spouse responds to what he/she *perceives* to be a violation of a fair exchange system. However, since the rules which govern the exchange system are rarely negotiated openly between prospective mates, it is possible that the two individuals hold vastly different views about the type of exchange rules which are to govern their marriage. It is easy to see how difficulties can come about between spouses in this area of distributive justice and sharing. For example:

First, in the early stages of relationship development (e.g., dating and courtship) the type of sharing and exchanges engaged in by the couple may be mutually satisfying. However, this exchange system may be socially patterned and determined by the stage of relationship itself. The highly novel and rewarding types of behaviors that are initially shared, the willingness to temporarily postpone one's own satisfactions for the sake of the developing relationship, and the lack of attention paid to future relationship costs result in a high proportion of positive interactions relative to negative ones (Jacobson & Margolin, 1979). How both partners share and exchange during this stage of the relationship may not be a reliable predictor of how each one will share and exchange after the marriage. In essence, both prospective spouses initially perceive their mates-to-be to have similar (if not identical) rules for exchange and distributive justice, and so there seems to be no perceived/ideal discrepancy on this dimension. However, after marriage each may use very different rules of exchange and the "idealized" expectations which were previously reinforced by the spouse may no longer realistically apply.

A shift in spouses' exchange behavior after marriage can be explained in a number of ways.

1. Premarital exchanges were strategically (consciously or unconsciously) designed maneuvers aimed at "winning over" the prospective mate. In this case, the spouse's true exchange orientation was masked.
2. With the change in context and relationship development (premarried to married) each spouse applies different rules of exchange. Here, no deception (conscious or unconscious) was planned. Spouses simply held a different set of expectations for exchanges after marriage than for courtship.
3. Spouses' exchange orientation may change with the passage of time, with the changing nature of the marital relationship, and with the incorporation of new sources of information from outside the marriage.

A second class of problems arise not because spouses apply different rules of exchange to their relationship but because they perceive that their mates are not sharing according to the rules. For example, one may disagree about the value of one's input into the relationship relative to that of the partner. An illustration of this would be the couple who agreed to share household tasks, parenting responsibilities, and a dual-career orientation. The wife's definition of sharing these tasks includes equal participation in house cleaning, cooking, and child care. The husband whose definition of equal sharing includes only taking out the garbage and mowing the lawn will be perceived by his wife as reneging on his part of the bargain.

Another class of difficulties arises when spouses are no longer able to provide resources which have been valued by their mates or when the resources that spouses have traditionally exchanged are no longer experienced as satisfying and they are unable to acquire new resources to use as exchange commodities. The former is illustrated by a spouse whose work schedule has changed so that she is no longer available for the couple's prized dinnertime conversation and they have been unable to find an alternative time to spend together. An example of the latter is the couple whose primary weekend activity together over the last ten years has been watching television together and "retiring early." However, the wife's enthusiasm for this activity has gradually declined over the years. The latter has been referred to as "reinforcement erosion" or the loss of novelty in a relationship (Jacobson & Margolin, 1979).

Rules for marital power sharing, influence, and leadership. According to Haley (1963), couples evidence either a complementary (one-up and one-down) or a symmetrical (equal) pattern of influence. Marital conflicts center around one or both spouses' dissatisfaction with the current interactional arrangement. A second consideration is the degree of flexibility or rigidity in the couple's interactional style. More flexible couples are able to alternate the one-up and one-down positions in different areas of the relationship (e.g., financial decisions; relationships with friends, neighbors and relatives; childrearing responsibilities; sexual practices; religious affiliations) or symmetrically share influence in some areas while allowing one or the other spouse to assume primary responsibility in others. The rigid adherence to a pattern perceived to be unacceptable to one or both partners is a major source of marital distress.

We also are attentive to alternate manifestations of complementary or symmetrical interactional rules. For example, distressed couples may evidence an "overfunctioner" (responsible, competent, healthy)-"underfunctioner" (irresponsible, incompetent, sick) dyadic arrangement (Bowen, 1978; Guerin & Guerin, 1976). Or distressed couples may symmetrically compete for the "underfunctioner" or sick role if both partners' personal mythology includes such strategies for meeting interpersonal needs.

Rules for communicating love, value and worth. Strayhorn (1978) has shown how behaviors exhibited by spouses carry important messages concerning the sender's evaluations of the receiver. For Strayhorn these messages convey much more to one's mate than the actual pleasurable or displeasurable value of the behaviors themselves; they signify love, value, and personal worth. Problems arise whenever the sender's rules and receiver's rules for the same behavioral message do not correspond. Three types of difficulties are identified.

The first type of difficulty involves *noncorrespondent rules for value messages*. Here the receiver's rules for the value message implied in a specific behavior does not correspond to the sender's rule and intention. Therefore, the receiver does not get the intended message. For example:

> *Sender's rule*: If you love me, you will show it by being concerned about my personal safety and whereabouts whenever I am late for an appointment.

> *Receiver's rule*: If you love me, you will always be prompt for appointments. Whenever I have to wait for you, it is proof that I really don't mean very much to you.

The second type of difficulty involves *reliance upon painful channels for communicating value messages*. In this situation, the sender's rules and the receiver's rules do correspond, but the channels necessitate pain on the part of one or both spouses. For example:

> *Sender's Rule*: If you love me, you will show it by being concerned when I am sick or hurt and by being jealous of other men/women when I flirt with them. I, in turn, will show my love for you by being concerned when you are hurt or ill and by being jealous of other men/women.

> *Receiver's Rule*: I will show my love for you by being concerned when you hurt yourself or when you are ill and by being jealous of other men/women. I know that you will show your love for me whenever I am sick or hurt and by being jealous of other men/women.

The third problem comes about whenever a spouse is extremely *sensitive to receiving devalue messages and has an inordinate fear of losing value messages*. For example, a spouse may respond immediately with coercion and retaliation to what he/she perceives as a devalue message. Or a spouse's intense fear of loss of love may drive him/her to resort to every increasing and dangerous painful channels in order to receive value messages.

Satir (1967) first called attention to some of the central individual dynamics involved in sending and receiving value messages. For her, all communications directed to another person are seen as carrying with them implicit requests for self-validation. The form that such requests take varies from individual to individual. For example, agreement with the sender of a message, sympathizing with the sender, and siding with the sender in a dispute are all seen as validations.

Self-Individuation

The important individual development task of emotionally and psychologically separating from one's parents and family of origin and developing an autonomous self and unique identity has long been recognized by psychoanalytic thinkers (e.g., Blos, 1967; Erikson, 1950, 1959, 1968, 1974). The failure of individuals to separate and individuate from their families of origin has been identified as a major factor in adolescents' adjustment problems (Anderson & Fleming, 1986a, 1986b, Fleming & Anderson, 1986) and as a major cause of marital/family dysfunction by intergenerational family therapists (e.g., Boszormenyi-Nagy & Sparks, 1973; Bowen, 1978; Napier & Whitaker, 1978; Bray, Williamson, & Malone, 1984). Bowen (1978) identified two highly correlated aspects of self-individuation: (a) the differentiation of emotional from intellectual functioning within the self, and (b) differentiation from one's family of origin. Bowen (1978) postulates that the more individuated the person's self, the less likely he/she will be to fuse emotionally and psychologically with another individual. Bowen (1978) has also postulated that persons tend to marry spouses who have the same level of self-individuation. Although no empirical data have been presented in support of Bowen's hypotheses, our clinical experiences seem to bear this out to some extent. Therefore, we have included self-individuation as another quality or trait that must be considered in the cognitive matching process of mate selection.

Unconscious Collusion and Agreements in the Fashioning of Conjugal Mythologies

Regardless of the matching strategies used, perfect congruence rarely occurs. Therefore, partners must somehow compromise and negotiate a mutually acceptable solution to this problem, a solution that will allow them to maintain a stable relationship in spite of the ideal spouse/perceived spouse discrepancies that exist. The agreements that they ultimately negotiate must make use of and incorporate the individual defenses of both partners to insure that each spouse receives some measure of protection in the marriage. For this mutual defense system to be maintained successfully over long periods of time, each spouse must become a willing participant in the personal mythology of his/her partner by playing out central thematic dramas and enacting key roles associated with these themes. *The integration of the personal mythologies of both spouses produces a superordinate, overarching mythology that we call the couple's "conjugal mythology." It is important to understand that neither spouse is able to see the totality of this conjugal mythology* for a number of reasons:

1. The mutually protective contracts that couples negotiate are similar to those described by Sager (1976) in that they are products of unconscious agreements.
2. The dynamics of the negotiation process whereby spouses collude to play out specific themes and enact certain roles also take place out of the conscious awareness (Dicks, 1967).
3. Each spouse can only perceive and experience his/her mate in ways consistent with his/her own personal mythology.
4. Spouses unconsciously agree to play out only those themes and enact only those roles in their mates' personal mythologies that are consistent with their characteristic interpersonal style and fit within the framework of their own personal mythologies.

In most cases, one's ideal spouse is expected to validate the self. However, difficulties arise whenever a mate is chosen because he/she is perceived as someone who will bolster a person's low self-esteem, alleviate a person's depression, reduce a person's anxiety, etc. This frequently is the motivating force behind mate selection for individuals with very low self-esteem or for those who do not possess a clear sense of self. Frequently such individuals are *blinded by their own ideals, which are projected onto their spouses-to-be;* therefore, they are unable to see their mates realistically. The ideal obscures the true nature of the spouse-to-be. In some cases, the spouse-to-be is seen as the ideal who possesses those desired traits and characteristics that the person lacks. Through intimate association and marriage, the person hopes to gain or share in the longed-for qualities. In other instances, one's spouse-to-be is seen as the ideal who is perceived as an extension of the self. When this happens, the person's self-esteem is elevated through his/her identification with the spouse-to-be.

In all these instances disappointment is inevitable, because the true nature of one's spouse has been obscured by projection. Conflicts arise whenever the discrepancies are realized and the person attempts to co-erce his/her mate into providing the much needed self-validation and self-esteem.

ASSESSMENT OF CONJUGAL MYTHS

We use a number of methods to gather and organize information about the central symbolic and affective themes that comprise a couple's conju-gal mythology. First, we conduct initial assessment interviews with both spouses to collect information regarding the couple's relationship history and the history of the presenting problem. In our approach, the couple's presenting problem is viewed as a condensed and highly symbolic repre-sentation of the central themes that will later be shown to comprise the couple's conjugal mythology. This initial assessment phase will often include seeing each spouse individually to conduct the Family Relation-ships History and the Personal Myth Assessment Interviews. Secondly, we often use a number of empirically derived instruments to help identi-fy major themes in a couple's mythology. Finally, we organize the infor-mation obtained from the initial assessment interviews, the empirical instruments, and any additional information obtained in subsequent interviews according to the four global indicators noted initially in Chap-ter 4. These include: (1) recurrent topics of concern, (2) redundant inter-action patterns, (3) repeated surfacing of specific affect-laden conflicts, and (4) the couple's predominant affective tone. Our use of structured assessment interviews and empirical instruments is discussed below. The use of the behavioral indicators to organize conjugal themes is illus-trated in Chapter 8.

Initial Assessment Interviews

Assessment usually begins with the therapist's meeting with both spouses to collect detailed information about the *couple's relationship his-tory and the history of the presenting present problem*. In conducting this interview, the therapist should not accept, as valid and reliable, only one spouse's account of the dating and courtship process, because each spouse's account represents only his/her own unique perceptions and recollections. Therefore, the therapist must allow ample time, in these initial sessions, for both spouses to discuss (from their own vantage points) how they first met, their first date together, and the subsequent developments in their relationship. The therapist should note any gross discrepancies and major differences in the spouses' accounts of the same experience and ask for their assistance in understanding how such major differences in perception might have come about, why they have continued for so long, and how these differences and discrepancies have affected their relationship together.

Couple's Relationship History

1. How did you meet?
2. Which one of you initiated dating?
3. a. Where did you go on your first date? How was this decision made? How would each of you describe this first date? Was it successful or unsuccessful? What is it about your spouse that made you want to date him/her again, after your first date?

   b. What traits, behaviors and characteristics about your spouse did you find most attractive when you first met?

   c. What traits, behaviors and characteristics about your spouse did you dislike most when you first met? How did you deal with these traits, behaviors and characteristics during your courtship? How did you deal with them after you were married? How do you deal with them now?
4. If you had sexual relations together before you were married, how long after your first date did you wait before having sexual intercourse?
5. How would each of you describe your first sexual intercourse together? Was it satisfying, disappointing, uneventful?
6. How frequently (on a weekly basis) did you have sexual intercourse during your dating and courtship together? How frequently (on a weekly basis) did you have sexual intercourse during the first year of your marriage? Has the frequency of your sexual intercourse changed substantially over the years?
7. When did you first notice the change?
8. How did you both feel about this change when you first noticed it? How do you feel about it now? Have you ever sought the help of a sex therapist for this change in frequency?

If the couple identifies a sexual problem during this part of the interview, additional interviews based upon the work of Masters and Johnson (1970) are conducted.

9. How long did you date before deciding to marry?
10. Were there any significant circumstances, in your personal lives, that you believed played a part in your decision to get married? For example: the death of a parent or sibling, disabling illness of a parent or sibling, graduation from school, personal illness (physical or emotional), loss of steady employment, personal trauma, etc.
11. Did you marry because of pregnancy? If yes, how was that decision made?
12. Which of you proposed marriage and how was the proposal received?
13. Did you have a formal engagement? How long was the engagement period before you actually married?
14. How did your respective parents respond to your decision to marry?
15. Were there any breakups before marriage? If yes, how many times did you break up? What were the reasons for these breakups? Did you date other people during these breakup periods? Who initiated reconciliation each time?
16. How did your parents respond to these breakups and reconciliations?
17. How was the decision made concerning where you were going to live in relationship to where your parents were living at the time of your marriage?
18. How did your friends respond to your decision to marry?
19. Do either of you still maintain friendships with people you knew before you began to date each other?
20. Do you continue to have relationships with individuals or couples whom you met together?
21. Do either of you have friends that your spouse disapproves of?
22. How was the decision made concerning whether or not to have children and the number of children you were going to bring into the world?
23. What legacy from your family of origin did you bring into this marriage? Does it affect your life as a couple? Examples: inheritances; values; spiritual or religious beliefs, traditions and commitments; emotional, psychological or financial debts; emotional or psychological loyalties; unresolved conflict or unfinished business with members of your family of origin?
24. What traditions did each of you bring to this marriage from your families of origin?

25. What rituals did each of you bring to this marriage from your families of origin?
26. Which of these traditions and rituals do you think are beneficial? Which are harmful to your marriage?
27. What traditions and rituals have you developed as a couple/family that are unique to your relationship?

History of the Presenting Problem

1. Describe the problem you have as a couple in your own words. (Be as behaviorally specific as possible.)
2. When did you first notice that there was this problem in your relationship? (How long has the problem been going on?)
3. What made you decide to seek professional help at this particular time?
4. What have you done, as individuals, to correct this problem in the past?
5. What have you done, as a couple, to correct this problem?
6. What remedy or remedies have been successful in correcting this problem? What remedies have been unsuccessful?
7. What significant people have been involved in helping you solve this problem in the past?
8. What significant people are now involved in trying to solve the problem with you or for you?
9. Do either of you use any nonprescribed drugs for alleviation of this problem (including alcohol, marijuana, hashish, cocaine, etc.)?
10. If one spouse is singled out as the identified patient or as having a problem, how does he/she feel about the problem and his/her role as the identified patient?
11. As individuals, what do you hope to accomplish in therapy?
12. Please describe, as best you can, what your relationship together will look like at the end of successful therapy? How will you both have changed at the end of successful therapy? How will you both remain the same after successful therapy?
13. How willing are each of you, on a scale from 1–10, to make changes in your own behavior so that you can function better as a couple and have a happier relationship?
14. Situational analysis (if necessary):
    a. In what situations does the problem occur?

b. In what situations does the problem never occur?
c. In what situations is the problem most severe?
d. In what situations is the problem least severe?
e. What situations, people, thoughts, feelings, etc., set off the problem?
f. How does each spouse behave?
g. How does each spouse feel at the time it is happening?
h. What does each spouse say to himself/herself at the time it is happening?
i. How does each spouse behave immediately after the problem behavior is exhibited?
j. How does each spouse feel immediately after the problem behavior is exhibited?
k. What does each spouse say to himself/herself immediately after the problem behavior is exhibited?
l. What happens later on, after the spouses have had a chance to think about what has transpired?
m. What are the conditions, in your environment, that you both believe contribute to maintaining this problem?
n. What are the conditions, in your environment, that you both believe can contribute to reducing the problem or solving it altogether?

15. What positive (reinforcing) behavior change strategies do each of you use to get each other to change your behaviors as they relate to the presenting problem?
16. What negative (coercive, punishing, negatively reinforcing) behavior change tactics do each of you use to get the other to change behaviors as they relate to the presenting problem?
17. Incentive analysis
    a. What *benefits* would derive for each spouse if the problem continued in its present form?
    b. What *benefits* would derive for each spouse if the problem became worse?
    c. What *benefits* would come about for each spouse if the problem were solved?
    d. What are the *disadvantages* for each spouse if the problem continued in its present form or intensity?
    e. What are the *disadvantages* for each spouse if the problem becomes worse?
    f. What are the *disadvantages* for each spouse if the problem were solved?

18. Is there anything else about the presenting problem that you think is important for the therapist to know?

Once the Couple's Relationship History and History of the Presenting Problem Interview sessions have been completed, individual interviews are scheduled for each spouse. During these individual sessions, Family Relationships Histories and Family Myth Assessment interviews are conducted. *The material gathered in these conjoint and individual interviews helps the therapist identify how the central themes in each spouse's personal mythology dovetail to form the basis for the couple's conjugal mythology.*

In our work with couples, during these initial interviews, we frequently use a variety of visual aids to stimulate memory and facilitate recall. For example, genograms are used to help spouses identify intergenerational themes and toxic issues (Corrales, Kostoryz, Rotrock, & Smith, 1983; Guerin & Pendagast, 1976). We frequently ask spouses to bring in photographs of their parents, siblings, extended family members (both living and deceased), and significant others as part of the interview process and as a complement to their genograms. We also ask couples to bring in any photographs of them as a couple that were taken during their courtship period. Couples who have been married for several years or more are also asked to bring in photographs taken during critical periods of their marriage.

With certain individuals and couples we have used Tarot Cards as a projective technique. When Tarot Cards are used, each partner is asked to select those Tarot card characters and symbols that have special significance for him/her because he/she can associate these archetypal characters with family members. The symbol cards chosen by a person are usually ones that represent significant themes in that person's life. When Tarot cards are used as an adjunct to the Couple's Relationship History and History of the Presenting Problem Interviews, each spouse is asked to tell his/her version of the dating and courtship process and to describe his/her perception of the presenting problem and its history by using Tarot character and symbol cards. An alternative projective technique, often effective during the Halloween season, is to ask partners which costume best represents each of them, as well as significant others from their respective families of origin.

Another routinely used visual aid involves diagramming each spouse's family of origin in terms of its structural characteristics as perceived by the individual. We make use of the structural symbols and characters suggested by Minuchin (1974). Here again intergenerational themes and family dynamics become evident. Once the structural diagram is completed, each spouse is asked to discuss the sub myths, family secrets, and shared family myths and beliefs that were used to help maintain his/ her family's particular structural arrangements. Spouses are also asked to consider the possible influences that their respective family structures might have had on their own marriage/family structure. Furthermore, they are asked to consider which of their families of origin seems to be serving as a model for their own marital/family system. Such questions often highlight conflicts between spouses over which type of marital/ family structure is to take precedence in their marriage. Similarly, such discussions allow the therapist to assess the degree to which the couple has been able to achieve a mutually satisfying integration of their respective families' structures. They also help the therapist assess the couple's ability to negotiate its own, unique structural arrangements and marital/ family system.

Using Empirically Developed Instruments

IMAGES. Earlier in this chapter we said that congruence between one's ideal spouse and one's perceived spouse plays an important role in determining one's satisfaction with one's mate. In order to gain some insight into the nature of the discrepancies perceived by spouses, we developed IMAGES (Anderson, Bagarozzi, & Giddings, 1986). This 35-item, self-report instrument consisting of 7 relatively independent sub-scales was empirically established through factor analysis. Each subscale represents a separate factor which identifies a specific set of behavioral traits. Each subscale factor has been statistically tested to determine its internal consistency. Cronbach alpha correlations for these subscales range from .70 to .87. Anderson et al. (1986) believe that IMAGES taps both conscious and preconscious dimensions of one's ideal spouse. These 7 dimensions include: emotional gratification and support (8 items); sex-role orientation and physical attraction (6 items); satisfaction with one's spouse in the areas of sexual, emotional and intellectual intimacy (3 items); parent; parent-sibling identification (4 items); emotional maturity (4 items); intelligence (3 items); and homogamy. This last factor, homogamy (7 items) deals with racial, ethnic, and social class compatibility. Additionally, two of these behaviorally worded items deal with spiritual intimacy.

A spouse is asked to rate, on a 6-point Likert type scale, the degree to which his/her actual spouse corresponds to his/her ideal spouse for each of the 35 behaviorally worded items. Each spouse is also asked to consider how important each of the 35 items is in determining his/her satisfaction with his/her chosen mate.[1]

By using IMAGES, the therapist can get direct information about which ideal/perceived spouse discrepancies might be a serious source of conflict in the marriage.

We also have stressed the importance of spouses' sharing the same, or at least similar, expectations concerning relationship rules and values in five distinct areas of marital behavior: interpersonal closeness-separateness; distributive justice and social exchange; power sharing, influence, and leadership; self-individuation; and communicating love, value and worth. We use the following empirically tested instruments to gain some insights into the first four sets of expectations.

Family Adaptability and Cohesion Scales III. FACES III is the third in a series of scales developed by Olson and his colleagues to assess the two major dimensions of the Circumplex Model of Marital and Family Systems (Olson, Portner, & Lavee, 1985). The two dimensions are cohesion and adaptability. FACES III is comprised of 20 5-point Likert type scale items describing specific behaviors that operationalize the two dimensions of cohesion and adaptability. Odd-numbered items assess each spouse's perceptions of cohesion in the marital dyad, while even-numbered items are used to operationalize the adaptability dimension. Although a number of studies have been undertaken to determine the reliability and independence of each subscale, results have been less impressive than expected. Cronbach alpha reliabilities for the cohesion dimension have been shown to be consistently acceptable, ranging from .75 to .77. Internal consistency reliabilities for the adaptability dimension have been between .58 and .63.

We use the cohesion dimension to operationalize each spouse's perceived need for interpersonal closeness and separateness. The total scale

---

[1]Discrepancy scores, in the form of percentages, are computed for all factors. The formula for arriving at this score is

$$D = \frac{\text{Number of actual discrepancies for a factor}}{\text{Number of possible discrepancies for a factor}}$$

For example: Factor I Emotional Gratification: 24/48, D = 50%
A total discrepancy score is calculated for the entire IMAGES scale in a similar manner. For Example:

$$D = \frac{\text{Total number of actual discrepancies}}{\text{Total number of possible discrepancies}} = \frac{105}{210} = 50\%$$

score can be contrasted with norms and cutoffs provided by the FACES III authors to determine which one of four categories best describes an individual's preferred interpersonal style. The categories are disengaged (at one extreme), separate, connected, and enmeshed (at the other extreme).

When FACES III is used in conjunction with the last factor of IMAGES, the therapist can develop a pretty good idea about each spouse's desires and expectations concerning interpersonal intimacy. Olson et al. (1985) also developed ideal spouse and perceived spouse versions of FACES III which can be used to help assess the extent to which ideal/perceived discrepancies are present in this critical dimension.

Relational Communication Coding System. Although the adaptability dimension of FACES III is meant to operationalize some aspects of marital rules for power sharing, influence and leadership, the validity of this subscale has been questioned (Brock, 1986; Schmid, Rosenthal, & Brown, 1988). Therefore, whenever time and circumstances permit, we also use the well researched Relational Communication Coding System (Rogers, 1972) to determine the couple's characteristic control and dominance interaction patterns. The Relational Communication Coding System operationalizes the two interaction styles of complementarity and symmetry first identified by Bateson (1935, 1936, 1949, 1961, 1972) and later reintroduced within the psychotherapeutic research context of the Palo Alto Group (e.g., Haley, 1963, 1964; Jackson, 1959, 1965; Watzlawick, Beavin, & Jackson, 1967). Since considerable time and training are necessary before a person becomes proficient in the use of this coding system, it may be inappropriate for use in clinical settings where video recording equipment is not readily available. However, once a person is trained in the use of these coding procedures, he/she is quite capable of making on-the-spot clinical judgments about the type of control and dominance patterns displayed by a particular couple. Essentially, the FACES III and the Relational Communicating Coding System enable us to operationalize relationship rules for closeness-separateness and power sharing, influence, and control in marital dyads.

Spousal Inventory of Desired Changes and Relationship Barriers. Bagarozzi and his associates (Bagarozzi, 1983b; Bagarozzi & Atilano, 1982; Bagarozzi & Pollane, 1983) have developed SIDCARB to help spouses evaluate the fairness of the social exchange dimension of their marriage. SIDCARB is a self-report factor-analyzed questionnaire consisting of 24 Likert type scale items. The first 10 items in factor I assess the spouses' perceptions of the fairness of the social exchange process in 10 areas of marital exchange (household chores, finances, communication, expressions of love and affection, in-laws, religion, recreation, sexual relations, friendships, and children). Questions 11–15, factor I, assess satisfaction with one's spouse, satisfaction with one's marriage, the strength of one's commitment. Questions 16–21 make up factor II. These questions assess internal psychological barriers to divorce and separation (e.g., obligations to children, commitment to marriage vows, religious beliefs, concerns about other family members' reactions). Questions 21–24 constitute the final factor and measure the strength of external, circumstantial barriers to divorce that spouses perceive (e.g., what friends and neighbors might say, job considerations, legal costs, and financial concerns).

SIDCARB is also another measure of power, influence, dominance and control in marriage. By comparing the husband's and wife's scores on all three factors, the therapist can easily identify which spouse has more power and ability to control and influence the other by virtue of his/her perceiving fewer barriers to relationship termination, operationalizing the exchange principle of least interest (Waller & Hill, 1951).

Personal Authority in the Family System Questionnaire. In order to get an indication of the extent to which spouses have successfully individuated from their respective families of origin, we have used the PAFS (Bray, Williamson, & Malone, 1984). Respondents are asked to rate, on a series of 5-point, self-report, Likert type scales, their current relationships with relevant family members from their families or origin. The Personal Authority in the Family System Questionnaire consists of eight statistically derived independent factors which are measured by 132 items. The eight subscale factors are: (1) spousal fusion/individuation, (2) intergenerational fusion/individuation, (3) spousal intimacy, (4) intergenerational intimacy, (5) nuclear family triangulation, (6) intergenerational triangulation, (7) intergenerational intimidation, and (8) personal authority. Subscales 2, 5, 6 and 7 (i.e., intergenerational fusion/individuation, nuclear family triangulation, intergenerational triangulation, and intergenerational intimidation) are most relevant for our purposes.

Assessing rules for communicating love, value, and worth. We are unaware of any empirically validated instruments developed specifically to measure these three constructs. The most frequently used paper-and-pencil measure of marital communication has been the Marital Communication Inventory (Bienvenu, 1978). However, the validity of this instrument as a measure of clear and open communication has been seriously questioned (Schumm, Figley, & Jurich, 1979). Furthermore, the practice of using self-report questionnaires as valid indicators of respondents' actual behaviors has also been criticized by clinical researchers on the grounds that, because of social desirability biases and experimenter effects, respondents' self-reports may in no way reflect their actual behavior (Bagarozzi & Rauen, 1981).

For these reasons, we assign any number of conflict negotiation tasks and problem-solving exercises to couples so that we can observe their actual behavior, typical interaction styles, and characteristic ways of sending and receiving value messages. In addition, we ask spouses to specifically send each other messages that convey love, worth, and valuing. We also ask each spouse to identify what he/she says and does that he/she believes his/her spouse perceives and experiences as an expression of love, valuing, and worth. Spouses are likewise asked to identify what they do or say that they believe their mates experience and perceive as devaluing and derogatory and as an attack on their self-esteem and self-worth. Finally, spouses are asked to discuss any differences in perception, attribution, and intention they have identified during these exercises.

It is important to remember that every message sent to one's spouse or family member carries with it both report and command components, as well as meta communicative qualifiers about the message itself, the sender, the receiver, and the relationship (Haley, 1964; Watzlawick, Beavin, & Jackson, 1967). Furthermore, every message sent carries with it an implicit request for validation of the sender's self. The highest form of self-validation one can receive is an empathic response from another. While agreement with the sender or compliance with the command component of a message is validating, it does not communicate the same level and depth of acceptance as does an accurate empathic response. Finally, we believe that it is crucial for therapists to understand that all behaviors exchanged between spouses and among family members have psychological and symbolic value. The importance of the symbolic psychodynamic component of human interaction in editing conjugal and family myths will be highlighted in subsequent chapters.

6

Selecting and
Preparing Couples

A T THIS POINT IN OUR WORK we have only preliminary clinical data to
support the effectiveness of our approach. Therefore, additional
empirical study is necessary in order to provide us with a better understanding of the types of presenting problems that best lend themselves
to treatment using this clinical method. We must also investigate what
types of relationship systems can profit most from the intervention strategies that have grown out of this approach. Finally, it is important for us
to explore at what stages of relationship formation and marital/family
development using our understanding of personal, conjugal, and family
myths is most beneficial. Given the current status of our clinical research, however, we can offer our readers only tentative guidelines and
suggestions.

CLIENT SELECTION

Preliminary Considerations

We view the myth approach as a broad clinical strategy to be used
under certain conditions and in certain circumstances. Our customary
mode of practice is to begin direct intervention only after a thorough
assessment has been conducted. Initial intervention usually begins with
a structured, cognitive, sociobehavioral-exchange and skills training approach (Bagarozzi, 1983a, 1983b; Bagarozzi & Giddings, 1983a, 1983b;
Bagarozzi & Pollane, 1983; Bagarozzi & Wodarski, 1977, 1978). We have
found skills training to be the initial treatment of choice when the presenting problem is seen as stemming from limitations in one or both
partners' social or interpersonal skills (Bagarozzi, 1985; L'Abate & Milan,
1985). We move to the use of our understanding of myths as the primary

99

mode of treatment whenever the more structured, cognitive sociobehavioral-exchange and skills training model proves to be ineffective or inappropriate for a given couple or family system. In this sense, we agree
with Stanton's (1981) recommendations that the therapist first use a
more structured behavioral approach and then switch to a predominantly strategic approach when techniques are not succeeding or are unlikely
to succeed. Although we do not consider our approach to be a strategic
one per se, we frequently use our understanding of myths strategically
(Anderson & Bagarozzi, 1983).

Selection Criteria: Presenting Problems

Individuals, couples, or family members who present with specific
behavioral problems that have been shown to respond well to behavior
modification techniques (e.g., phobias, anxiety), biofeedback procedures (e.g., stress), or medication are not considered appropriate candidates for this approach. Referral to qualified practitioners who specialize
in the use of these techniques and procedures is advised. However,
individuals, couples, and families who have availed themselves of these
services and have found them to be ineffective, unsatisfactory, or unsuitable for their personal needs may be accepted for treatment.

Dyadic or family systems whose presenting problem is substance
abuse are considered for treatment only after the substance-abusing
member(s) have been detoxified and have become actively involved in a
drug or alcohol rehabilitation program. In such instances, our approach
can be used to complement these other forms of treatment.

When the presenting problem is spouse abuse, child abuse (including
incest), domestic violence, etc., the couple or family is not seen as ready
for this method. Only after the violence, abuse, etc., have been completely discontinued is the system able to use this approach (Bagarozzi,
1982b; Bagarozzi & Giddings, 1982, 1983a).

Selection Criteria: Systems Characteristics

Couples and family members who have been unable to benefit from
behavioral marital/family therapy or have been unable or unwilling to
use skills acquired in these therapies outside the confines of the therapist's office can make use of this approach. Essentially, these people are
unable to change the destructive interlocking cycles of mutual coercion
and punishment that characterize their relationships. In some instances,
both spouses are more concerned with defeating each other than with

improving their relationship. With such couples and family systems we frequently find themes of conquest, vanquishing one's spouse who is seen as "the enemy" or a "monster," mistrust of members of the opposite sex, fear of interpersonal intimacy, fear of abandonment, etc. On rare occasions, both spouses have joined in collusion to defeat the therapist, rendering behavioral techniques and behavioral practitioners helpless. The Family Relationships Histories of such individuals should alert the therapist to such themes and defensive systems at the outset of treatment. With such couples, a more indirect, analogical/symbolic approach may be the treatment of choice.

Couples and families that have made modest or even considerable gains through behavioral marital therapy and contingency contracting procedures sometimes continue to experience inequity in their conjugal/ familial exchange systems in spite of the objective reality that both spouses and family members have made substantial behavioral changes. Such couples and families are good candidates for our approach if they are able to understand that there is deeper meaning to their dissatisfaction, disappointment, disillusionment, and frustrations.

Frequently couples realize that the difficulties they are having with their spouses and other family members stem from unresolved, long-standing conflicts with significant others in their families of origin. They enter therapy with the intention of unearthing these conflicts and resolving them to the point where they no longer interfere with their marriage and family life. Couples and families presenting this type of insight into their presenting problems are excellent candidates for a mythological approach.

If couples have not been able to benefit from traditional behaviorally oriented sex therapy and continue to experience inhibited sexual desire, hypoactive sexual desire, and serious desire discrepancies, they are appropriate candidates if they have been medically screened to rule out physical causes for these difficulties (Bagarozzi, 1987).

Couples who have been married for a considerable amount of time yet present long-standing problems of poor communication or an inability to understand each other are also able to benefit from this approach.

We have come across a number of marriages where both spouses recognized, from the onset of their relationship, that there were serious perceived spousal/ideal spouse discrepancies. Nevertheless, they chose to marry in spite of what seemed to be irreconcilable differences in critical areas of their relationship. Frequently, one spouse has spent an enormous amount of time, energy, and effort in an all-out crusade to change the mate's personality. These couples are also appropriate candidates for this approach if they are willing to explore the unconscious motives for choosing their mates and if they are also willing to investigate the nature of their conjugal dynamics. Usually, in such marriages both spouses' central conflicts revolve around what we have come to call "Pygmalion" and "Frog Prince" themes that no longer seem to serve their original homeostatic purpose. These couples are actually searching for a new conjugal myth to replace the one that has outlived its usefulness. Often the dissatisfied partner is hard pressed to identify a specific behavioral change that his/her spouse could make to improve the sorry state of affairs. SIDCARB scores on Factor I frequently show little dissatisfaction for the distressed spouse, and neither spouse perceives the marriage as nonvoluntary (Factors II and III). Nevertheless, one spouse is thoroughly unhappy, frustrated, or exasperated with his/her mate.

We first encountered this phenomenon during our early work with myths. A couple who had been married for 46 years (and whose two children had long since left home to establish families of their own) came in for marriage counseling. The presenting problem was outlined by the wife, who said that she was extremely frustrated because she had been unsuccessful in her endeavors to get her husband to "actualize himself and fulfill his true potential as a feeling person." The husband agreed that his wife had been making valiant attempts to help him experience and discover "his true nature" and that she had not been very successful. He added that, although he was very comfortable with himself and who he had become, his wife must be correct in seeing this latent potential of which he was unaware. He was genuinely distressed, because after 46 years of marriage she was threatening to divorce him if he did not "become actualized."

We have used this approach with a variety of ethnic and racial groups and with relationship systems from all levels of socioeconomic strata (Bagarozzi & Anderson, 1982). We also have been able to apply our knowledge and understanding of myths and myth-making in both long-term and short-term therapy. We have found that, if we are able to carry out our assessment procedures, then we have gathered sufficient information to implement this approach. However, some marital/family systems seem ill suited for this method:

1. Systems whose members refuse to take part in the assessment process.
2. Systems that are so chaotic and disorganized that it is difficult, if not impossible, to conduct thorough assessments.

3. Systems whose members are not psychologically-minded, who lack the capacity for insight, who have very poor impulse control, or who cannot delay immediate gratification and expect quick or magical solutions to long-standing, serious problems.
4. Systems which operate according to a crisis mode and whose members are unable to formulate realistic treatment goals, personal goals, or marital/family goals.
5. Systems whose external boundaries are poorly defined, porous, and permeable, and therefore so highly susceptible to outside influences, that the therapist is unable to determine which persons are permanent members or which participants will continue to attend therapy sessions with any degree of regularity.

We have used the myth approach with couples and families who are at all stages of relationship formation (dating, courtship, remarriage, etc.) and marital/family development. At this point in time, we have no reason to believe that this clinical approach is inappropriate for couples and families at any stage of relationship development.

COUPLE PREPARATION

In the first interview the couple is prepared for what is to take place in therapy. The induction procedure is designed to underscore several points.

1. *The distinction between individual psychotherapy and marital therapy.* This is done in order to help the couple understand what types of goals and outcomes are realistically achievable and what can be expected from successful marital therapy. The following differences are reviewed for the couple.

a. The goals of marital therapy are to help the couple learn new and more functional ways to communicate, resolve conflicts, solve problems, set goals, and achieve these goals. Unlike individual psychotherapy, the focus of marital therapy is the marital relationship and not the individual spouse.
b. The purpose of individual psychotherapy is usually to bring about changes in a person's self system, psychic structures, and intrapsychic dynamics. Accomplishing these ends usually takes a considerable amount of time, frequently years. Marital therapy, on the other hand, is not concerned with changes in the individual spouse's

personality organization and intrapsychic structure. The major focus is modification of dysfunctional interaction patterns in the marital system.

Though personality changes are possible, spouses entering marital therapy should not expect such changes in themselves or their mates. If intrapsychic changes and modifications in personality are sought, individual, long-term psychotherapy should be considered as an alternative.

c. Since marital therapy focuses on the couple's characteristic ways of interacting, it is considered to be a short-term affair. The average length of therapy for couples who are able to work together cooperatively is 20 weekly sessions (Gurman & Kniskern, 1981).

d. Marital therapy, by its very nature, tends to be more behaviorally focused than traditional individual psychotherapy, but it is not as rigidly behavioral as behavior modification. In marital therapy, couples' goals are behaviorally specified. In traditional individual psychotherapy, changes in the self system and personality structures are often difficult for the client to evaluate for himself/herself. Therefore, the therapist usually plays a greater role in determining when such changes have taken place and whether therapy should be brought to a close.

2. *Distinction between the roles of the therapists.* Differentiating between the roles of marital therapists and more traditionally oriented individual practitioners is done in order to educate couples as to what they can expect from the therapist, to prepare them for how the therapist will treat them, to demystify the psychotherapeutic process, to model open, clear and functional communication, and to involve the couple (as much as possible) in a collaborative psychotherapeutic endeavor. The following differences are discussed:

a. Traditional therapists tend to be passive and reflective. Their primary concern is to help the client gain insight and understanding. Traditional therapists tend to offer little direction and usually do not give homework assignments. They tend to believe that insight into one's problems is a necessary prerequisite to behavior change for all individuals. Marital therapists, on the other hand, tend to be quite active and directive in their work with couples. Education and social skills training in such critical areas as communication, problem-solving, conflict negotiation, contingency contracting, goal-setting, goal attainment, and goal evaluation are central elements of marital therapy. Homework assignments, where couples practice the skills learned in the therapist's office, are used to facilitate generalization. These too are an integral part of marital therapy. Marital therapists tend to focus more on cognitive understanding than psychological insight. *However, marital therapists realize that psychological insight may be a necessary prerequisite to behavior change for some couples and that understanding the symbolic significance of one's actions and behaviors may be necessary before behavior change can occur for some couples.*

Marital therapists expect spouses to become actively involved in the therapeutic process and to learn how to collaborate so that they can resolve their differences without the therapist's help in the future.

Engendering Hope and Creating Positive
Expectancies for Successful Outcome

After the couple has been prepared and briefed concerning what is to take place, the therapist explains that the success or failure of therapy depends, to a large degree, upon the spouses' sincere desire to continue in their marriage and to improve their relationship. The spouses are then told that the degree to which they are seriously committed to improving their marriage will be demonstrated by their willingness and ability to: (a) learn functional communication, problem-solving and conflict negotiation skills; (b) carry out in-session directives; (c) complete homework assignments; and (d) implement and utilize the social skills learned in therapy in their day-to-day lives. Spouses also are told that their willingness to cooperate, collaborate, compromise, negotiate differences, and make specific behavioral changes in how they relate to each other are additional, concrete examples of their commitment to improving their marriage. *Couples are told that, if they can do these things, their relationship should improve. They are also advised that, if they are unwilling or unable to do these things, they should not expect their feelings toward their spouses and their marriage to change or for their relationship to improve appreciably. The therapist is direct and frank with the spouses and tells them that lack of commitment simply means that they may not be ready for the changes that successful therapy may produce.*

At this juncture, spouses are asked to evaluate whether they are ready to begin marital therapy. If either spouse is undecided or unwilling to begin treatment, the couple is permitted as much time as is needed to make a decision. However, no additional interviews are scheduled and further contact is left up to the spouses. If the couple decides to begin treatment, we inform the partners that we will begin intervention by using a very straightforward sociobehavioral-exchange skills training approach (Bagarozzi, 1983a, 1983b; Bagarozzi & Giddings, 1983b; Bagarozzi & Pollane, 1983; Bagarozzi & Wodarski, 1977, 1978). However, if the couple has already been involved in behavioral marital therapy and has found this approach to be unsuitable, we begin with an exploration of the couple's unconscious contracts, mutually protective collusive agreements, unresolved intrapsychic conflicts, developmental delays, perceived spouse/ideal spouse discrepancies, dysfunctionally related themes, and dysfunctional conjugal myths.

When couples enter therapy with no prior experience in a sociobehavioral exchange-social skills training approach, we clearly explain that if the spouses have difficulty keeping scheduled appointments, learning the skills taught to them by the therapist, carrying out in-session directives, completing homework assignments, or using the skills learned in sessions outside the confines of the therapist's office, that this is an indication that the therapist and the couple need to reevaluate the decision to continue marital therapy. If such an eventuality does come about, spouses are asked to consider a number of options. For example, they are asked whether they would prefer to: (a) make a renewed effort to use the straightforward sociobehavioral exchange-skills training approach; (b) explore some of the unconscious reasons for their not being able to work together in therapy and to develop a more satisfying relationship (e.g., unconscious contracts, mutually protective collusive agreements, unresolved intrapsychic conflicts, dysfunctionally related themes, dysfunctional conjugal myths); (c) have a referral to another therapist whose theoretical/clinical orientation may be more suitable for them; (d) postpone therapy temporarily, until they are ready to proceed; or (e) terminate treatment completely.

Through this process, the couple is thoroughly prepared for therapy. Spouses know that they will be fully involved in determining their fate and that the therapist will be forthright and direct with them and that he/she has no hidden agenda.

7

Assessing Couples' Mythologies

Roy and Marian

R OY, AGE 34, AND MARIAN, age 32, had been married for only 15 months when they decided to seek professional help for their failing marriage. Both had had some previous experience with individual counseling during their college years—Marian for anxiety attacks and Roy for periodic depression. They had a ten-month-old daughter who was conceived four months before the couple married. Since both partners were born and raised as Roman Catholics, Marian's out-of-wedlock pregnancy caused a considerable amount of consternation in both spouses' families of origin.

Presenting Problem

As is sometimes the case, Roy and Marian were not able to identify specific behavioral changes that each desired of the other, but both spouses complained of growing dissatisfaction and disappointment. When urged to become more behaviorally specific, however, Marian disclosed that she had experienced Roy as having become increasingly less responsive, more distant, and less emotionally available to her ever since the birth of their daughter. She added that he seemed to be taking little or no initiative in their relationship. She noticed that, the more she pressed him for involvement with her, the more he tended to withdraw. Roy agreed that he had become more withdrawn and removed from Marian and that he had been feeling depressed for some time.

Each spouse was allowed to discuss the presenting problem in his/her own words and to describe the problem from his/her own unique perspective. Then the couple was given its orientation in preparation for the treatment that was to follow. At the end of the first interview, the couple was given: IMAGES, SIDCARB, FACES III, and the Personal Authority in the Family System (PAFS) questionnaire to complete and return to the therapist for scoring and interpretation before the second session. The scores and interpretations of these instruments are presented below.

Assessment Findings and Interpretations

I: IMAGES

DISCREPANCY SCORE ROY	IDEAL/PERCEIVED CATEGORIES (FACTORS)	DISCREPANCY SCORE MARIAN
7/48 = 14%	I Emotional gratification	16/48 = 33%
5/36 = 14%	II Sex-role orientation and physical attraction	7/36 = 19%
4/18 = 22%	III Spousal satisfaction	6/18 = 33%
1/24 = 4%	IV Parent-sibling identification	2/24 = 8%
2/24 = 8%	V Emotional maturity	6/24 = 25%
4/18 = 22%	VI Intelligence	0/18 = 0
10/42 = 23%	VII Homogamy	10/42 = 23%
33/210 = 16%		47/210 = 22%

As can be seen from the above scores, neither partner can be said to be consciously aware of perceiving substantial ideal spouse/perceived spouse discrepancies. Overall percentage scores are relatively low: Roy = 16% and Marian = 22%. However, Marian's greatest discrepancies appear in three related areas reflecting the concerns she verbalized in her description of the presenting problem (i.e., Emotional Gratification, Spousal Satisfaction, and Emotional Maturity). The variables identified as problematic for these three factors were:

1. My spouse encourages me to grow and to be myself.
2. My spouse is affectionate.
3. My spouse is loving.
4. My spouse is caring.
5. My spouse shares his feelings with me.
6. My spouse confides in me.
7. My spouse is understanding.
7. My spouse is empathic.
15. My spouse satisfies me sexually.

16. My spouse satisfies me emotionally.
17. My spouse satisfies me intellectually.
23. My spouse is emotionally healthy and stable.
24. My spouse had good interpersonal skills.
25. My spouse has a good self-concept.

In all 14 areas cited by Marian she indicated that she wanted her husband to increase certain behaviors (to encourage her to grow and to be herself; to be more affectionate, loving, caring and empathic; to share his feelings and to confide in her) and to develop specific traits and skills (e.g., to become more emotionally healthy and stable, to develop better interpersonal skills and a better self-concept) in order to approximate more closely her ideal.

Although Roy did not experience the same degree of perceived spouse/ideal spouse discrepancies, he did agree with Marian in two areas: Spousal Satisfaction and Homogamy. He too perceived his spouse as being less sexually, emotionally and intellectually satisfying than he desired, but to a lesser degree than Marian.

Both agreed that Homogamy was a problem for them. Although being approximately the same age was not a concern for Marian, it was for Roy. He believed that if his spouse had been considerably younger than himself, she might not have made as many demands upon him. Although both were Catholic, Roy considered Marian to be too rigid in her beliefs; he wanted her to take a more liberal, less dogmatic view of Christianity. Marian, on the other hand, wanted Roy to become more spiritual and to initiate more couple involvement with organized religion. Marian came from an old, established, well-respected southern family. Both her parents were professional people who were socially active and highly visible in the community. Roy's background was considerably different. He was a northerner whose parents had immigrated from a Mediterranean country. Although his parents had had little formal education, his father became a successful businessman. When he died, Roy and his two older brothers received a considerable inheritance.

The ethnic, regional, and subcultural differences between Roy and Marian were the source of periodic conflict. Each spouse complained that the other had little understanding, tolerance, or empathy for his/her own cultural heritage. These differences made it extremely difficult, and sometimes impossible, for Roy and Marian to interact with their in-laws in any meaningful way. Even though his father had prospered financially, Roy considered himself to be a product of a working-class home. He felt uneasy with and inferior to Marian's upper-class family and could not identify with most of the members of her extended kinship network.

II: SIDCARB

		standard scores (Mean = 50, sd = 10)	
		ROY	*MARIAN*
Factor I	Fairness of the social exchange process (Amount of Behavior Change Desired of One's Spouse, Satisfaction with One's Spouse, Satisfaction with One's Marriage, Strength of One's Commitment).	54	64
Factor II	Internal Psychological Barriers to Divorce and Separation.	52	55
Factor III	External-Circumstantial Barriers to Divorce and Separation.	52	40

The first factor score reveals that Marian perceived the couple's social exchange system to be unbalanced and inequitable. As a result, she desired a substantial amount of change in Roy's exchange behavior toward her. Communication, Expressions of Love and Affection, and Sexual Relations were areas where she desired a great deal of change. Recreation, Friendships, and Relationships with Children were three additional areas where a moderate degree of change was requested. Even though these six areas cover a wide range of marital behaviors, only one theme permeated all of Marian's requests for change, i.e., that Roy take more *initiative* in (a) communicating with her, (b) sharing his feelings, (c) making sexual overtures, (d) planning recreational activities, (e) making friends with other married couples, and (f) playing with their child.

Roy, on the other hand, perceived the exchange system to be fair and just and to his liking. He desired few changes in Marian's overall behavior toward him in this area of exchange. However, Roy identified two areas where he desired moderate degrees of change in Marian's behavior: Sexual Relations and Religion. As far as their sex life was concerned, Roy said that he wanted his wife to be more responsive to his needs and not to attempt to orchestrate their sexual behavior. He experienced Marian as attempting to "direct" and "control" their lovemaking. In the area of Religion, Roy expressed his desire to find a new church that the couple could attend together. He said that he had been unhappy with the priests in their current church for some time. He perceived them to be too "old world" and "too authoritarian" and wanted to avoid their "rigidity." It is important to know that the church Roy and Marian had been attending was Marian's family's church, the church to which her parents belonged. Frequently, the couple had attended religious services and church events with Marian's parents.

Factor II shows that both Roy and Marian experienced approximately the same level of constraint. Internal–Psychological prohibitions against leaving the marriage (e.g., obligation to one's children, commitment to marriage vows, religious beliefs and concerns about what family members might think, say and do if the couple separated) were not very strong, and both spouses perceived approximately the same degree of barrier strength.

However, factor III scores (perceptions of External-Circumstantial Barriers, such as what friends and neighbors might say, job considerations, legal costs and financial concerns) were noticeably different for the two spouses. Roy perceived these barriers to be as strong as those in the second factor. Marian, on the other hand, did not. This discrepancy in barrier strength is important for two reasons. First, it is uncharacteristic for women to have lower scores on this factor. Typically, most women who are not employed and who have small children are dependent upon their husbands for financial assistance. In Marian's case, however, she knew that she could always turn to her parents for financial support. Second, it identified Marian as the more powerful spouse according to the principle of least interest (Waller & Hill, 1951); i.e., she is less dependent upon the relationship and more likely to terminate the marriage if things do not improve. This interpretation is supported by Roy's written comments (on SIDCARB) concerning his feelings about divorce and separation: "I would have serious doubts about my self-worth if I left my wife and child. If the marriage doesn't work out, I know I will blame myself for its failure. I don't know if I could ever live with the guilt and depression that would result."

III: FACES III

As we said in Chapter 5, the FACES III Cohesion scale is used to investigate the intimacy dimensions of relationships. Perceived/ideal Cohesion data for Roy and Marian are reported below:

ROY		MARIAN	
PERCEIVED	IDEAL	PERCEIVED	IDEAL
Separate	Connected	Separate	Enmeshed

These findings show that both Roy and Marian experienced their relationship as one where more interpersonal closeness was desired. However, Marian wanted much more closeness than Roy. Our clinical experience in using the FACES measure (i.e., FACES I, II, and III) with distressed couples consistently shows that family members who perceive their relationships as either disengaged or separate tend to *overcorrect* when asked to represent their ideal levels of closeness; thus, frequently they receive extreme scores that place them in the Enmeshed category. It is difficult to know whether such overcorrection reflects a deficit in scale construction, the nature of clinical samples, or an interaction between the two. However, we have come upon this phenomenon too frequently to accept such scores at face value. Therefore, we tend to interpret them simply as the person's request for a greater degree of closeness and intimacy than he/she is currently experiencing.

To augment these data, we frequently ask the spouses to draw their perceived/ideal levels of closeness. The drawings depicted in Figure 1 were made by Roy and Marian. Based upon these drawings, we can see that there are some major differences in the ways Roy and Marian per-

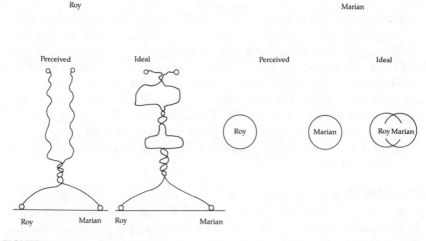

FIGURE 1

ceived their ideal relationship. Roy's drawing represents how he sees their marriage developing over time, if it were to continue on its current course. His drawing of the progression and development of an ideal marriage portrays the ebb and flow of a relationship over time and graphically demonstrates the fluid nature of interpersonal intimacy. Marian's view is more static. She sees herself as distant and cut off from Roy. Her drawing of the ideal relationship vividly shows her desire to merge with him, to become enmeshed. These drawings strengthen the validity of FACES III scores for Roy and Marian. Both perceive their relationship to be more separate than they both would prefer. Roy's ideal allows for flexible patterns of separateness and connectedness. However, Marian's static view of marriage and her desire to merge with Roy cannot be seen merely as an artifact of the measuring instrument, nor can it be seen as an intentional overcorrection. In this instance, FACES III does accurately tap Marian's wish to establish an enmeshed relationship with Roy.

IV: PAFS

In Chapter 5, we said that we use only four of the eight subscales from the Personal Authority in the Family System Questionnaire (Intergenerational Fusion/Individuation, Nuclear Family Triangulation, Intergenerational Triangulation, and Intergenerational Intimidation) to measure the extent to which a person has successfully individuated from his/her family of origin. The scores on these four subscales for Roy and Marian were:

Subscales	ROY	MARIAN	RANGE OF SCALE		
			LO	MID	HIGH
INFUS	30	19	8	24	40
NFTRI	45	25	10	30	50
INTRI	50	20	11	33	55
INTIM	100	65	29	87	145

KEY: INFUS = The higher the score, the higher the individuation
NFTRI = The higher the score, the lower the triangulation
INTRI = The higher the score, the lower the triangulation
INTIM = The higher the score, the lower the intimidation

These data show that Roy seems to have been more successful in emotionally separating from his family of origin. Conversely, Marian appears to be still quite involved with intergenerational issues. However, Roy's responses to PAFS are suspect. The reasons for this will become clearer when we review his Family Relationships History and profile his personal mythology.

V: COMMUNICATION PATTERNS AND CONFLICT NEGOTIATION SKILLS

The couple's characteristic styles of communicating and resolving interpersonal conflicts were also assessed during the initial interview. These patterns and processes were elicited in response to the therapist's in-session directive to: "Identify an area of conflict in your relationship that you both consider to be of some importance. Once you have done this, try to resolve this conflict in a way that you both feel is fair, just and mutually satisfying."

Observing Roy and Marian's behavior during this diagnostic exercise also made it possible to assess the two remaining dimensions of marital behavior identified in Chapter 5: rules for marital power-sharing, influence, and leadership; and rules for communicating love, value, and worth of one's spouse.

Based upon observations of Roy and Marian's interactions, it was evident that they did not communicate clearly and that they had not developed flexible relational control patterns. The predominant type of relational communication interaction style observed during their problem-solving and conflict negotiation attempts consisted of a fairly rigid, complementary control pattern (Rogers & Bagarozzi, 1983), with Marian in the dominant, one-up position. Symmetrical interaction sequences were infrequent and there was no indication that Roy and Marian had developed a parallel style of interaction.[1]

Both Roy and Marian were very tentative in their speaking styles, and Roy seemed to be overly sensitive, aware, and cautious about sending messages that might be considered devaluing. He also seemed likely to perceive Marian's statements as devaluing.

Roy and Marian tended to problem solve and negotiate their conflicts in a very rigid, zero-sum complementary fashion, with Roy usually giving in to Marian's requests or suggestions. From these observations, it

---

[1]Complementary interactions consist of behavioral exchanges of logically opposite behaviors. Symmetrical interactions are made up of exchanges of identical behaviors. Parallel interaction control patterns, however, are characterized by the exchange of different behaviors. For example, a spouse's empathic response to his/her mate's anger would be considered a parallel response; reciprocating a spouse's anger would be a symmetrical response, and cowering in response to anger would be considered complementary.

was determined that modification in the couple's communication system was required.

VI: HISTORY OF THE PRESENTING PROBLEM

Both Roy and Marian agreed that they first noticed a problem in their relationship when Marian became pregnant. Although the couple had announced their decision to marry to both friends and relatives and wedding preparations had already begun, Roy felt that the option to change his mind, to postpone the wedding, or to lengthen the engagement had been unilaterally taken from him. He expressed some "resentment" about being subtly manipulated, while acknowledging that both he and Marian had become lackadaisical in their birth control practices once they had decided to marry. When the announcement of Marian's pregnancy did not meet with overt hostility by either set of parents, Roy's "resentment" (which manifested itself as depression and withdrawal) "disappeared," as did Marian's feelings of dread and anxiety. However, Roy's "depression" returned with the birth of their daughter, and he became more withdrawn as time went by. Although his sexual needs and desires remained strong, he no longer initiated sexual contact with Marian. As a matter of fact, he frequently rejected any of her sexual overtures. Masturbation had become his only sexual outlet. One evening, shortly after Marian's sexual advances had been rebuffed by Roy, she found him masturbating in their bedroom. When she confronted him, a conflict ensued. The next day Marian called the therapist for an appointment.

VII: COUPLE'S RELATIONSHIP HISTORY

Marian and Roy met at a social function that had been organized by a local political organization. Marian approached Roy and introduced herself to him. They spent much of that evening together and before the social gathering ended Marian had invited Roy to her apartment for a "nightcap." Soon after they arrived at Marian's apartment, she asked Roy if he would like to spend the night with her, and he agreed. Although they slept together that evening, they did not engage in sexual intercourse. Both Marian and Roy concurred that, although the suggestion not to be sexual was made by Marian, Roy was relieved not to have to "perform for her." They also agreed that this first experience together was pleasant, successful, and nonstressful.

Marian said that she found Roy's "laid back style" most appealing. All her previous relationships with men had been extremely intense. In these relationships she had felt that she was "out of control" and "at their mercy." She revealed that a few weeks prior to meeting Roy she had ended a longstanding and heated relationship with a black man. She characterized this relationship as being intensely sexual but highly anxiety-producing. In Roy she had found a man whom she could influence. Being with Roy offered her an opportunity to have equal power and leverage in a relationship for the first time in her life, and she knew that he was the type of man she wanted to marry. The only negative quality of which she was aware was Roy's lack of initiative; however, she accepted this trait as part of his "laid back" posture.

Roy's feelings about Marian were ambivalent from the start. He liked her straightforward and direct manner but found that her directness could sometimes evolve into pushiness and controlling behavior. Similarly, he appreciated her energy and her "take charge" manner, because they relieved him of the responsibility for always taking the lead in their relationship; however, he sometimes experienced Marian's assertiveness as domineering and her "take charge" manner as discounting him and his desires, needs and wishes. When Roy and Marian first met, Roy was also recovering from a relationship that had ended badly. The woman with whom Roy had been living had recently left him because Roy had found himself unable to make any type of long-term commitment to her.

Roy and Marian described their first attempt at sexual intercourse (several days after their first meeting) as a complete disaster. Both were extremely anxious and Roy felt a lot of self-generated pressure to perform and to take the lead in their lovemaking. This was the first and only time in Roy's life that he experienced erectile failure. In response to Roy's inability to achieve an erection, Marian was sympathetic, patient, and understanding. Their next attempt, the following morning, was described as mutually satisfying. Neither partner had any difficulty becoming sexually stimulated and both were orgasmic. No further sexual difficulties were experienced until the incident that precipitated the couple's entry into treatment.

Roy was the first man Marian ever considered marrying; i.e., he was the only person she had dated whom she believed would be acceptable to her parents, especially her mother. Shortly after they began to date exclusively, Roy's father was involved in a near-fatal automobile accident which left him partially paralyzed. The realization that his father might not have long to live proved to be a turning point in Roy's life. Several weeks after his father was released from the hospital, he asked Marian to marry him. Although this was something that she had hoped for, Marian did not accept his offer immediately. Instead she asked for some time to think the matter over (so that she could discuss this possibility with her parents and sisters). Weeks passed, but Roy never brought up the subject of marriage again. One evening, Marian told Roy that she had given the matter a lot of thought, and she had come to the conclusion that marriage was a good idea. Roy's response to her acceptance was unanticipated. He was ambivalent and suggested that perhaps they should reconsider. Marian was dismayed. She became depressed and tearful. To console her, Roy agreed to go through with the marriage.

Both sets of parents were pleased with their children's decision to marry. The engagement period was uneventful except for Marian's pregnancy, which made the couple's plans to marry irrevocable. Marian's conception came at an extremely significant time in her life, but neither she nor Roy had realized its importance until they discussed her pregnancy during the Couple's Relationship History interview. It seems that Marian had conceived shortly after the death of her maternal grandmother, a woman whom Marian called her "second mother." Shortly after their daughter was born, Roy's father died.

PHASE II: INDIVIDUAL ASSESSMENT OF SPOUSES' FAMILY RELATIONSHIPS HISTORIES, CENTRAL THEMES AND PERSONAL MYTHOLOGIES

Roy: Family Relationships History Summary

Here is Roy's first memory:

> I was about four years old. My parents and I were visiting my father's parents who lived in the apartment above us. My father was ridiculing me and scolding me for something I had failed to do. My grandfather gently told my father not to frighten me and to leave me alone. I was frightened by my father and felt protected by my grandfather.

The circumstances surrounding Roy's parents' courtship and marriage were common knowledge and were a source of conflict throughout their married life. Roy's father dated and married Roy's mother against his parents' wishes. Until the day Roy's grandmother died, she did not accept her son's marriage. Roy's grandparents did not attend their son's wedding. All preparations, arrangements, etc., were made by Roy's mother's parents. Roy's paternal grandparents thought that Roy's mother was "not good enough" for their son.

Roy's parents were Catholic and did not use birth control. Therefore, the number of children they had was not planned. After the birth of their third son, Roy, Roy's mother was hospitalized for psychosis. She was diagnosed as "schizophrenic" and was hospitalized periodically for this "condition" throughout the rest of her life. After her first hospitalization, however, she did not become pregnant again. Roy was not sure if his parents began to practice birth control at that time or whether they resorted to abstinence to prevent pregnancy. Nevertheless, Roy was the last child born to the couple.

Roy guessed that he and his two brothers had been conceived as a matter of course and that the sexes of the first two children did not matter to either parent. However, Roy remembered hearing his mother remark that she had hoped that her third child would be a girl who would take care of her in her old age.

Roy's given name was "Charles," but his oldest brother called him "Roy" and that name remained with him. Roy saw this nickname as a sign of love and caring on the part of his older brothers. Roy's parents seemed to have no particular expectations for him. His father's attentions were focused on the oldest child. His mother, on the other hand, favored the second son. Roy was left "pretty much on my own" from an early age. Roy knew, from a number of things that his father had said, that his father did not expect him to "amount to much" in life. Overall, Roy felt that both parents were indifferent toward him.

Roy recalled having no particular role in his family of origin. Most of his time was spent alone. He avoided his father as much as possible and tried to console his mother whenever she became "depressed" or "emotional," but his efforts all seemed to be in vain.

Roy found it difficult to pinpoint what he would have to do to be loved by his parents and siblings. His major concerns were trying to stay out of his father's way and not upsetting his mother. If he did this successfully, he would be left alone—this was the closest thing to feeling loved by his parents.

There was very little open conversation or "give and take discussions" in Roy's family. Mother's remarks were often "irrelevant" or "self-centered," and one never knew how father was going to react to any given topic of conversation. Frequently, his father became angry at something his sons said; these angry outbursts were unpredictable and frightening.

When asked to identify any personal secrets that he felt he should keep from his parents, Roy said that "his entire life was a secret." He rarely divulged what he was thinking or feeling to either parent. He said that there were two family secrets that he was aware of: (a) "My father married my mother to defy his father," and (b) "my father felt inadequate and relied on my mother for approval and acceptance." He knew the latter to be a fact because recently he had come across a number of love letters that his father had written to his mother during their courtship. In these letters his father had said that he was "worthless" and that he existed only for Roy's mother's love.

Roy was explicit when describing the secrets that his family had to keep from outsiders. He said that all members were not to show "the outside world how we really feel about our family unit."

Roy was unable to identify any particular values, beliefs, or rules that played a significant role in shaping his self-image. However, he was able to articulate how his reactions to his parents' behavior and his family life had affected him as a husband and father. He said that, as a reaction to his upbringing, he believed that parents should be kind, gentle, patient, and polite with their children and with each other. It was especially important for children not to be afraid of their parents and not to feel responsible for taking care of their parents' emotional and physical well-being.

Unwritten rules in Roy's family of origin were seen as being the same as the family's secret of never showing the outside world how they truly felt about the family as a unit.

The motto, coined by Roy, to describe family functioning was, "We remain silent, but we are constantly watching for others' pain so that we can offer solace."

Roy described his parents' relationship as "distant" and "cautious."

Roy singled out his oldest brother, James, as the person he liked the most, confided in, was closest to, identified with, and tried to emulate in many ways. James was also Roy's protector. Roy was unwilling to identify any family member as a person he disliked. He did admit, however, that he had the most difficult time with his father. He was terrified of him and did whatever he could to avoid any confrontation with him. His father was a fanatically religious man who demanded obedience from his children. He ruled with unquestioned power. This power had two distinct sources: physical and financial. Roy recalled a number of instances where his oldest brother had stood up to their father. These confrontations resulted in physical violence between James and Roy's father. Roy vowed never to be like his father; he also vowed never to confront him. He was afraid that such a confrontation might have dire consequences.

Mother was portrayed as the person who owned Roy emotionally. Her fears, her vulnerability, and her susceptibility to depression and emotional upset "sucked" him into her emotional sphere. When she would become "ill," he "hurt for her." He found it difficult to separate his own "pain" from "her pain." His conscious identification with her "passivity" and "depression" overshadowed his life. He was totally unaware of his unconscious identification with his aggressive father. His use of reaction formation, intellectualization, denial and withdrawal, defenses against his own deeply hidden feelings of rage and his desire for violent retaliation, gave him the appearance of a calm and gentle person.

Roy characterized his parents' relationship as lacking any vitality, as dead, and as devoid of any emotion except sadness. This relationship did not seem to change over time. Roy cited two changes that he would have liked to have seen in his family of origin: (a) that his family would have been less isolated, and (b) that his parents would have shown more warmth and caring toward each other and their children.

Roy: Personal Myth Assessment Summary

Sometimes a person is not able to select a story, film, etc., that has special significance for him/her, but he/she may identify with a character type that is the hero of a number of different stories, films, books, etc. This was the case for Roy. When asked to identify his favorite fairy tale, book or play, he chose three different characters from three separate books. The characters were: *Steppenwolf* (Hermann Hesse), Plucky Purcell from a book entitled *Another Roadside Attraction* (Tom Robbins), and Stephen Dedalus, the protagonist in *A Portrait of the Artist as a Young Man* (James Joyce).

These characters were picked for very special reasons; all were "loners" and "metaphysically on the mark." They all kept themselves "apart from others and guarded their individuality." All were "outrageous" and were not afraid to "live life to the fullest." None of these men was "afraid." All three authors were admired for their "irreverence" and "mockery" of organized religion.

In his characteristic manner, Roy would not single out any persons in these novels as individuals he disliked. His identification with the protagonists in each book was based upon their "uniqueness," "differentness," and "aloneness," and the fact that they were all treated with respect by others, especially the women with whom they were involved. Another aspect of these novels was that the main characters came to "no definite end" at the close of the novels. They just seemed to "go on."

Roy: Personal Mythology and World View Summary

The major themes that emerged for Roy were:

1. Aggression = Destruction. Any type of assertive behavior may become aggressive and lead to terrible consequences (especially aggression against father). Aggression of any kind is wrong and bad. I am bad if I am aggressive. I am afraid of what I might do if I were to become aggressive.

2. In order to deal with my aggressive impulses I must avoid all confrontation. I must become very passive and not assert myself.

3. I must be constantly vigilant in life, and I must find someone who can protect me. I am barely able to take care of myself, and I am totally inadequate when it comes to taking care of others. Having any type of responsibility for another person's health and welfare frightens and angers me. I experience their helplessness as abandonment. I am very sensitive to other people's suffering, but I am powerless to do anything to help them in their suffering.

4. I am very ambivalent about close, intimate, interpersonal relationships with men. Because of my relationship with my father, I see other men as aggressive, frightening, and dangerous. I cannot compete with other men. I am totally inadequate to face them. It is best to avoid all contact with males where there is the potential for conflict. On the other hand, some men (like my grandfather and my brother) will protect me and take care of me. I am drawn to such men and I will submit to them homosexually, in order to gain their protection.[2]

5. I am also ambivalent about close, intimate, interpersonal relationships with women. I want them to take charge and to take care of me, but I don't want them to overpower and control me. I am also afraid that they will expect me to take care of them or to take charge. I am afraid that women will reject me or retaliate if I am unable to satisfy their wishes, desires, and sexual needs.

6. Closeness with women is also dangerous because it simulates the fusion I experienced with my mother when I was a child and which I sometimes still experience when she is physically present. It requires all my strength to maintain my separateness.

Roy's personal mythology and world view can be summarized as follows:

---

[2]Roy had had a number of homosexual encounters as an adolescent and young adult and considered himself to be "potentially bisexual."

I must avoid confrontation with anyone, at all costs. Confrontations with men will result if I am too assertive or aggressive. If I cannot avoid confrontation, two outcomes are possible: destruction or submission. Submission is more acceptable and allows me to avoid confrontation. It also offers a certain amount of protection. In order to avoid confrontations with men, I must become a loner. As a loner, I can drift from woman to woman, who will shelter and protect me and not demand much from me. However, I must not get too close or become too dependent upon these women, because they will begin to expect too much from me. They will want to engulf me and control me. They may even want me to take care of them, to meet their needs, etc., and I am not capable of doing this. Eventually they may engulf me and I will lose all sense of self, of who I really am. Being a loner also protects me from this fate.

Marian: Family Relationships History Summary

Marian's first memory was:

I remember my father taking me and my two older sisters to visit my mother at the hospital. She had just given birth to my youngest sister. Because my sisters and I were too little (I was four years old and my sisters were six and eight at the time), we could only wave to my mother from the street below her hospital window. We were not permitted to visit her in her room.

Marian's parents were strict Catholics who had been high school sweethearts. The parents on both sides approved of their dating each other and may have had some hand in encouraging them to date. They married shortly after graduating from the same college. Since Marian's parents were devout Catholics, they did not use birth control or plan the number of children they had. Sex, pregnancy, childbirth, etc., were not discussed in her family of origin. Marian said she never knew what her father's true feelings about sex and sexual intercourse were, but she thought he might be more accepting and "less Puritanical" about sexual matters than her mother, since it was her father who had been responsible for telling her all about "sexual reproduction." When Marian first began to menstruate, there was no discussions of her menstruation with her mother. Her mother simply provided her with a book on the subject. Based upon Marian's experiences and observations of her parents' behavior, she came away with the perception that her mother disliked sex but tolerated her father's sexual advances and that pregnancy was the price one pays for being sexual. Childbirth was a painful ordeal—again, a natural consequence of being sexual.

Marian was the third of four daughters. She believed that her parents had no preferences concerning the genders of their first two children but that her father had hoped that she would be a boy. She guessed that her youngest sister, the last born, represented her parents final attempt to have a son. Since her parents were "orthodox Catholics," she guessed that they probably used natural family planning and abstinence to avoid any additional pregnancies after the birth of their fourth child.

Marian knew that all of her mother's pregnancies produced turmoil in her family. Her mother was bedridden most of the time during each pregnancy, and recuperated only slowly after each delivery. She guessed that her mother's response to finding out she was pregnant with Marian was no different from that to any other pregnancy, i.e., "the beginning of another ordeal and long convalescence."

Marian believed that her parents' reaction to seeing her for the first time was that she was a "cute" baby. However, their response to finding out that she was female was less positive. Her father, she thought, was probably disappointed. Her mother, she knew, must have been upset because the birth of another female meant that she would have to become pregnant again.

Siblings' reactions to her birth were "fairly standard." There was much rivalry, jealousy, and competition among the sisters. This was the state of affairs that characterized her life in her parents' home. Sibling rivalry continued into the present.

Marian was named after her mother and was expected to be mother to her younger sister. Marian was openly acknowledged as her mother's favorite, and as she grew older she became her mother's confident. She was expected to think, feel, and be like her mother. They had become so close by the time Marian was an adolescent that sometimes Marian found it difficult to differentiate between her own feelings and thoughts and those of her mother.

Marian's father was considered an enigma. Distant and detached from the family, he seemed to have been always out of reach. She had no idea what his hopes and aspirations for her might have been. He was gentle and polite, staid and reserved, even tempered and matter-of-fact. After 32 years, she still did not know him at all.

In order for Marian to be loved by her mother, she had to "think like her, feel like her, and be like her." There was no room for differentness. She believed her father loved her—she could "feel his love"—but he never verbalized his feelings or demonstrated his caring. Marian knew that she was not loved by her older sisters because of her relationship with her mother. She knew that there was nothing she could do to gain their love. She thought that her younger sister depended upon her and loved her, and she really did not have to do anything to win this sister's love.

Sex was the topic that could never be discussed openly in Marian's family. She and her sisters felt extremely guilty for having sexual thoughts and feelings.

Marian recognized a number of family secrets that could not be discussed openly and could not be divulged to outsiders. The first was that she was mother's favorite. The second was that the family was fragmented. This fragmentation took several forms, depending upon the circumstances. The three configurations in Figure 2 were common. However, whenever mother got upset by one or more of the children, father would be called in to discipline. At such times the structural arrangement looked like Figure 3.

The final family secret was that the family was not a happy one. The motto that Marian chose to describe her family encompasses all these secrets, i.e., "The family that looks perfect isn't." She added, "You can't tell a book by looking at its cover."

Unlike her husband, Marian kept no secrets from her mother. She told her mother everything. She said she would feel very guilty if she kept anything from her mother. She did not confide in her sisters, and the idea of confiding in her father never crossed her mind. The only thing about herself that she dared not share with her mother was her sexuality.

An important value that Marian retained from her family of origin was to respect other people. Because of this value, Marian was able to get along with most of the people with whom she came in contact. This value also allowed her to appreciate others. Carried to an extreme, however, this value prevented her from speaking her mind and asserting herself with her parents.

Marian gave considerable thought before answering the question having to do with the existence of unwritten family rules. She could think of many prohibitions that were verbalized by her parents, but unearthing nonverbally communicated rules was difficult. Finally, she decided that the closest she could come to identifying an unwritten rule had to do with the children's relationship with their father. As she put it, "We were not allowed to become too close to our father."

Marian identified her maternal grandmother as the person she liked most. She singled out her oldest sister as the family member she liked least of all. She attributed this mutual dislike to intense sibling rivalry. Marian felt closest to her younger sister.

Marian singled out her father as the one person she feared in her

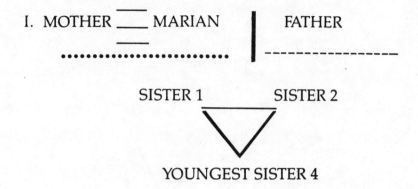

I. MOTHER ⎯ MARIAN   FATHER

      SISTER 1   SISTER 2

      YOUNGEST SISTER 4

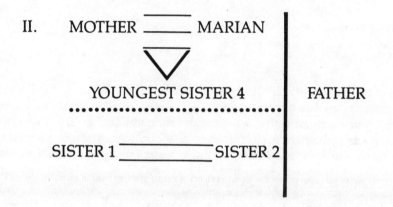

II.   MOTHER ⎯ MARIAN

      YOUNGEST SISTER 4   FATHER

      SISTER 1 ⎯⎯⎯ SISTER 2

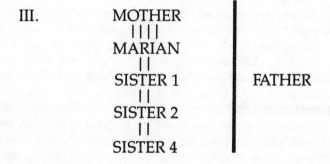

III.   MOTHER
        | | | |
      MARIAN
       | |
      SISTER 1   FATHER
       | |
      SISTER 2
       | |
      SISTER 4

FIGURE 2

125

IV.   MOTHER ＿＿＿＿ FATHER

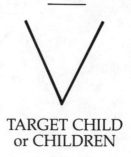

TARGET CHILD
or CHILDREN

FIGURE 3

family. He was the disciplinarian. Whenever her mother could not force her children to obey her commands, father was called in to "do her dirty work." Marian recalled that on many occasions he had pulled down her underpants and spanked her on her bare buttocks. These experiences produced two very conflicting feelings: humiliation and sexual excitement. Being spanked represented the only time that Marian recalled being physically close to and touched by her father. He was not very demonstrative. Later in life, when she became sexually active, spanking became an extremely pleasurable/painful prelude to sexual intercourse. Sometimes spanking resulted in orgasm. However, Marian never revealed this aspect of her sexuality to her husband.

Mother was seen as the person wielding the power in Marian's family. She controlled everything "from her sick bed." Several strategies were used to keep her children in line: guilt, becoming physically ill in response to her children's misbehavior, calling her children sinful and warning them that they would go to hell for their evilness. Threatening to tell their father about their transgressions was the strategy used by Marian's mother when all other attempts failed. On rare occasions, Marian's mother had severe anxiety attacks which frightened her children. Marian was not sure what triggered these attacks, but they functioned to bring all the sisters to their mother's side. All rivalry and scapegoating among the children halted whenever mother had these anxiety "episodes." Physical illness was the power tactic used by Marian's mother to gain leverage in her relationship with her husband.

There was no doubt in Marian's mind that she was owned emotionally by her mother. She had always been ambivalently tied to her mother and feared her mother would die if Marian were not close at hand to console her, to offer her emotional support, and to agree with her. This ambivalent tie still existed when she and her husband came in for marital therapy.

Marian's description of her parents' relationship was simple: "Mother spent most of her time chasing my father and trying to get him to do what she wanted him to do for her."

When asked what changes she would make in her family of origin and the way it functioned, Marian was very clear. She said she would make her mother "healthy" and that she and her sisters would get along together. Finally, she said: "I would get to know my father better, and he would take an interest in me as a person."

Marian: Personal Myth Assessment Summary

Unlike her husband, Marian did very little reading, but watched television a great deal. She chose "The Cosby Show" as her favorite story. Her responses to all the questions dealing with the program's plot, its characters, and the relationships among family members were short and concise. These are summarized as follows:

> Although this TV series is too goody-goody, I still like it, because it is very much how I would have liked my family to be—a caring father, a vital mother, and happy siblings. I am drawn to the father because he is strong, involved, caring, but yet maintains a sense of humor. He loves his wife, but not to the exclusion of his children. All family members treat him with respect. They love him and tolerate his foolishness. He stands for the moral and ethical things in his life, but has an open mind. He listens to his children and invites discussion. Sometimes, he is wrong. He is not perfect.
>
> At the end of each episode, he always helps his family get on the right track.
>
> I dislike the oldest sister. She has no character and does not stand up for herself. She loves and respects her father, but there seems to be little depth in their relationship.
>
> If I could be any character in this story, I'd be the mother. She adores and at the same time tolerates her husband. She is a mother. Her children love her, and she is a career woman. My mother gave up her career when she had children. The mother on "The Cosby Show" does it all and has it all.

If I could change anything, I would introduce some conflict. Things don't get resolved at the end of each day as they do in a sit-com. You have to live with your mistakes and profit from them. There is no pain in this show. It should show that there is joy in life in spite of the pain. Pain and joy go hand-in-hand in real life.

Marian: Personal Mythology and World View Summary

The major themes that emerged for Marian were:

1. Love=sameness. Separateness and difference (especially from mother) are unacceptable and wrong. The threat of separateness leads to anxiety, panic and depression. It is bad to be different and it is wrong to be autonomous from someone who loves you. Therefore, I am bad if I am different and/or autonomous.
2. I must be loyal to my family even if I dislike some of them, like my older sisters. I must be especially loyal to my mother.
3. Relationships with men are forbidden if they in any way pose a threat to the primary mother–daughter relationship. This is especially true for father–daughter relationships. Relationships with men are acceptable only so long as they don't threaten the mother–daughter bond.
4. Any type of sexual behavior outside the confines of marriage is wrong, bad, and evil. Sexual behavior for pleasure is bad and evil. Sexual behavior in marriage is only acceptable for the procreation of children. Sexual behavior for pleasure should be punished. I am sexual, therefore, I am bad and should be punished if I engage in sex for pleasure.
5. Men rarely take the initiative unless women cause them to do so. One way to get men to take the initiative is to be sexual with them, because men are sexual creatures. However, men are also potentially violent and should be feared.
6. Sickness, illness, and pain are part of every interpersonal relationship. Illness is one way to regulate interpersonal closeness and distance.

Marian's personal mythology and world view can be summarized as follows:

Life is a constant struggle to find my independence and autonomy from my mother. Being a separate person from my mother is risky business, because either she might become ill and die or I may not be able to exist without her. All my life I have been looking for a man who will help me separate from my mother. I wish my father would have been strong enough to help me develop independence. One way to attract men who will help me is to be sexually active. However, I have ambivalent feelings about being sexual. When I am sexually active, I must find some aspect of the experience which gives me some punishment or pain for my sexual feelings and behaviors. I can find someone who hurts me, I can become ill, or I can get pregnant. Pregnancy is the ultimate punishment for being sexual.

If I find a man who is passive and distant, like my father, I can be in control of the relationship, especially the sexual part of the relationship. If I marry such a man, I can enjoy sex as long as we continue to use sex for procreation. When I don't want to be sexually involved, I can become ill, like my mother.

8

Profiling the Couple's Mythology

THE FAMILY RELATIONSHIPS HISTORY and the Personal Mythology Assessment Guidelines of both spouses are invaluable sources of information. They enable the therapist to identify each spouse's particular needs, motives, and unresolved developmental conflicts that appear as central themes in their personal mythologies. Once these themes have been identified, the final phase of assessment can be accomplished. This last phase consists of two interrelated processes:

1. Understanding how the spouses' personal themes are organized and woven together to form central marital themes in the couple's conjugal mythology.
2. Understanding how each spouse's needs, motives and unresolved developmental conflicts and personal themes manifest themselves in the spouses' responses to the four assessment instruments, the way the spouses interact as a couple system, and their typical styles of communicating, solving problems, and resolving marital conflicts.

The therapist must also evaluate which conjugal themes are growth-producing for each spouse and the relationship, and which themes curtail the growth and development of the conjugal system as a whole and/or prevent the self-realization and self-actualization of the spouses as individuals.

OUTLINING THE THEMES OF ROY AND MARIAN'S CONJUGAL MYTHOLOGY

It is important to remember that the individual themes that make up each spouse's personal mythology can appear to stand in relationship to those of his/her mate in a variety of ways. For example, individual themes may appear clearly complementary to each other and dovetail neatly. Table 2 outlines the central themes derived earlier from assessing Roy's and Marian's personal mythologies and family histories.

In Roy and Marian's marriage, the following themes appeared to be complementary and merge together harmoniously:

1. Roy's unresolved conflicts concerning his own aggressive impulses, his confusion of assertive behavior with destructive aggression and his defensive passivity (themes 1 and 2) were complemented by Marian's search for a father substitute (theme 5) who did not threaten her relationship with her mother (theme 3).
2. Marian's loyalty to her family of origin and her mother (theme 2) and her ability to find a husband who did not threaten the mother-daughter bond (theme 3) appeared to complement Roy's theme of closeness with women being dangerous because it threatens fusion and intense struggle in order to maintain a separate sense of self (theme 6).

Individual themes can also appear to be incompatible, competitive, and antagonistic. For example:

TABLE 2 Summary of Roy's and Marian's personal themes

Roy	Marian
1. Aggression = Destruction	1. Love = Sameness
2. Passivity vs. Assertiveness	2. Loyalty to Family of Origin (especially mother)
3. The Search for the Protector (failure to protect and nuture others)	3. Men as Saboteurs of Mother-Daughter Bond
4. Retreat from (or Submission to) Male (father) Figures	4. Sexual Pleasure = Evil and Punishable (ultimately by pregnancy and childbirth)
5. Caretaking of vs. Subservience to (or retaliation from) the Female (mother) Figure	5. Men are Unpredictably Violent or Passive (but can be tempted toward initiative with sex)
6. Fusion with Female (mother) Figure vs. Aloneness	6. Illness as Interpersonal Distance Regulator

1. Roy's quest to find a female who would take charge of the relation-ship and who would not become dependent upon him for physical and emotional support during times of illness (theme 3) appears to be in direct conflict with Marian's theme of illness and sickness as a way to regulate interpersonal closeness (theme 6).
2. Roy's fears of being overpowered and controlled by a female and his reactive distancing and isolation (theme 5) appear to be antago-nistic to Marian's theme that equates love with sameness, symbio-sis, and enmeshment (theme 1).

However, at a broader, more abstract level of analysis, these individual personal themes become interwoven into a fabric that is highly interde-pendent and complementary. There are several important considerations to note regarding these apparently incompatible themes.

First, *spouses' individual themes generally involve ambivalent, conflicting feelings. In most instances, one side of the ambivalence may be more conscious than the other*. For instance, Roy's desire to be taken care of by a woman (theme 5) is also accompanied by fears of rejection, retaliation (theme 5), and engulfment (theme 6). Marian's desire for men to take the initiative with her (theme 5) is accompanied by fears of men becoming potentially violent (theme 5) or expressing differentness rather than sameness, which she would equate with loss of love (theme 1). Additionally, if Roy took initiative with Marian sexually, she would be faced with potential feelings of guilt and punishment for sexual pleasure (theme 4). These examples illustrate clearly the conflicting elements often present within each theme. The above examples also illustrate the interdependence among clusters of spouses' personal themes.

Second, *The unconscious elements of these individual themes are displaced or projected onto the spouse so that aspects of each spouse's self are manifest in the conscious personal themes of the other*. Thus, Roy's search for a woman who would take care of him physically and emotionally without asking for anything in return and Marian's illness behaviors, which are designed to elicit closeness from Roy, can be viewed as highly compatible if we con-sider that:

(a) Marian's illness behaviors and bids for emotional closeness protect Roy from feeling rejected by a female (wife/mother) figure as he is repeatedly placed in a position of being approached and needed.
(b) Roy's press for Marian to become the "all-giving" woman (wife) protects Marian from facing her disappointment in her own father for never having been available to her and never needing anything from her.

In addition to offering a shared protection for one another, these inter-dependent themes may offer potential solutions to each spouse's unresolved conflicts.

   (a) Roy's desire for a supportive, nurturing relationship with no personal costs to himself offers Marian the opportunity to learn to give freely and to be needed by a significant yet emotionally distant male figure.
   (b) Marian's personal theme of illness and neediness offers Roy the chance to revise his view of himself as inadequate to care for others.

Similarly, Roy's fear of being overpowered and controlled (theme 5) could be viewed as compatible with Marian's theme that love equals sameness, symbiosis, and abandonment (theme 1). Here we may view Roy as playing out the part of the couple's shared ambivalence, which perpetuates distance and separateness. In contrast, Marian assumes the counter position of perpetuating fusion, oneness, and togetherness. Each partner's part keeps the spouse's unacknowledged needs for emotional closeness and/or autonomy alive in the relationship and thus available for reclaiming by the self at some point in time.

For Roy and Marian, the potential solutions available in their reciprocal themes had not yet been actualized. As a result, their individual themes continued to appear antagonistic and competing. When spouses' individual themes are considered less as digital elements and more as analogical wholes, we find that the fit between conflicting elements of an individual theme and among clusters of certain themes becomes a coherent representation of the couple's conjugal mythology.

Finally, some spouses' themes seem to be totally unrelated and independent of each other. For example, Roy's ambivalence about close interpersonal relationships with men (theme 4) appeared initially to have a separate and independent existence from any of Marian's personal themes. This theme seemed to follow its own developmental course.

However, the relationship between and among spouses' personal themes are not static, even in the most distressed marriages and dysfunctional relationships. Any significant developmental transitions, life changes, or changes in one spouse's personal themes will necessitate a reactive change in those themes with which they were associated or with which they have become associated. For example:

As Marian began to interact with other married women who had children her daughter's age, she learned that Roy had no desire to become involved in any type of social interactions with these women and their husbands. Roy's potential involvement with these men activated personal themes of competitive aggression (theme 1: aggression = destruction) and ambivalence about intimate contact with males (theme 4). Similarly, as their daughter grew older, Marian encouraged her husband to become more involved with her so that her daughter would not feel that a relationship with her father was forbidden or that intimate associations with men were unacceptable (Marian's theme 3). However, Roy experienced Marian's encouragement to become more involved with their child as an indication that he was being asked to take full responsibility for another person (theme 3: inadequacy in caring for others). The more she urged him to "do things" with his daughter, the more anxious he became.

Similarly, as Marian and Roy began to develop an autonomous couple system and to reduce the amount of contact and interaction that they had with Marian's family, the primacy of the mother-daughter relationship (theme 3) was threatened. Marian found herself torn between her loyalty to her mother and her loyalty to her husband. The realization and the conflict associated with it caused Marian to have acute anxiety attacks. In order to reduce her anxiety, she began to visit her parents, especially her mother, more frequently. Roy experienced Marian's increased visits to her parents' home as neglecting her duties and responsibilities toward him and their marriage. This triggered Roy's feelings of being abandoned, uncared for, and unprotected (theme 3). As a result, he became enraged, but the fear of his own violent aggression frightened him. He internalized this anger, became depressed (theme 2), and began to withdraw from Marian. On the evening before this couple sought therapy, Marian had attempted to bring Roy out of his depressed mood and to make some type of contact with her husband. She did this in the only way she knew how, by approaching him sexually (theme 5). Unfortunately, Roy perceived Marian's sexual advances as her attempts to control him (theme 5). In order to demonstrate his autonomy, Roy rejected Marian's sexual overtures. Furthermore, he used masturbation (which Roy referred to as "self-abuse") as a symbolic gesture to express his pent-up rage.

As one can see from this discussion, the personal themes of spouses stand in fluid and changing relationship to each other. The balance between and among various themes is delicate and complex and not as simple as it first appears. Themes that were once independent may suddenly come into direct and intimate contact. Sometimes these themes fit together neatly and flow together in smooth harmony. In other instances they appear to clash violently and crises develop. As is the case with ambivalent, competing, or antagonistic symbolic/affective themes in one's personal mythology, the conflict will persist until there is some sort of reorganization or synthesis of these themes (through the give and take processes of assimilation and accommodation) or a new superordinate theme is created that allows these apparently antagonistic personal themes to remain intact with a greater sense of harmony. In situations where an antagonistic personal theme of one or both spouses undergoes revision, the relationship between the two themes that stood in conscious opposition may change in such a way as to cause them to become totally unrelated (e.g., more autonomous and differentiated). In other cases, the two consciously antagonistic personal themes, once modified, may become compatibly joined within the context of a larger, superordinate theme. The unsuccessful resolution of spouses' consciously competing themes, however, is seen as pivotal to the development of psychiatric symptoms. In the case of Roy and Marian, the symptoms were depression, anxiety, withdrawal, and a breakdown in the couple's sexual relationship.

The Emergence of Central Personal Themes in Response to Assessment Instruments

In Marian's responses to IMAGES, we can see the emergence of theme 3 (her desire to have an intimate relationship with a father figure that would not disrupt the primary mother-daughter bond) and theme 5 (her attempts to get a man to take more initiative and responsibility in their relationship). Theme 1 is also evident in Marian's response to IMAGES (love = sameness; separateness and difference are unacceptable and wrong in an intimate relationship). However, this theme is graphically seen in Marian's response to FACES III and her drawing of her desired relationship with Roy.

Marian's responses to PAFS graphically underscores her struggle to separate and individuate from her family of origin (themes 1 and 2).

Finally Marian's SIDCARB scores, as we said in Chapter 7, all underscore her desire that Roy take more initiative in their relationship in the areas of communication, sexual relations, expression of love and affection, recreation, making friends, and interaction with their daughter.

Roy's responses to IMAGES reflect his desire that Marian be more responsive to his needs and more understanding and tolerant of their differences as individuals. While Marian pressed for the reduction of their differences, Roy guarded his differentness and wanted Marian to "respect" his differentness and accept his need to be "alone" and to himself. He wanted Marian to see these traits as "strengths" that signified "autonomy." Marian's need to reduce the differences between them as much as possible (theme 1) came into direct, conscious conflict with Roy's lifestyle and need not to be intruded upon (theme 5). Since Roy was much more comfortable with intellectual and spiritual intimacy than Marian, he urged her to read more and "develop her mind," so that she could become more involved with him intellectually. Similarly, his desire to find a less traditional church was an attempt to have them develop and share a more self-styled spirituality which would bring them together in a spiritual way. It also allowed Roy to break away from the authoritarian, dogma-oriented church which he identified with his father (themes 1 and 4).

Roy's responses to FACES III only underlined his need to maintain interpersonal distance, but still to be taken care of to some degree (theme 5).

Roy's responses to PAFS showed him to have successfully separated from his family of origin. However, because of the tenacity with which he held onto his separateness and his autonomy, and because he would recoil whenever anyone "invaded his personal space," we interpreted his responses to PAFS as defensive. These responses can be seen as Roy's use of denial, one of the four defenses used by him to deal with anxiety (i.e., denial, intellectualization, reaction formation, and avoidance of or withdrawal from conflict).

Finally, Roy's SIDCARB responses indicated that he desired fewer changes in his marriage than did Marian. He cited only two areas of concern: sex and religion. As we said earlier, religion seemed to be a fairly autonomous and independent theme in Roy's personal mythology, having to do primarily with his ambivalent feelings and unresolved conflicts with his father. However, as we shall see below, this theme later came into direct conflict with themes 2 and 3 in Marian's personal mythology. Sexual relations were tangentially related to Roy's ambivalent feelings toward women (theme 5), but did not seem to arouse any concern during the courtship and dating process.

Summary of the Couple's Conjugal Mythology

The themes which comprise a couple's conjugal mythology can be complex and difficult to grasp concretely. However, we have found that the central themes in the couple's mythology can be condensed by the therapist into an abbreviated, more easily retained cognitive representation. Others have referred to this process as therapeutic mythmaking (cf. Roberts, 1989; van der Hart et al., 1989). To aid us in the development of this constructed version of the couple's mythology, we rely on the four behavioral indicators referred to initially in chapter 4 and briefly in Chapter 5. These indicators include: (1) redundant interactional patterns, (2) repeated surfacing of specific affect-laden conflicts, (3) the couple's predominant affective tone, and (4) recurrent topics of concern. Applying these indicators to Roy and Marian resulted in the following portrayal of the couple's mythology.

Wedded throughout this couple's conjugal mythology are themes of *closeness* (love, fusion, lack of differences) versus *distance* (aloneness, withdrawal), *dominance* (control) versus *submission* (*loss of control, loss of self*), assertiveness (*aggression, initiative*) versus *passivity*, and *caretaking* (protection, support, nurturance) versus *dependency* (needing protection, support and nurturance).

In many of the above themes, one spouse typically enacted one end of the dichotomy while the other enacted the complementary pole. Thus, Marian's part in the interactional dance included behaviors related to control, dominance, assertiveness, parental caretaking and protection. She frequently pressed for and sought emotional closeness from Roy. Her behavior included frequent requests for Roy to "change." In contrast, Roy's part in the interactional dance included behaviors related to passivity, submission, withdrawal, and the maintenance of aloofness and emotional distance.

The couple's conjugal script included a number of painful, *recurring affects*. Marian often felt dissatisfied with the marriage, overtly angry, and disappointed in Roy. She frequently felt anxious, especially in her dealings with her mother and other members of her family of origin. Roy's part in the script included feelings of depression, inadequacy, and low self-worth, but less overt dissatisfaction with Marian or their marriage and less desire for either the marriage or Marian to change. While the above affects rested frequently with one spouse or the other, many of these affects were at times shared. For instance, Marian could at times feel inadequate (e.g., in the area of sexuality) and Roy at times could feel angry toward Marian (though his more typical style was to deny, project, or displace such feelings). The *predominant affective tone* that characterized Roy and Marian's interactional dance and relationship toward one another was disappointment and frustration. *Recurrent topics of concern* around which these affects generally revolved included *religion* (how conservative or modern to be in their religious worship, whether to attend the same church as Marian's parents or a different one), their *sexual relationship* (where issues of submission/control, initiative/passivity were played out), and *parenting* (would both spouses or just Marian be responsible for parenting their daughter?).

When the data from our assessment interviews, the empirical assessment instruments, and the four indicators were combined and reviewed, we arrived at the following condensed version of the couple's mythology:

> MARIAN   I will be your caretaker, assume primary responsibility for the marriage, parenting and family responsibilities.
>
> ROY   In return, I will remain emotionally distant and not challenge your primary loyalty and commitment to your mother, father and siblings.
> I will be passive, avoid all major confrontations with you and others, and allow you to take initiative in most matters.
> You will press me frequently to take more initiative, to become more involved, which will enable you to reenact your unresolved experiences with your father. I will not submit to your pressure because I would equate this with a loss of my sense of self, my uniqueness. Furthermore, to submit would be to realize my fear of being engulfed and overwhelmed by a woman (my mother).
>
> MARIAN   Although I am ambivalent about this, I do not want you to submit to my demands for you to be more assertive (to take more initiative) because if you did I would have to deal with my mother, my disappointment in my father, my conflicts with my sisters, and my unresolved feelings about sexuality.

However elegant this arrangement was in enabling each spouse to reenact major themes in their personal mythologies and in protecting them from their worst fears, the arrangement also restrained each spouse's personal development and the growth and development of the entire nuclear family system. Inhibition of Roy's personal development was evidenced in his depression, lack of assertiveness, and low self-worth. These were problems he readily acknowledged for himself. For Marian, constraints to her personal development were associated with conflicting loyalties to others (e.g., mother, Roy) which left her other-directed (versus self-directed) and less able to attend to her own personal needs. To acknowledge a clear sense of self with needs which were different from her mother's was to risk losing her mother's love. The developmental delay for the family as a whole was most evident in the couple's ambivalence surrounding the decision to have another child before Marian's "biological clock" expired.

INTERVENTION

Roy and Marian were seen in therapy for approximately 14 months. However, their treatment extended over a period of two and one half years. In our work, we routinely schedule individual therapy sessions with both spouses as part of our overall treatment design. It is not uncommon for us to arrange for a specific block or series of individual therapy sessions with spouses throughout the course of treatment. The movement from couple focused interviews is strategically designed and timed. Such shifts in focus may be used to de-escalate nonproductive conflicts (Bagarozzi & Giddings, 1982, 1983a), to precipitate a crisis, or to unbalance the system. Most often, however, blocks of individual sessions are used to help spouses: (a) become aware of previously unrecognized ideal spouse/perceived spouse discrepancies, unverbalized assumptions, expectations and disappointments; (b) crystallize personal needs, motives, drives and desires; (c) edit personal themes; and (d) modify or reorganize central aspects of the self and/or ideal images.

We begin this phase of treatment by meeting with both spouses together to discuss our assessment findings and to answer any questions they might have about the instruments (IMAGES, FACES III, SIDCARB, and PAFS), the Family Relationships History or the Personal Myth Assessment interview. Next we explain the scoring procedures used for each instrument and discuss the meanings of the various scores and our interpretation of these scores in terms of the couple's presenting problems. For example, in this meeting with Roy and Marian, we discussed each instrument separately and then summarized our findings in terms of "major issues to be considered" by the couple. A brief description of this process is described below.

Feedback Session

First we focus on IMAGES. This is done to give the couple very concrete and tangible feedback about ideal spouse/perceived spouse discrepancies. This provides the couple with a context for discussing heretofore unverbalized expectations, disappointments, unmet needs, etc., that have become the source of resentment and conflict. With Roy and Marian we indicated that Marian perceived more ideal spouse/actual spouse discrepancies than did Roy. In order not to induce a negative expectancy, we added that both Roy's and Marian's ideal/perceived discrepancies were small (16% and 22% respectively). We then proceeded to identify the factors or factor items where discrepancies were noted.

Next we moved to a discussion of SIDCARB in order to help spouses focus on those areas of marital exchange where rule discrepancies and conflicts are perceived. We discuss the meaning of each factor score after explaining that each score is a standard score having a mean of 50 and a standard deviation of 10. The first SIDCARB factor is discussed in terms of each spouse's perception of the fairness of the social exchange process and his/her satisfaction with the rules governing conjugal exchanges. The higher the score, the higher the dissatisfaction with this process and the more one desires changes in his/her spouse's behavior in the particular areas identified. Spouses are then asked to focus on their responses to items that measure spousal commitment to the marriage. *We believe that it is important to have spouses openly acknowledge and discuss their willingness to make specific behavioral changes in order to improve their marriage.* The higher the scores on this factor, the more distressed the marriage and the harder the spouses will have to work in order to improve their relationship. We also note the correspondences between items identified on factor I of SIDCARB and items identified on IMAGES.

Factor II is usually interpreted as a satisfaction with one's spouse and with one's marriage. We distinguish between satisfaction with one's marriage and one's mate, on the one hand, and satisfaction with the exchange process, on the other. These two factors are independent. We also talk about "barriers" to divorce and separation (factors II and III) in a positive sense. Rather than interpreting these scores as "barriers," we refer to them as "responsibility items," i.e., how responsible one is in the marriage. *We do not interpret these scores in terms of a power dimension, even though that is what these scores actually represent, because we do not want to underscore the power struggle that exists between spouses.*

SIDCARB scores for Roy and Marian were interpreted to them as showing Marian to be more concerned with inequities in the couple's exchange system rules and her wanting more changes in Roy's exchange behavior than he desired of her. We interpreted their commitment and willingness to improving the exchange system and their relationship. In our discussion of barrier scores, we stated that Roy and Marian appeared to share approximately the same degree of "responsibility" for the relationship, with Roy perceiving himself as having more financial responsibilities than Marian. We then pointed out how ideal spouse/perceived spouse discrepancies on IMAGES corresponded with each spouse's desires for specific behavioral changes on factor I of SIDCARB.

We next discuss FACES III and PAFS scores under the broad rubric of intimacy (i.e., closeness and separateness) in familial relationships. We explain that in all close relationships individuals continually negotiate their own comfort levels of "interpersonal space." Individuals have different "need levels" and these "need levels" change with the passage of time and the development of the marriage. We explain that for most people there are two primary groups for which changing needs for closeness and separateness present special problems, i.e., one's family of origin and one's family of procreation. Some of the most frequently experienced problems in these two primary groups are then outlined:

1. One's attempts to separate from one's family of origin and one's struggles to develop an autonomous self and separate identity.
2. The process of negotiating (from time to time) mutually acceptable levels of intimacy (physical, sexual, emotional, psychological, intellectual, spiritual, aesthetic, social, and recreational) with one's spouse, with one's children, and with one's parents.
3. Conflicting or competing commitments, responsibilities, and allegiances to one's family of origin and one's family of procreation.

For Roy and Marian, we did not have to do much interpreting of FACES III scores, because the spouses' drawings of their desired levels of closeness and separateness were graphic representations of their differing expectations.

PAFS scores required a bit more discussion. Marian's Intergenerational Fusion/Individuation score was interpreted as showing her to still have some unresolved issues of separation-individuation, while Roy's scores appeared to show him as "less fused and more differentiated." Similarly, we indicated that Marian seemed to have been (and still appeared to be) very much involved in her parents' marriage. We also said that her responses to items dealing with Intergenerational Triangulation showed that she was experiencing some anxiety concerning dual allegiances and conflicting loyalties between her responsibilities to Roy and responsibilities to her parents. Marian agreed that this was indeed the case and that her mother was "driving her crazy" by telephoning her daily to complain about Marian's father and sisters.

Roy, on the other hand, received high scores on Nuclear Family Triangulation and Intergenerational Triangulation, which indicated that he did not perceive himself to have been triangulated as a child. He also was very clear about his role vis-à-vis his mother after his father's death. His older brothers, who lived in the same northern city with his mother, had the responsibility for his mother's care. His main responsibility was

142   *Personal, Marital, and Family Myths*

to himself, his wife, and his child. He rationalized his position by explaining that his oldest brother was a confirmed bachelor and his middle brother and his wife did not plan to have children. Therefore, both brothers were in much better position than he was to care for mother.

Finally, scores for Intergenerational Intimidation were also quite different for Roy and Marian. The intimidating figure in Roy's life, his father, was now dead. However, Marian's parents were seen as formidable. She acknowledged that she still felt like a "little child" whenever she was with her parents for any length of time.

Our feedback to couples about their communication patterns and conflict negotiation skills is done in nontechnical language. We simply indicate whether their communication and problem-solving style are functional or dysfunctional and whether communication skills training and conflict negotiation training are necessary before the couple can hope to improve the relationship and resolve central conflicts. In-depth analysis might be detrimental in highlighting a couple's competitive struggle, crystallizing dysfunctional interaction patterns, or solidifying zero-sum attitudes and cognitive sets. Similarly, we do not identify dysfunctional ways of communicating love, value and worth, because this is perceived as a direct assault upon the couple's collusive system. Finally, we do not comment upon any unconscious contracts and agreements that have become apparent to us in our observations of the couple's communication/interaction style and conflict negotiation attempts. Any such interpretation would be premature and would only serve to heighten the couple's defenses or, even worse, drive the couple out of therapy.

Summary Feedback

Our summary comments to Marian and Roy were simple and straightforward. We indicated that both Marian and Roy were dissatisfied because their mate's actual behavior did not correspond to their unverbalized expectations on a number of important dimensions. Next we said that, although both Marian and Roy desired specific changes in the rules governing their exchange system, Marian was more dissatisfied with this process than Roy, and she wanted more changes in his behavior than he desired of her. Targeting the dimension of intimacy as an area of central concern, we said that both spouses had quite different expectations for intimacy in the marriage and that these differences seemed to permeate the relationship. We extended our discussion of intimacy to include conflicts with each spouse's family of origin. As we pointed out to them, our findings showed that Roy and Marian had come into treatment at a critical period in their relationship and that issues having to do with conflicting loyalties between Marian's relationship with Roy and her relationship with her family of origin were just beginning to surface. Finally, we gave Roy and Marian feedback about their communication skills, saying that they needed skills training in functional communication, conflict negotiation, and problem-solving. Training in these areas would begin with their next therapy session.

9

Couples' Mythologies
in Marital Therapy—Part I

ONCE FEEDBACK IS completed and any questions raised by the spouses have been answered, we begin our formal treatment program. The sequence presented below is typical.

MODIFICATION OF SPOUSAL IDEALS

Our first treatment goal is to help spouses begin to reduce ideal spouse/perceived spouse discrepancies. We begin this lengthy process under the guise of communication skills training. Training in functional communication is the most logical place to begin, both from an empirical basis (Lewis & Spanier, 1979) and from a practical standpoint. Couples coming in for marital therapy frequently, if not always, cite poor communication as a problem in their marriage. All assessment instruments ask couples questions about their satisfaction with communication, and responses on one or more of these questionnaires usually show communication as an area of the relationship in need of modification. This is especially true for IMAGES and SIDCARB.

Each spouse is given a copy of the Structured Guidelines for Establishing Functional Communication in Marital Dyads. These guidelines are presented in Table 3.

After the spouses have read these guidelines, any questions they might have about them are answered. The remainder of the session is spent teaching the couple these skills. The therapist uses modeling, positive reinforcement, and shaping to bring the couple to a point where the skills have been mastered. The reader will recall that in the treatment of individuals (Chapter 4) we stressed that the ability to role take (step back, decenter, reverse perspectives) and the ability to become empathic

were considered to be important skills for the client to develop if individual therapy was to be effective. A similar statement can be made for marital
therapy. However, in marital therapy, the therapist helps the spouses
develop and use these skills in their relationship with each other.

We also stressed that the development of trust between the individual
client and the therapist is central to the treatment process and is necessary for achieving positive therapeutic outcome. Again, a similar statement can be made for marital therapy. Both spouses must be able to trust
the therapist. However, in marital therapy, the therapist must also create
a climate conducive to the development of trust between the spouses. In
individual treatment, we rely heavily upon the use of nondirective, client-centered interviewing techniques to establish trust and develop rapport with the client. In marital therapy, on the other hand, the therapist
cannot afford to be nondirective and passive. Such a stance would be
counter-therapeutic (Pinsof & Catherall, 1986). In marital therapy, trust
in the therapist comes about when the spouses see the therapist as one
who can structure the session, give definite direction, teach specific
skills, reduce reciprocal punishments between the partners, offer concrete suggestions when appropriate, prevent negative reinforcement patterns from escalating out of control, help the couple set realistic goals,
etc. In addition, trust in the therapist is also dependent upon the therapist's ability to remain neutral, to maintain an objective stance, to avoid
forming coalitions or unconsciously colluding with one spouse against
the other, and to not become triangulated in the couple's power
otruggleo.

By doing this, the therapist not only establishes trust but also provides
the couple with a safe environment. The therapist's office often becomes
the only tranquil port in the couple's self-generated and self-maintained
storm.

Once the spouses have mastered these communication skills, they are
asked to practice them at home in order to insure transfer and generalization.

At the beginning of the next session, the therapist assesses the
spouses' progress in using their newly acquired communication skills
before moving to the next step in the process, i.e., the reduction of ideal
spouse/perceived spouse discrepancies. Using the Structured Guidelines for Establishing Functional Communication in Marital Dyads as a
foundation, the therapist asks the couple to discuss ideal spouse/per-
ceived spouse discrepancies identified on IMAGES. Spouses are directed to focus on those ideal spouse/perceived spouse discrepancies that
they consider to be of central importance. At this juncture, some addi-

tional guidelines are introduced into the structural communication exercise:

1. Discuss how you *perceive* your mate whenever he/she behaves in a way that is *consistent* with your ideal mate. Next, tell your mate how this makes you feel about him/her and your relationship.
2. Discuss your *attributions* (i.e., your interpretations of your mate's behavior, motives, intentions, and how you interpret his/her caring and valuing of you) whenever your mate behaves in a way that is *consistent with* or *closely approximates your ideal.*
3. Next, discuss how you *perceive* your mate whenever he/she behaves in a way which is *inconsistent* with your ideal. Tell your mate how this *inconsistency* makes you feel about him/her and your relationship.
4. Finally, discuss your *attributions* (i.e., your interpretations of your mate's behavior, motives, intentions, and how you interpret his/her caring and valuing of you) whenever your mate behaves in a way that is *inconsistent* with your ideal.

When spouses are asked to discuss ideal spouse/perceived spouse discrepancies using these guidelines, *we explain that the goal of this exercise is not to change one's spouse's behavior but to help both spouses become aware of their own and their partner's unverbalized expectations, disappointments, and disenchantments and how these have led to misunderstandings, resentments, and conflicts in the past.* We stress the importance of each spouse's taking full responsibility for explicitly stating his/her expectations, for verbalizing his/her assumptions, for acknowledging one's own unique perceptions and experiences, for recognizing one's own attributions and for understanding how one's perceptions, expectations and attributions influence how one treats one's spouse.

The following is an excerpt from Roy and Marian's discussion of ideal spouse/perceived spouse discrepancies. The discrepancies under consideration have to do with Marian's expectations that Roy share his feelings with her and that he confide in her more than he has in the past (IMAGES items 5 and 6 of factor I: Emotional Gratification).

MARIAN   Roy when you come home in the evening and you are silent and you don't share your thoughts and your feelings with me, I get frustrated.

ROY   (Reflects Marian's statements back to her)

MARIAN   When you do share your thoughts and feelings with me, I feel close to you. I feel connected. I feel good. I think that we are really a couple. I don't feel isolated and I also feel loving toward you.

ROY   (Reflects Marian's statements back to her)

MARIAN   When you don't share your thoughts and feelings with me, you seem so distant. I get anxious, because I don't know what is wrong. Sometimes I think you are angry with me or disappointed in me or something. I'm not sure what is going on in your mind.

ROY   (Reflects Marian's statements back to her)

MARIAN   Many times I feel that if I don't ask you questions about your day that the entire evening could be spent in silence and that you will not volunteer anything. Could you please tell me why you don't share your thoughts and feelings with me or confide in me unless I question you?

ROY   (Reflects Marian's statement and then replies) "Sometimes I am silent because I really have nothing to say, and sometimes I am silent because I am mentally struggling with a problem or a concern that I have.

MARIAN   (Reflects Roy's statements back to him)

ROY   When something is troubling me, I don't usually tell you immediately. I have to think it out for myself first. I also don't want to burden you with my personal problems.

MARIAN   (Reflects Roy's statements back to him)

ROY   Sometimes when you question me about what I am thinking, I feel invaded by you. I think you are trying to intrude upon my privacy. I think you know that I have always been a solitary individual.

MARIAN   (Reflects Roy's statements back to him)

This brief passage offers a typical example of how spouses use the Structured Guidelines to address ideal spouse/perceived spouse discrepancies. Once the spouses have learned to use these skills proficiently, the therapist begins to help them become aware of their personal themes and how these themes are manifesting themselves in their marriage. For example, at the conclusion of this verbal interchange, the therapist made the following comments.

THERAPIST   (to Marian) It seems very important that Roy share his thoughts and feelings with you. When he keeps to himself, you feel anxious and the differentness between you, your separateness causes you to feel unloved (Marian's theme 1). It seems like it is always your responsibility to make contact with Roy (Marian's theme 5).

THERAPIST   (to Roy) You really seem to cherish your separateness and your individuality. This gives you a sense of independence and freedom. You also seem very concerned not to overburden Marian with your own personal problems. I think you would like both you and Marian not to become too dependent upon each other for caretaking and support (Roy's theme 5). By you not sharing your problems with Marian, you are actually trying to strengthen her and your relationship.

The reader will note that positive connotations are used when underscoring personal themes, even if the themes that are highlighted appear to be antagonistic.

The therapist continues to use this approach to flag personal themes in all the couple's discussions of ideal spouse/perceived spouse discrepancies. However, no direct statement of personal themes or their relationships is made during this phase of treatment. We assume that the continual underscoring of themes will register unconsciously with both spouses. There is no need for a blatant interpretation, since more subtle methods will be used to modify these themes later in therapy.

Frequently, when spouses are confronted with their ideal spouse/perceived spouse discrepancies they express disappointment. Sometimes they experience a sense of loss and depression which is similar to a grief reaction. Such responses should not be considered pathological. They frequently signify that some type of cognitive restructuring is in progress and that one's *ideal spouse* may be undergoing revision or modification.

Using Behavioral Exchanges to Further Reduce Ideal Spouse/Perceived Spouse Discrepancies

Exchange contracting is the next skill taught each couple as a routine part of the therapeutic process. Whereas the Structured Guidelines were used to affect changes in spouse's ideals, behavioral exchanges are used to help spouses change their own behavior so that it is brought more closely in line with the mate's ideal image. The model of behavioral exchange outlined in Table 4 is a modified version of the behavioral exchange paradigm first proposed by Rappaport and Harrell (1972) and revised by the first author (Bagarozzi, 1983a; Bagarozzi & Wodarski, 1977).

Spouses are asked to take turns discussing IMAGES items and ex-

TABLE 4 Modified behavioral exchange model

---

1. Using IMAGES as a guideline for identifying ideal spouse/perceived spouse discrepancies, select one behavior of your spouse that you would like him/her to change.
2. Once you have done this, propose an alternative behavior that your spouse could substitute for his/her problem behavior. Select a behavior that would make your spouse behave in a way that more closely resembles your ideal.
3. If your spouse agrees to make the behavioral change you have suggested:
   (a) Identify the times, locations, contexts and environments where this change is to occur.
   (b) State specifically the frequency of behavioral performances, the rate of increase or decrease of the behavior and the duration of behavioral performances.
4. If your spouse does not wish to make the behavioral change you have suggested, ask him/her to propose three alternative behaviors (to the problem behavior you have identified) that he/she would be willing to make.
5. Once your spouse has proposed these three behavioral alternatives, you are to select one behavioral alternative that you are willing to accept. Then:
   (a) Identify the times, locations, contexts and environments where this change is to occur.
   (b) State specifically the frequency of behavioral performance, the rate of increase or decrease of the behavior, and the duration of behavioral performances.

---

changing problematic behaviors until they have gone over all ideal/perceived discrepancies. Ideal spouse/perceived spouse discrepancies that cannot be negotiated satisfactorily between the spouses are acknowledged, but no further attempt is made to deal with them at this time.[1]

---

[1]Frequently, one finds couples who have been very successful resolving ideal/perceived discrepancies through the use of symbolic contracting procedures unable to follow through on what appears to be a simple, straightforward behavioral contract. When this occurs, one should suspect that the consciously negotiated contract (in some way) poses a serious threat to the system's equilibrium which is being maintained by a previously negotiated unconscious contract.

Negotiating Symbolically Meaningful
Behavioral Contingency Contracts

Symbolic contingency contracting was first developed by the first author to help couples overcome their resistance to behavioral contracting and behavior modification practices (Bagarozzi, 1981). We introduce this procedure at this time in therapy because it is a logical extension of the behavioral exchange procedure the couple has just mastered. It also allows the couple to make a smooth and natural transition from discussing and negotiating isolated behaviors to dealing with much broader thematic concerns. We teach the couple this process by helping spouses negotiate those ideal spouse/perceived spouse discrepancies that were identified earlier but which the couple was unable to resolve through simple behavioral exchange procedures. Essentially, the procedures used to teach spouses how to negotiate symbolically meaningful contingency contracts encourage each spouse to become more aware of the broader personal thematic meaning of specific behaviors. The following guidelines in Table 5 are used.

This intervention strategy usually produces a number of significant outcomes: (a) it helps spouses become aware of the symbolic significance of behaviors exchanged between them; (b) it sensitizes spouses to the underlying themes in their personal mythologies that are operating in their marriage; (c) it reduces projective identification and transference distortions between spouses; (d) it brings to light each spouse's negative attributions, interpretations, perceptions, expectations, and distortions of the other's intentions and behaviors; (e) it encourages spouses to become more empathic and to role take, thus strengthening the empathy and role taking skills acquired in communications training; and (f) it facilitates mutual trust and understanding and makes both spouses more likely to exchange behaviors and negotiate contracts to resolve some of the ideal spouse/perceived spouse discrepancies that still remain.

A brief description of how behavioral exchange procedures and symbolic contracting were used with Marian and Roy is offered below.

One of the ideal spouse/perceived spouse discrepancies that Roy and Marian had some difficulty resolving had to do with both spouses' perceptions of their mate's religiosity and spirituality. As we said earlier, Roy perceived Marian to be too rigid and orthodox in her religious beliefs. Marian, it will be recalled, wanted her husband to become more spiritual and more involved in organized religious practices. In their discussions about this issue, the therapist commented on Marian's need

TABLE 5 Contract negotiation guidelines

---

1. Once you have identified an ideal spouse/perceived spouse discrepancy, select a specific behavior of your mate that you would like him/her to change and propose a behavioral alternative for that problem behavior.
2. Explain to your spouse the meaning you associate with the problem behavior. Discuss:
    (a) how it makes you feel when your spouse exhibits the problem behavior.
    (b) your interpretation of this behavior in terms of how much your spouse values you, loves you, and sees you as worthwhile.
3. Describe to your spouse what memories and associations come to mind from your experiences in your family of origin whenever he/she exhibits this problem behavior. If you can identify this particular behavior as being associated with a particular family member, share this with your spouse.
4. Now, explain to your spouse the meaning you associate with the alternative behavior you would like him/her to exhibit. Discuss:
    (a) how it makes you feel when your spouse exhibits the behavior you desire.
    (b) your interpretation of this behavior in terms of how much your spouse values you, loves you, and sees you as a worthwhile person.
5. Describe to your spouse what memories and associations come to mind from your experiences in your family of origin whenever he/she exhibits the desired behavior. If you can identify this particular behavior as being associated with a particular family member, share this with your spouse.

---

to have her husband subscribe to the "same" religious convictions that she held and that any "difference" in their religious beliefs "seemed to pose a serious threat to the couple's oneness and togetherness" (theme 1). On the other hand, the therapist's comments to Roy focused on his ambivalent feelings concerning his relationships with authoritarian and overpowering parental figures (themes 4 and 5) as symbolized by the Roman Catholic Church and the clergy. The therapist underscored these themes by commenting on Roy's fears of being "dominated and controlled by authoritarian figures" who "stifled his attempts to think for himself, become autonomous and develop independence." The therapist then used the following phrases, taken directly from Roy's Personal Myth Assessment, to describe Roy's dilemma: "It seems that organized religion prevents you from living your own life to the fullest, stifles your individuality. You seem to believe that the Church is not metaphysically on target." Finally, the therapist commented on Roy's "irreverence" and "outrageousness" as being a sign of his "courage" in the face of "over-whelming odds."

Again, the reader will note that no direct statement about the antago-nistic relationship between elements of the spouses' personal themes is made. The therapist simply underscores the themes without calling the couple's attention to them.

Since this issue was one that Marian and Roy had considerable diffi-culty negotiating and resolving, symbolic contracting was used. The following is an excerpt from the contracting session:

ROY   When you ask me to go to church with you on Sundays, I feel anxious. I think you are trying to make me conform to your way of thinking. I think that you don't value my opinion and my way of seeing the church. I don't think you respect my opinion. I know you love me, but there is one part of me that you don't seem to accept.

MARIAN   (Paraphrases Roy's statements and reflects them back to him)

ROY   I remember when I was growing up, my father would ask me and my brothers to stand in line for inspection every Sunday morn-ing before we would go to church. He'd inspect our hands and fingernails to see if they were clean. He'd inspect our clothes. We always had to wear starched shirts and ties. I used to get this sick, sinking feeling in my stomach.

MARIAN   (Paraphrases Roy's statements and reflects them back to him)

ROY   I hated to go to church with my family. The priests' sermons were always about sin, Hell and punishment for not following God's word. My father would sit there and say nothing. Sometimes he would nod his head in agreement. Sometimes he would look at us in disgust.

MARIAN   (Paraphrases Roy's statements, reflects them back to him and asks a question) Roy, didn't you ever have a positive experi-ence with the Church?

ROY   Well, on a few occasions I went to church with my grandfather and grandmother. My grandfather was not as strict as my father.

He never talked about the sermons and after the service he took me and my grandmother for ice cream sodas.

MARIAN   (After paraphrasing and reflecting Roy's statements back to him) Sunday mass was a happy occasion in our family. When we went to church, I got a chance to sit next to my father. It was one of the few occasions we got to do things as a family. I really liked the closeness going to church brought to our family. Sometimes, before my sister was born, when church was very crowded, I would sit in my father's lap.

ROY   (Paraphrases Marian's statements and reflects them back to her) I know we have very different feelings about the Church and Sunday mass, but I know that it is a source of peace for you. Maybe I would not feel the way I do if we attended another church, one that was more modern, less old world.

At this juncture, the therapist asked the couple to consider a contract where both spouses might "compromise a little in order to improve their relationship." With the help of the therapist, Marian and Roy worked out the following contract.

1. Marian agreed to attend a different church with Roy, if he would take the initiative to find one that was more "modern" and "less old world."

2. Roy agreed to do this in exchange for Marian's not pressuring him to accomplish this task immediately. She was to agree to let him move at his own pace and not to question him about his progress. Once he had found one or two churches that he believed would be acceptable to him, he would ask Marian to accompany him to church services so that she could decide whether she would be comfortable with the priests, the services, etc.

The therapist must take responsibility for helping couples negotiate contingency contracts that have symbolic significance for both spouses. He/she must be able to guide the spouses in such a way that they select for exchange those behaviors that represent central themes in both spouses' personal mythologies. For example, in this contract negotiated between Roy and Marian, several issues were taken into consideration:

1. This contract permitted Roy to play out the themes of rebelliousness with male authority figures in a way which did not bring him into direct conflict with them (theme 4). He was able to assert

himself with a woman and prevent her from controlling him (theme 5). This contract offered him an opportunity to act as a competent male capable of taking care of a woman without being overwhelmed. It also made it possible for him to take charge of a heterosexual relationship. Here we see how Roy's personal themes begin to undergo modification and how his self-concept was affected by this newfound competence.

2. Marian began to perceive Roy as active and involved with her as a result of this contract. She began to see that men could take their own initiative without being prodded or seduced (theme 5). It also offered her the possibility of establishing more closeness with a paternal figure (theme 3).

From the spouses' perspectives, it appears that the therapist has simply been teaching them a series of concrete skills that enable them to communicate more effectively, to solve problems more efficiently, to negotiate their conflicts more satisfactorily, and to see each other in more realistic and meaningful ways. They are not consciously aware that major changes have been taking place in their typical communication-relational pattern (Ericson & Rogers, 1973; Rogers, 1972; Rogers & Bagarozzi, 1983), and the manner in which they convey love, value and worth (Strayhorn, 1978).

For example, Marian and Roy continued to practice the communication skills at home using the Structured Guidelines for Establishing Functional Communication in Marital Dyads. As a result, they were able to develop a more flexible communication-relational interactional style. The rigid complementarity (with Marian in the domineering, one-up, superior position) observed during the assessment phase of treatment gradually gave way to more flexible styles of interaction, which included (a) alternating patterns of complementarity, (b) symmetrical escalations, and (c) parallel interactions. As Marian and Roy incorporated the communication guidelines for discussing ideal spouse/perceived spouse discrepancies into their everyday interactional patterns, they tended to use painful channels to communicate value messages less frequently and to achieve a greater correspondence in their rules for sending and receiving value messages (Strayhorn, 1978). In addition, both Marian and Roy became less tentative in their communications with each other, they appeared to be less sensitive to perceiving devalue messages, and they reduced the tendency to interpret each other's behavior negatively. The couple's willingness to negotiate symbolically significant contracts also reinforced the changes made in their communication-relational control patterns. For example, Roy and Marian were better able to use quid pro quo contracts than they had been in the past. Zero-sum standoffs, however, still occurred in those areas where their personal themes resulted in direct conflict.

Using Contingency Contracts to Edit Conjugal Themes

The therapist continues to help spouses work out symbolically meaningful contracts to resolve any ideal spouse/perceived spouse discrepancies that they are both willing to negotiate. Throughout these negotiations, the therapist continues to highlight personal themes that undergird particular IMAGES items or groups of items. However, the therapist now begins to underscore how these personal themes appear to be aligned and related to form specific conjugal themes.

When spouses have completed negotiating IMAGES items to their mutual satisfaction, they are ready to tackle discrepancies in the area of rules for distributive justice and social exchange. The first ten items of SIDCARB factor I are used to help couples identify discrepancy areas. Usually we begin these contract negotiations by having the couple first attempt to resolve exchange rules discrepancies in those areas where both spouses believe that a successful resolution is possible. The success experienced as a result of these initial attempts serves as a positive incentive to work on more difficult and complex areas of conflict and discrepancy. It is at this juncture that the therapist begins to help the couple negotiate contracts that will edit dysfunctional conjugal themes. Initial attempts to edit conjugal themes will tend to be successful if the themes targeted for modification are related to ideal spouse/perceived spouse discrepancies that have already been negotiated successfully by the spouses. Since Marian and Roy had identified religion as an area of concern on both IMAGES and SIDCARB, and since they had already achieved some degree of success negotiating ideal spouse/perceived spouse discrepancies in this area, the therapist suggested that the couple build upon this positive experience and continue to negotiate religious issues.

The reader will recall that we identified four behavioral indicators that signaled the presence of an underlying conjugal theme: (a) recurrent topics of concern; (b) redundant interaction patterns; (c) repeated surfacing of specific affect-laden conflicts; and (d) the couple's predominant affective tone.

Religious issues were a recurrent topic of concern for Roy and Marian.

Typically, Roy and Marian would avoid discussing this topic until it was time to attend church. Then they would become cautious and tentative. An air of somberness and feelings of tenseness characterized their discussions. The redundant theme was Roy's disappointment with Marian's parents' church and clergy and Marian's complaint that Roy would not take any initiative to explore other possibilities. Arguments over this issue usually left both spouses feeling frustrated, disappointed, and angry.

On the surface, Marian and Roy were discussing a religious concern. However, they were actually attempting to resolve a deeper conflict that came about when their daughter's birth produced an antagonistic relationship between two personal themes that had once been harmoniously aligned and integrated. Prior to their daughter's birth, the following two themes had been complementary:

ROY'S THEME 3 & 5   The desire for a woman who would take care of him and take charge of the relationship without overpowering him. The desire for a woman who would not make him feel inadequate by asking him to take the initiative or to take care of her when she was ill.

MARIAN'S THEME 3   The desire to have a relationship with a man which would be acceptable to her mother because it would not threaten the mother-daughter bond.

Sager's (1976) pioneering work on unconscious contracts has been helpful in the development of our formulations about how some personal themes become joined to produce conjugal themes. Essentially, spouses nonverbally and unconsciously negotiate quid pro quo contracts that permit both partners to maintain treasured personal themes intact. Such contracts always allow the spouses to continue behaving in ways that are comfortable and consistent with their interpersonal styles. Sometimes, as Dicks (1967) describes, these contracts may require that spouses play and act out specific roles and scripts from their partner's personal mythologies. Such contracts often offer spouses the illusion and the promise of providing them with an opportunity to relive, rework, master and correct unresolved developmental conflicts and past wrongs through transference acting-out and projective identification. While such clauses may be part of many contracts that couples make, they are not a necessary component of every contract that is negotiated, as we conceptualize this process.

Roy and Marian's unconscious quid pro quo contract for the above two themes was originally formulated as follows:

Marian agrees to take care of Roy and to take charge of their relationship without overpowering Roy. Marian agrees that she will not test his adequacy by asking Roy to take care of her or to take the initiative in their marriage.

In exchange for this:

Roy agrees to marry Marian and not to interfere with the enmeshed mother-daughter relationship.

When couples develop such unconscious contracts, they may incorporate a number of false assumptions. First is the assumption that the terms of the contract (i.e., the manner in which themes are related and joined together) are immutable. Second, there is a lack of recognition that one's own personal themes and those of one's mate will undergo revision with the passage of time. Finally, no consideration is given to the effects that changing life circumstances may have upon personal themes and contractual agreements.

With the birth of their daughter, the above contract was no longer viable. Marian was required to spend a considerable amount of time ministering to the child, and she could not take care of Roy in the way she had in the past. She began to spend more time with her mother and sisters who "simply adored Marian's child." Not only was Marian neglecting Roy, but she was also requesting that he become a more active parent and husband. She wanted Roy to help her with their daughter and to take more responsibility for their relationship as a family. After the birth of their daughter, Marian became more susceptible to colds, flus, viruses, etc., and she fell ill more frequently than had ever been the case during the couple's courtship. Her illnesses did not have the effect of drawing Roy closer to her. As a matter of fact, they drove him further away and increased his feelings of inadequacy, frustration, and despair.

Rather than confront these issues, the couple argued about religion. Each Sunday the couple would attend mass with Marian's parents. After church services, the couple would return to Marian's parents' home for Sunday dinner. The incident that brought them in for therapy had taken place on a Sunday evening shortly after they had returned from a day spent with Marian's parents.

Within the context of helping Roy and Marian resolve their conflicts about religion, several contracts were devised over a six-week period. Each contract was designed to edit specific aspects of this particular theme, the goal being to produce structural and process changes in the couple's system (Bagarozzi, 1983).

The first contract negotiated between Roy and Marian was based upon the agreement struck during their IMAGES negotiations. Roy had identified three new churches whose clergymen were relatively young and who appeared to be fairly modern in their approaches to Catholicism. Roy had shared these activities with Marian, and she had kept her part of the bargain by not pressuring him, by not questioning him, and by allowing him to proceed at his own rate of speed. This having been accomplished successfully, the couple was now ready to move on to the next step in this process. As part of their original agreement, Marian said that she would accompany Roy on his visits to meet with prospective pastors once Roy had taken the initiative to arrange for appointments with them. As Roy and Marian were discussing possible times to meet with the various clergymen, the therapist suggested that the couple also attend Sunday services at each church in addition to meeting with the pastors. Both agreed that this was a good idea. The session ended with Roy agreeing to arrange for meetings with the three prospective church leaders and Marian agreeing to be the one responsible for telling her parents that she and her husband would not be attending Sunday services with them on those Sundays when the couple was visiting other churches.

This contract was designed to help the couple begin to define its own boundaries as an independent, dyadic system separate from Marian's family of origin. It also was meant to be the first step in the direction of helping Marian separate from her mother. Knowing that such a separation would produce a great deal of anxiety, feelings of isolation and guilt for Marian, the therapist encouraged Roy and Marian to negotiate a second contract designed to increase the couple's "spiritual and recreational intimacy." These were two areas of their marriage where the therapist knew Roy would not feel uncomfortable becoming more intimate with his wife. It was hoped that this newfound closeness with Roy would offset, to some degree, Marian's movement away from involvement with her mother and her family of origin. The terms of this second contract were that Marian would take the initiative to engage Roy in weekly discussions about religious issues, concerns, topics, etc., in exchange for Roy's agreeing to become more actively involved with Marian in recreational activities (e.g., jogging, tennis, bicycling).

In addition to offering Marian some compensation for separating from her mother (by providing her with greater opportunities to become more intimately involved with Roy), this contract also addressed other important issues. For example, it required Marian to take the initiative in the marriage in a way which Roy did not experience as intrusive or overpowering. It relieved Roy of any pressure he might have felt to take the lead or to be in charge of these areas of their relationship. It also had an impact on Marian's self-concept, because she began to find that she could get her husband to become intimately involved with her without having to be sexually seductive. Similarly, this new experience also had an effect upon how she perceived her husband (her ideal) and men in general (her attributions, expectations, assumptions, etc., about all men).

These contracts became the basis for the development of a new conjugal theme, which allowed Marian to experience increasing degrees of separateness (from Roy) while at the same time offering her alternative ways of being intimately involved with him that did not threaten him or cause him to feel overpowered or pressured to perform. This new theme permitted Roy to have the separateness he needed but also provided him with the opportunity to take the initiative and become involved with his wife in those areas of the relationship where he felt most competent and least vulnerable. This theme also paved the way for the modification of themes from Roy's and Marian's personal mythologies. For Roy, this involved the differentiation of aggression from assertion. For Marian, the theme of separation-individuation from mother was addressed.

The final agreement negotiated during this contracting phase of treatment demonstrates how contracts can be used to establish what we call *procedural rules*. As the name implies, these rules represent agreed upon procedures that spouses and family members will be expected to use to guide their actions in certain key areas of family functioning. For example, rules can be devised to aid in the development, maintenance, and modification of marital/family structures; to modify dyadic interactions and alter family patterns; to help couples and families progress through developmental transitions and life cycle stages more smoothly, etc.

The simple and straightforward procedural rule presented below was suggested to Marian and Roy by the therapist as "one way to begin to define themselves as a system that was separate and distinct, yet still connected to both their families of origin":

In any dealings with either spouse's family of origin, both spouses must agree upon a course of action to be taken before discussing the decision with the family in question. No decision that will affect one's spouse, one's marriage, or one's family can be made unilaterally. *Once the couple has arrived at a mutually agreed upon decision or course of action, the spouse is responsible for relating this decision to his/her own parents.* This is especially important when the decision or course of action agreed upon by the couple may have a negative impact upon one's parents or extended family members. In dealing with one's parents, the spouse must be sure to make it clear that the responsibility for the decision is one that is mutually shared.

Using this procedural rule as a guideline, Marian agreed that she would be the person to inform her parents about the couple's decision to join a different church, once they had found one that was acceptable to both of them. Roy, on the other hand, agreed to take the responsibility for breaking this news to his mother and his two brothers.

Consequences of these Contractual Agreements

Watzlawick, Beavin, and Jackson (1967) stated, in their *Pragmatics of Human Communication*, one of the basic tenets of family systems theory: "The behavior of every individual within the family is related to and dependent upon the behavior of all the others. All behavior is communication and therefore influences and is influenced by others" (p 134). The change in one spouse's behavior toward his/her mate, therefore, will necessitate a change in how that mate responds. It is important to keep this axiom in mind when helping couples negotiate behavioral exchanges, because any change made by a spouse (vis-à-vis his/her partner) has the potential to disrupt the system's homeostatic balance. In work with couples, it is possible to arrange for behavioral exchanges that remain within the system's fixed range of variation and tolerance without threatening the stability of the system's equilibrium. Such contracts produce gradual changes and recalibration in specific areas of the marriage. The three contracts outlined above are examples of how first-order changes were brought about in this couple's marriage.

While the therapist might have some power to arrange for a couple to make stepwise changes that allow spouses to assimilate and accommodate to changes in their mate's behavior, the therapist has virtually no power to orchestrate how larger groups (e.g., family systems) will react to changes in the behavior of one or more of their members. For example, one could not foretell how Marian's parents were going to react to the couple's attempt to erect definite boundaries between the two systems and the decision to leave Marian's parents' church. Although the couple was asked to speculate about possible reactions by Marian's parents, no one was prepared for what actually occurred.

One evening, shortly after Roy and Marian had joined their new church, Marian received a telephone call from her oldest sister (the sister identified as least liked by Marian in her Family Relationships History). Marian was asked to come to her parents' home because her mother was having a "severe anxiety attack." When Marian arrived, her two older sisters accused her of causing their mother's anxiety attack. They said that this episode was brought on by Marian's decision to leave her parents' church. Her sisters' attacks then became personal and destructive, and a number of unresolved childhood conflicts having to do with sibling rivalry, favoritism, and jealousy resurfaced. During this confrontation, Marian's oldest sister attempted to assault her. However, her father intervened and prevented any violence from taking place. After this incident, Marian returned to her own home. Roy's response to this turn of events was to be understandably upset, but also supportive of Marian.

At the next therapy session, the couple asked the therapist for help in dealing with Marian's family of origin. In response to the couple's request, the following goals, dealing primarily with Marian's theme 2, were outlined:

1. To strengthen the couple system's boundaries vis-à-vis Marian's family of origin.
2. To help Marian set appropriate limits with her siblings, especially her oldest sister.
3. To reduce intergenerational intimidation from Marian's parents, especially Marian's mother.
4. To help Marian become detriangulated and end her role as scape goat.
5. To help Marian continue the process of separation/individuation.

Both conjoint and individual sessions were used to achieve these goals. In the next section, we outline some of the clinical strategies developed to accomplish these ends.

Conjugal Role Playing

Conjugal role playing is a technique which requires each spouse to enact roles from their personal mythologies vis-à-vis each other and/or vis-à-vis their families of origin. Like the role playing techniques used in individual therapy and described earlier in Chapter 4, conjugal role playing also fosters changes in the spouses' self-structures, self-concepts, cognitive ideals, and behaviors in relation to each other and their families of origin.

When the focus of concern is a spouse's family of origin, the therapist asks the couple to invoke the procedural rule outlined earlier in this chapter. The couple is coached, by the therapist, to function as a team. Defining systems boundaries and setting limits with the spouses' families of origin are presented to the couple as superordinate goals to be achieved and developmental tasks to be mastered if the couple is to function successfully as an autonomous system.

In some instances, couples who are unable to negotiate relationship differences can be taught the skills necessary to negotiate exchange contracts if they first learn these skills while attempting to solve a problem that they perceive as being external to their relationship (e.g., establishing boundaries and setting limits with their families of origin). When viewed in this way, the external problem becomes a superordinate goal. After several successful attempts at solving problems external to the relationship, the therapist can help couples conceptualize some of their less severe problems as external to their relationship, i.e., as superordinate goals (e.g., establishing boundaries and setting limits with their children).[2]

A number of intervention strategies used in our work with individuals have been adopted for use with couples as part of conjugal role playing. Some of these include: developing self-instructed and couple-instructed performance models in the form of roles and scripts, constructing cognitive-behavioral response chains and jointly shared secret mantras, couple rehearsals and practices, conjugal in vivo exposures and ritual prescriptions.

In order to achieve goals 1, 2, and 4, the following interventions were devised:

First, Roy and Marian agreed to adopt the roles of Mr. and Mrs. Huxtable (Bill Cosby and Phylicia Rashad). They were then directed to write a script for "The Cosby Show." In her role as Clair Huxtable, Marian was charged with the task of defining the couple's boundaries and explaining the couple's relationship to her parents. She was to do this by expressing the couple's feelings and viewpoints concerning religion and involvement with the church. Using the procedural rule established earlier, Roy (in his role as Mr. Huxtable) was to become Marian's steadfast backup, who continues to give her encouragement and support in her dealings

---

[2]In dysfunctional family systems, "curing" the identified patient can be seen as a superordinate goal shared by all family members.

with her parents. A key element in this procedure was for both Roy and
Marian to maintain a sense of humor.

Once the script was developed, the therapist acted as "acting coach"
and "ghost script writer." In this role he helped Roy and Marian develop
their respective roles, cognitive-behavioral response chains, and internal
dialogues specifically tailored for dealing with Marian's parents. Rehearsals were held with the therapist playing the roles of both of Marian's parents. In order to strengthen the couple's sense of "weness" and
"teamwork," the therapist helped Marian and Roy devise a secret mantra
that they could recite (subvocally) whenever the "going got tough." This
mantra was constructed from themes taken from each spouse's personal
mythology and was meant to be the basis for a new, consciously acknowledged conjugal theme. Roy and Marian's secret mantra was *"From
the separate strengths of the two the one draws threefold sustenance and
power."*

Second, in order to help Marian set limits with her two older sisters,
two separate scripts (based upon characters from Marian's Family Relationships History and Personal Myth Assessment Interview and Roy's
Personal Myth Assessment Interview) were developed.

The couple agreed that it would be easier to deal with each of Marian's
sisters separately and that her eldest sister should be approached only
after Marian had been successful in setting limits with her second eldest
sister. Environmental planning and stimulus control considerations fig-
ured prominently in the development of the scripts created for use with
Marian's eldest sister because of this woman's potentially violent behavior. Approaching Marian's sisters was conceptualized as a graded performance task that was to be mastered by Marian and her husband. In both
scripts, Roy was to be present whenever Marian met with one of her
sisters. His role in these meetings was to be "a silent but strong physical
presence" serving as a deterrent to any physical violence.

As part of the conjugal role plays, symbolic rituals were prescribed by
the therapist. These rituals were designed to strengthen the conjugal
system's boundaries and to reinforce the theme of autonomy and separateness within the context of "weness" and "togetherness." The rituals
drew their significance from symbols taken from Family Relationships
Histories of both spouses. For example, Roy and Marian had agreed that
the meetings with Marian's sisters should be held at their home on those
evenings when Roy could be present. The ritual was to begin on the
morning of the day of the scheduled meeting. Roy and Marian were
asked to identify treasured objects from their personal lives that could
serve as "strength-giving, inspirational reminders"; these were to be

carried on their persons throughout the day and during the meetings with Marian's sisters. Roy selected a photograph of his paternal grandfather (the protective grandfather recalled in his first memory); Marian chose some rosary beads that had been given to her by her maternal grandmother (the person identified as liked most in her Family Relationships History).

On the morning of the meeting, Roy and Marian were to remove these objects from their "places of honor" in their home. Each spouse was to keep the object with him/her throughout the day. They were asked to think about the person to whom the objects had belonged and to remember the "strength, warmth, acceptance and protection" that this person offered them as they were growing up. Roy was asked to call Marian during the day in order to verbalize his support. The couple was to meet for dinner (at a restaurant of their choice) on the evening of the meeting. After dinner, the couple could proceed to their church. Here they would pray the rosary and ask the Lord for strength and guidance in their undertaking. The couple was then to return home to await Marian's sister.

When Marian's sister arrived, she was greeted at the front door by Roy, who escorted her into the living room where Marian was waiting. Roy would then retreat to the adjoining room where he would remain, "in case he was needed." The length of time for each meeting was predetermined by Roy and Marian. At the agreed upon time, Marian was to terminate the meeting with her sister and Roy was to enter the living room. He would then accompany Marian's sister to the front door. After the meeting was over, Roy and Marian were to spend as much time as they needed to process what had taken place. Before retiring for the evening, the couple would return their inspirational reminders to their places of honor.

Throughout the entire process, the therapist continued to underscore Roy's "silent strength," his "supportive caring," and his "initiative." The therapist also focused on Marian's "growing autonomy" and "self-reliance," as well as the couple's "cooperative teamwork" and "different, yet complementary interpersonal styles."

With the successful completion of these conjugal role plays, the couple was ready to evaluate their progress and to set a future course. Marian and Roy agreed that their couple system's boundaries (as well as their personal boundaries) had become more clearly defined and that they had been able to work as a team in their attempts to set limits with Marian's parents and her two older sisters. However, Marian said she had not been successful in her efforts to detriangulate herself from her parents' relationship, and she still felt "tied to her mother" and "intimidated by her parents." Although the spouses felt less anxious about their sexual relationship and had become more sexually active than they had been before entering treatment, Roy indicated that the sexual area of their relationship still required attention. He acknowledged that the couple's sexual difficulties might be related to both his and Marian's intrapsychic conflicts and that this was an area to be explored after Marian resolved her difficulties related to her family of origin. The therapist responded to Roy's statement by describing him as a "very sensitive husband" who had his "wife's best interest" in mind, as well as a "man who understands his wife and does not wish to exploit her sexually." Roy and Marian decided to suspend marital therapy for a while so that Marian could work individually, with the therapist, to address those issues related to her parents.

Summary of Individual Series #I: Marian

The first block of individual therapy sessions with Marian lasted for approximately five months. During this time treatment focused on helping Marian gain more autonomy from her family of origin, especially from her mother. Most of the treatment strategies outlined in Chapter 4 were employed to bring about changes in those themes and cognitive structures associated with Marian's relationship to her mother (specifically themes 1, 2 and 3).

1. Love = sameness. Separateness and difference (especially from mother) are unacceptable and wrong. The threat of separateness leads to anxiety, panic and depression. It is bad to be different, and it is wrong to be autonomous from someone who loves you. Therefore, I am bad if I am different and/or autonomous.
2. I must be loyal to my family even if I dislike some of them, like my older sisters. I must be especially loyal to my mother.
3. Relationships with men are forbidden if they, in any way, pose a threat to the primary mother-daughter relationships. Relationships with men are acceptable only so long as they do not threaten the mother-daughter bond.

During this period of treatment Marian became increasingly disenchanted with "The Cosby Show." She said that it bore little resemblance to "real family life." She also said that people would always be disappointed if they tried to model their lives after television shows and that "people just have to make the best of it with what they've got." When asked if she could think of any other fairy tale, story, book, movie, television show, etc., that had had an impact upon her as she was growing up, Marian recalled that she had always been fascinated by the story of Rapunzel. The major features of this fairy tale, as Marian related them, were:

> There was this couple who could not have children, no matter how hard they tried. One day, the Lord smiled upon them and the woman conceived. At the back of their little house was a beautiful garden that belonged to a witch. In this garden were all sorts of beautiful vegetables. The wife longed to have some rampions to eat, and she asked her husband to steal some rampions from the witch's garden. As he was stealing the rampions, the witch caught him. The witch threatened to harm him and his wife unless they gave her their child (to raise as her own) once the wife delivered her baby. The child was born and named Rapunzel (which means rampion). She was given to the witch when she turned 12. The witch shut her up in a tall tower which stood in the forest. It had neither staircase nor doors. The only way to get up to Rapunzel's tower was for Rapunzel to let down her beautiful hair and the witch would climb up.
>
> One day the king's son, who was riding through the forest, heard Rapunzel's sad and lonely song. He fell in love with her immediately, but did not know how to reach her. He would come to the forest everyday to watch Rapunzel at her window. One day he saw the witch climbing up the tower wall, using Rapunzel's hair as a ladder.
>
> The next day the prince called out, pretending to be the witch, "Rapunzel, Rapunzel, let down your hair." She did and he climbed up to meet her. They fell in love and the prince came to see her every evening, because the witch came to Rapunzel during the day time. The witch did not know of Rapunzel's relationship with the young prince until one day Rapunzel asked the witch why she was so much heavier to draw up the tower wall than her young prince. The witch called her a "wicked child" and cut off her beautiful hair. She hid Rapunzel in another part of the forest. That evening, when the prince came to the tower, the witch let down Rapunzel's hair for him to use as a ladder. When he reached the tower window, the witch put a spell upon him and he became blind. He wandered about blind for many years until he reached that part of the forest where Rapunzel was living with her two children, a boy and a girl. When Rapunzel saw him she began to weep. Her tears fell upon his eyes and he could see again. He then took her and the two children back to his kingdom where they lived "happily ever after."

The Rapunzel theme was used extensively in Marian's individual treatment. The more insight she developed into the nature of her relationships with her mother, father and sisters and the more she understood the reasons behind choosing Roy for a husband, the more realistic and pragmatic she became in her dealings with her parents and Roy.

A critical turn of events took place when Marian informed her parents that she would no longer play the role of their "family counselor." She said that they should seek "professional help" and that it was "unfair and inappropriate" for her to be asked to take on such a responsibility. In response to Marian's suggestion that her parents become involved in marital therapy, her mother asked Marian for the name of her therapist so that she and her father could consult him. Marian saw this as another attempt by her mother to intrude upon her relationship with a man whom her mother perceived as threatening the mother-daughter bond. In response to her mother's request, Marian asked her therapist for a list of therapists to whom she could refer her parents. She then gave this list of names to her mother and explained that she did not want her parents involved with the therapist she and her husband were seeing. She stood her ground firmly against her mother's protestations. Eventually, her parents did find a therapist of their own choosing, a pastoral counselor.

With her parents' entry into marital counseling, Marian began to feel less guilty and less responsible for her mother's welfare. She and Roy then decided to reenter marital therapy (after a brief hiatus) in order to begin work on their sexual relationship.

10

Couples' Mythologies
in Marital Therapy—Part II

WHEN THE COUPLE RESUMED therapy, there were some noticeable differences in the relationship. Marian seemed less threatened by her husband's need for separateness; with the progressive development of her own autonomy, her desire for closeness lessened. Roy appeared to be more secure in his role as husband and father, and he had begun to assert himself more frequently in his dealings with Marian. As a matter of fact, it was Roy who suggested that the couple focus on their sexual relationship. He reiterated his initial request that Marian become more responsive to his sexual needs. This time, however, he said that he felt more comfortable taking the initiative in their sexual relationship. He also indicated that he did not see Marian's assertiveness in the sexual arena as the threat it once was. He verbalized the importance of both partners being "active and creative in lovemaking."

The consciously agreed-upon decision to deal with the sexual aspect of their relationship had a number of unsuspected consequences for Roy and Marian.

First, it activated a number of unresolved thematic issues from both spouses' personal mythologies which had lain dormant for most of the couple's time together. For example, this goal brought Roy face to face with theme 6 (ambivalence about close and intimate relationships with women) and theme 1 (his lifelong fear and confusion of assertive behavior and violent aggression). Similarly, Marian was once again required to confront her own sexuality, theme 4 (sexual behavior is bad and evil and should be punished. Even within the bonds of marriage, sexual intercourse is only acceptable for the procreation of children).

Second, it changed the relationship among several themes which had previously been complementary. For example, as Roy became more active and assertive with Marian, and as he began to differentiate between assertive responding and aggressive behavior (Roy's themes 1 and 2), he no longer represented Marian's passive father substitute (Marian's theme 5) and became a serious threat to the mother-daughter bond (Marian's theme 3). In addition, his requests for Marian to become more responsive to his sexual needs forced Marian to come to grips with the guilt associated with her own sexual behaviors, thoughts and desires.

Roy and Marian spent the first few sessions mapping out changes that they would like to make in their sexual relationship. Roy reiterated these two requests for change made during the couple's initial sessions.

1. I would like Marian to be more responsive to my sexual needs.
2. I would like Marian not to attempt to orchestrate, direct or control our lovemaking.

Marian's request was in keeping with her central complaint about her husband:

1. I would like Roy to take more initiative in our sexual behaviors and in our lovemaking.

The couple was directed to discuss these three concerns using the Structured Guidelines for Establishing Functional Communication in Marital Dyads in order to help each spouse gain an empathic understanding of his/her partner's perspective. As they discussed these concerns, several issues became apparent. First, as was characteristic of his interpersonal style, Roy's sexual advances and his requests for sexual intercourse were rarely communicated openly and directly to Marian. He usually sent "nonverbal signals." Unfortunately, Marian did not understand his "signal system." Furthermore, Roy's signals were intentionally vague and faint, so that he could avoid being punished for speaking his mind, expressing his feelings, and asking for something he desired (Roy's themes 1, 2, and 3). Second, Marian's seductive behaviors, which Roy experienced as demanding, controlling, and overpowering (Roy's theme 5), were actually Marian's attempts to engage Roy and bring about their interpersonal closeness (Marian's theme 5). This activity on Marian's part was also a way for her to gain mastery over the anxiety and guilt she frequently experienced whenever she became sexually stimulated and aroused (Marian's theme 4).

Before any qualitative work could be done in the sexual area, Roy and Marian first had to learn how to relax and develop more functional ways of communicating sexual feelings and desires, making sexual requests, and initiating sexual interactions. Therefore, sensate focus procedures were introduced (Masters & Johnson, 1970). Sensate focus procedures are routinely used by sex therapists and form the basis for progressive integration of verbal and nonverbal skills into the couple's sexual activities. All sensate focus exercises assigned to couples are to be completed in the privacy of their own homes. In the initial stages of these exercises, spouses are instructed to abstain from intercourse and genital stimulation. This is done to reduce anxiety, to give the spouses permission to enjoy the experience of being sensual, and to enable them to develop new patterns of nonverbal and verbal communication. Finally, it heightens their sensory awareness (Kolodny, Masters, & Johnson, 1979).

> In order to achieve optimum effect, sensate focus should be used as a means of physical awareness by the partner doing the touching and not specifically or solely for the sensual pleasure or even sexual excitation of the partner being touched. . . . By specifically structuring the sensate focus opportunities at the onset of therapy, it is usually possible to significantly reduce the constraints imposed by old habit patterns of sexual interaction. Concomitantly, removing stereotyped expectations of what sexual interaction should be often leads to an awakening of spontaneous natural response that has long been forgotten and was sometimes never recognized (p. 504)

The couple gradually moves through various levels of sensate focus touching that is done in a simultaneous, mutual manner. Touching gradually progresses from nongenital touching, to touching that includes breasts and genitals. Finally, touching is extended to allow for the possibility of intercourse.

The model of sensate focus used in our work is divided into three distinct stages:

1. Didactic education.
2. Observation of videotaped instructions and human models using sensate focus procedures.
3. Sensate focus practice exercises that the spouses carry out in the privacy of their own homes.

During the educational stage, couples are assigned written materials to read which explain the purpose of sensate focus exercises and describe the entire sensate focus procedure that they will be asked to follow. In the second stage, couples are asked to view a series of professionally produced, sexually explicit educational videotapes of human models progressing through the graded stages of the sensate focus process (Edcoa, 1976). After viewing these videotapes in the privacy of their own homes, couples meet with the therapist to discuss these tapes and to ask any questions they might have concerning the procedures. Finally, couples are assigned the first in a series of four sensate focus exercises to complete in the privacy of their own home. After each exercise is completed, couples meet with the therapist to discuss their progress, ask questions, etc. The third stage is thought to be completed when couples have successfully mastered all sensate focus exercises.

Under the guise of teaching couples skills that will enable them to communicate their sexual needs and desires more effectively, we frequently use modified versions of sensate focus exercises to edit personal and conjugal themes that are sexual in nature. We incorporate into the sensate focus model many of the treatment procedures outlined in Chapter 4. In addition, we use intervention techniques designed specifically for editing conjugal themes (e.g., reattribution of responsibility to the therapist, character reversal role plays, character blending role plays, conjugal script editing assignments, character compromise dilemmas, multifocused contracts, and behavioral assignments to foster cognitive and/or response differentiation).

We shall now describe, in outline form, how we used these procedures with Roy and Marian.

SENSATE FOCUS PROCEDURES AS A CONTEXT
FOR EDITING PERSONAL AND CONJUGAL THEMES

Before beginning these exercises, couples are asked to refrain from having sexual intercourse for the duration of the sensate focus procedures (Masters & Johnson, 1970). This is done for a variety of reasons:

1. To eliminate the demand characteristics, anxiety and performance expectations that usually accompany such sexually intimate experiences.
2. To facilitate verbal and nonverbal communication.
3. To help couples distinguish between sensual feelings and sexual feelings.
4. To help couples learn how to give pleasure and receive pleasure, i.e., sexual exchange and reciprocity.
5. To teach couples that one can experience pleasure through giving as well as through receiving.
6. To help spouses become comfortable adopting active and passive roles in lovemaking.

7. To help couples adopt a nonlinear model of sexual behavior.[1]

Roy and Marian were assigned the sensate focus materials to read and were asked not to engage in sexual intercourse until they had completed all exercises. As part of this first assignment, they were asked to share their thoughts, feelings, etc., about the reading materials and the sensate focus procedures using the Structured Guidelines for Establishing Functional Communication in Marital Dyads. These instructions are standard procedures in our work with sex therapy clients; however, when sensate focus is used as a context for altering personal and conjugal themes, additional directives and comments specifically tailored to edit personal and conjugal themes are introduced. For example, the therapist stressed the nondemand aspects of these exercises and underscored the importance of the spouses' developing their own nonverbal and verbal sexual signal system. He talked about how it was important for both Roy and Marian to distinguish between sexual and sensual feelings. This comment was especially important for Roy, because differentiation of feelings was difficult for him. The therapist also made a point of discussing the concept of sexual exchange and reciprocity; it was important for Roy and Marian to become comfortable in the roles of active giver and passive receiver. Finally, the therapist charged Roy with the responsibility for initiating the couple's discussions of the sensate focus materials.

Having completed this first homework assignment successfully, Roy and Marian were asked if they thought they were ready to move on to the second stage of the process: the observation of videotaped models progressing through the various sensate focus exercises. Both agreed that they were ready to do so. However, Marian said she felt somewhat anxious in anticipation of what the couple was going to observe and how she would react to the videotaped presentation.

A two-hour session was arranged for the next meeting so that the couple could meet with the therapist immediately after viewing the videotapes to ask questions and discuss any feelings, concerns, etc.

It was at this point in the treatment that part of Marian's theme 4 (sexual behavior is bad and evil and should be punished) became activa-

---

[1]The linear view of sexual behavior is held by most lay people (no pun intended). It assumes that any type of sexual activity engaged in by two people is always a prelude to sexual intercourse and must culminate in sexual intercourse in order for it to be fulfilling and satisfying to the participants. The nonlinear model of sexual behavior, which is subscribed to by most sex therapists and sex educators, postulates that sexual behavior does not always have to end in sexual intercourse and may be discontinued during any stage of the sexual response cycle.

ted. The prohibition against having sexual intercourse throughout the course of the sensate focus procedures was effective in suppressing the second part of theme 4 (even within marriage, sexual intercourse is only acceptable for the procreation of children). However, it did not address the first part of theme 4. Keeping in mind Marian's need to be in charge of her sexual experiences and in control of her relationship with Roy, the therapist put Marian in charge of the second stage of the process. She was asked to monitor her own anxiety while watching the videotapes and told that any time she felt herself becoming uncomfortable she could stop the tape and discuss her feelings with Roy, whose "empathy and understanding" would be there for her "support." Marian was also told that, if she so desired, she could also ask the therapist to preside over their discussions.

USE OF TRANSFERENCE IN MARITAL THERAPY

In our presentation of individual psychotherapy, we spent some time discussing the dynamics of transference phenomena and how these can be used by the therapist to edit personal themes. In marital therapy, however, transferences to the therapist are usually not encouraged; when they do occur, they are not interpreted unless the transferential distortions are impeding therapeutic progress. In our experience as clinical trainers and supervisors, we have found that intense transference reactions to the therapist are more likely to occur in marital therapy when the therapist (a) encourages the spouses to talk to him/her rather than to each other, (b) acts as a go-between who interprets or explains the behavior of one spouse to the other, (c) remains silent, passive and nondirective, (d) does not structure the couple's interaction and allows punishing and negative exchanges to continue, and (e) takes sides with one spouse against the other.

With some couples, however, intense negative or positive reactions occur in the very early stages of therapy (within the first few sessions). When this happens, the therapist may be overvalued and idealized or undervalued and treated with contempt by both spouses. In some instances, the therapist may be praised by one spouse and derided and chastised by the other. Usually, these outbreaks of intense emotion are totally inappropriate and have little or nothing to do with the realities of the therapist-client situation or the therapist's actual behavior. However, our clinical experience has shown that such emotional responses are diagnostically significant. They frequently indicate that object splitting has taken place and suggest that either one or both spouses have a borderline personality organization. Regardless of the form this intense emotional reaction takes, the therapist should see it as the spouses' collusive resistance to change.

For the most part, it is the spouses' negative projections and transferences to each other that become the focal point of the therapist's interpretations. However, the therapist does make use of the spouse's positive transferences to him/her in order to modify cognitive structures and themes. For example, in positive transferences the therapist is perceived and experienced as a good parental introject, an idealized part of self that has been projected, a nonpunitive superego, etc. In the context of sex therapy, the therapist provides the spouses with a corrective emotional experience with a permissive and accepting parental figure. For Marian, this was particularly important. The therapist's matter-of-fact acceptance of Marian's sexuality as normal, healthy and good, as well as his frank discussions of sexual matters with her and Roy, offered Marian an accepting and permissive parental model (who did not view sex as bad or her as evil) with whom she could begin to identify. The use of the client's positive transference to the therapist, in this case, paved the way for Marian's redefinition and acceptance of herself as a sexual being (Marian's theme 4).

RELABELING AND REFOCUSING: STRATEGIES FOR MODIFYING SPOUSES' COGNITIVE STRUCTURES

A large part of our work with individual clients is devoted to modifying the client's cognitive structures (e.g., internal representations of significant others in the form of cognitive ideals, cognitive-behavioral response chains, person perceptions, cognitive classification and categorization systems). In marital therapy, we frequently relabel a spouse's behavior so that it can be perceived as being more closely in line with the mate's cognitive representations of his/her *ideal spouse*. This technique differs from positive reframing and positive connotation in that no attempt is made to attribute positive motives or intentions to the spouse's behavior and no effort is made to alter the couple's contextual setting. However, the goal of relabeling is to broaden (or to produce greater elaboration in) the spouse's cognitive classification system to include new behaviors not previously considered to be part of that particular system or cognitive category.

For example, after viewing the videotaped sensate focus exercises, Marian and Roy were asked to discuss their thoughts and feelings about these observations. Throughout the course of these discussions, the therapist would comment on Marian's ability to empathize with Roy as being "sensitive to his sexual needs and concerns." Marian's ability to listen to her husband, to reflect verbal content, and to pick up on his underlying feelings about sexual matters was gradually assimilated into Roy's "sexual sensitivity" classification schema. Similarly, the therapist would relabel Roy's requests for clarification as his "taking the initiative" with Marian. Whenever he disagreed with Marian, this disagreement would be labeled as "assertiveness." When done tactfully, used judiciously, and timed appropriately, relabeling can be a very effective means of altering cognitive structures and modifying personal perceptions.

Refocusing is another technique used to change cognitions. In refocusing, the therapist calls to a spouse's attention behaviors of his/her mate which usually go unnoticed. Again, behaviors that are consistent with a spouse's ideal are acknowledged and reinforced through the therapist's selective attention to them. For example, Roy's suggestions that the couple take a short vacation trip was cited by the therapist as Roy's "taking the initiative." Marian's willingness to become involved in sensate focus exercises was used as another example of her being "sensitive to Roy's sexual needs."

The final stage of the sensate focus procedure (active participation) was begun three weeks after Roy and Marian had first received the written materials outlining all sensate focus exercises. Roy and Marian were instructed to proceed at their own pace and to discontinue any exercise immediately if either felt uncomfortable or anxious. For the first non-genital pleasuring exercise, Roy was asked to take the more active role of giver and pleasurer. For the second part this first exercise, Marian would then be responsible for adopting the giver and pleasurer role and Roy was to adopt the receiver position. The couple was asked to repeat the exercise three times before returning for the next session. When Roy and Marian returned the following week, they had been able to complete only one exercise session. Their second practice session had to be terminated because Marian became extremely anxious in her role as less active receiver and pleasurer. The couple's third attempt to complete this first exercise also had to be terminated because of Marian's mounting anxiety in her role as receiver of pleasure.

We have found that when a person experiences overwhelming anxiety, guilt, or shame during sensate focus exercises, this frequently indicates that strong sexual taboos, prohibitions and inhibitions have been activated. In other instances, being asked to become a passive recipient of another's sexual advances precipitates severe anxiety, panic attacks, and dissociative reactions (e.g., depersonalization, estrangement, fugues) in some individuals who have been able to repress or defend against (up to this point) sexual traumas experienced during infancy and childhood. Because of Marian's intense reaction to the sensate focus homework, individual interviews were scheduled for her and Roy, in addition to their conjoint sessions with the therapist. During these individual interviews, detailed sex histories of both spouses were taken (Masters & Johnson, 1970).

SUMMARY OF INDIVIDUAL SERIES #2: MARIAN

This series of individual interviews proved to be most enlightening, because it shed some new light on themes 4 (sexual pleasure is evil and punishable) and theme 6 (illness as interpersonal distance-regulator) from Marian's personal mythology. From material gathered in the detailed sex history (Masters & Johnson, 1970), it became evident that Marian's first experience with sexual intercourse, during high school, was actually "date rape." She unwillingly submitted in order to maintain a relationship with an older boy whom she liked (theme 5: men are unpredictably violent or passive but can be tempted toward initiative with sex). It is difficult to say whether the experience was actually "rape" (because she continued to date this boy and continued to have sexual relations with him for more than a year) or whether being "forced" to submit to his sexual advances made it easier to engage in sexual intercourse without experiencing debilitating guilt. Nevertheless, Marian experienced all their sexual encounters as "forced." In order to deal with the anxiety and guilt associated with sexual intercourse, Marian learned to "hurry through" the sexual act. The faster she could make her partner and herself achieve orgasm, the quicker the sexual act would come to an end and the less she would experience the guilt and anxiety associated with any sexual pleasure. As she grew older, punishment as a prelude to intercourse (in the form of mild spanking) or as an aftereffect (in the form of extreme fears of venereal disease or pregnancy) took the place of forced submission. In her relationship with Roy, sexual intercourse resulted in her becoming pregnant (a punishment for her premarital sexuality).

The sensate focus exercises required that Marian submit, willingly, to the sexual advance of another. Furthermore, these exercises required that she become a willing participant whose goal was to achieve sexual enjoyment. Obviously, this had a tremendous impact upon theme 4, which categorized any type of sexual enjoyment as "bad" and "evil" and branded Marian as "bad" and "evil" for engaging in such behavior. Similarly, the experience of pain in the form of anxiety, guilt, fear of pregnancy, etc., was also used to draw her male partners closer to her (theme 6). Without the painful and punishing aspects of her sexuality, Marian would lose a valuable strategy for securing love, physical closeness, intimacy, nurturance, etc., and she would have to learn new ways to bring about interpersonal closeness.

Marian was not consciously aware of the contents of these two themes. Nor was she aware of how these themes were related to her husband's personal mythology. The therapist, accepting Marian's first sexual experience as a "date rape," used this information and the material gathered from Roy's individual sessions to alter the sensate focus exercises in ways designed to bring about changes in one of this couple's central conjugal themes.

The basic thrust of therapy with Marian throughout these sessions was to help her become more accepting of her sexuality. The therapist, using the power of a positive maternal transference, was able to bring about additional modifications in theme 4 so that she was cognitively able to view sexual pleasure as acceptable within the confines of marriage.

SUMMARY OF INDIVIDUAL SERIES #1: ROY

In addition to gathering information pertinent to Roy's sexual history, the therapist used these sessions to edit themes 3 and 5 from Roy's personal mythology. The reader will recall the content of these themes as being:

3. I must be constantly vigilant in life, and I must find someone who can protect me. I am barely able to take care of myself, and I am totally inadequate when it comes to taking care of others. Having any type of responsibility for another person's health and welfare frightens and angers me. I experience their helplessness as abandonment. I am very sensitive to other people's suffering, but I am powerless to do anything to help them in their suffering.
5. I am also ambivalent about close, intimate, interpersonal relationships with women. I want them to take care of me, but I don't want them to overpower and control me. I am also afraid that women will reject me or retaliate if I am unable to satisfy their wishes, desires and sexual needs.

Treatment began with an exploration of Roy's relationship with his mother and how his experiences with her had shaped his views about women, himself, his gender, his self-esteem, his self-confidence, and his feelings of adequacy. As a result of treatment, Roy was able to differentiate between his experiences with his mother and his subsequent experiences with other women, especially his experiences with Marian. In order to help Roy gain a more realistic appraisal of himself and his capabilities, refocusing was used to help him recognize the progress he had made (e.g., by taking the initiative and asserting himself with Marian) throughout the course of marital therapy. A very significant cognitive change occurred when Roy began to understand that it had really been impossible for him to take care of and nurture his psychotic mother when he was a child, but that the kind of care, nurturance and protection that his wife needed and desired were not at all inappropriate. Furthermore, he began to realize that he did possess the skills and resources to satisfy some of Marian's needs.

It would be inaccurate to claim that this brief series of eight sessions was responsible for dramatically altering theme 3 and 5 of Roy's personal mythology. However, his confidence did begin to develop and he began to picture himself as more competent, adequate and assertive. This newfound confidence took dramatic form when Roy joined a neighborhood health spa (without any urging from Marian) and enrolled in jujitsu classes. This was a prelude to his individual work on personal themes 1 (aggression = destruction) and 2 (passivity vs. assertiveness).

This series of individual interviews made it possible to see how a number of themes from the spouses' personal mythologies had coalesced to produce this particular dysfunctional conjugal theme. For example, Marian's theme 6 (sickness, illness and pain are part of every relationship; illness is one way to regulate interpersonal closeness) was antagonistically paired with Roy's theme 3, which involved perceptions of inadequacy when caring for others. Similarly, Marian's theme 4 (sexual behavior for pleasure is evil; sexual behavior in marriage is only acceptable for the procreation of children; sexual behavior for pleasure should be punished, etc.) stood in antagonistic relationship to Roy's theme 5, which involved ambivalence about close relationships with women. While these pairings made it difficult for Roy and Marian to enjoy a fulfilling sexual relationship, they also served protective functions for both spouses. Seen in this light, the unfulfilling sexual relationship represents an overt symbolic manifestation of an unconscious contractual agreement that allows Roy and Marian to maintain intrapsychic equilibrium while simultaneously maintaining the integrity of the marital system.

We used this understanding to formulate a series of ritual prescriptions, framed within the context of the final sensate focus procedure, that were designed: (a) to edit the dysfunctional themes of both spouses, and (b) to provide them with a different context for developing a (new or modified) more functional conjugal theme that incorporated the edited personal themes of both spouses in a more harmonious, less conflictual fashion.

PRESCRIPTIVE ASSIGNMENTS

When Roy and Marian felt ready to resume the sensate focus procedures, they approached this task with edited versions of those personal themes that were part of the larger, conjugal theme having to do with sexual relationships. They also came to this assignment with altered concepts of themselves, each other, and each spouse's self-in-relationship to a more reality-based version of his/her mate, i.e., a more congruent match between ideal spouse/perceived spouse in the sexual realm of their relationship. During the couple's conjoint sessions, Marian had disclosed her date rape experience to her husband. Roy was understanding and very supportive of Marian. He demonstrated a considerable amount of empathy and sensitivity to her pain. Once the couple had discussed the date rape experiences, the therapist was able to use this shared information to change the context of the sensate focus exercises themselves. By doing this, the therapist created an environment in which Roy and Marian could work together to produce changes in the conjugal theme that governed their sexual behavior.

Before prescribing any homework assignments, an acceptable rationale must be given to the couple explaining why particular roles are being assigned and why certain procedures are being introduced. The rationale given for the final group of sensate focus procedures was "to use desensitization techniques to help Marian work through the past traumatic effects of her date rape trauma." Having set the stage in this manner, the following roles were prescribed.

Marian was assigned the role of "giver" and "pleasurer" which she would take throughout the entire third stage of sensate focus. The reasons for doing this were explained to the couple as:

> To help Marian master the anxiety she experienced during sexual encounters that she associated with date rape. By playing the role of active initiator, she now could relive and orchestrate the sexual situation so that she no longer had to become a passive victim who was helpless to influence the course of events or their outcome. She could move at her own pace and terminate the exercise whenever she desired. She had complete control.

The reader will be aware that the prescription actually required Marian to behave in a manner that was similar to the "orchestrating" behavior that Roy identified as a problem in his SIDCARB responses. However, the prescription was intended not to be paradoxical, but to help Roy accept Marian's taking the initiative in their lovemaking without feeling controlled by her or experiencing performance anxiety. It also allowed him to take a passive role in lovemaking, where he could feel taken care of by a woman (Roy's theme 5). In addition, this prescription was designed to help Roy perceive and experience Marian's active behavior as her being "sensitive to his sexual needs."

For Marian, the therapist's matter-of-fact acceptance of her sexuality as normal, healthy, and desirable and his frank and open discussion of sexual material presented her with an accepting and permissive parental model for the first time in her life. The positive transference to the therapist as a permissive mother who viewed sex positively, who supported her relationship and involvement with her husband (men), who encouraged her separation-individuation, etc., had a mollifying effect upon her severe, punishing, and guilt-engendering maternal ideal (superego). Furthermore, putting Marian in charge of these exercises also allowed her to become more accepting of Roy's passivity.

In another effort to alter Roy's and Marian's cognitions about themselves and each other, the therapist relabeled Roy's role as receiver of pleasure as one of "passive activity," because he was being asked to be "deliberately passive" and to behave "as if" Marian were in complete control of their lovemaking without taking any "overt responsibility." Marian's role, as active pleasurer, was also relabeled as "active passivity," because she was to become extremely attentive to Roy and responsive to his "slightest nonverbal cues" throughout the course of the procedure. This was especially true for the first assignment, which required that the participants communicate their needs and desires *nonverbally*. Since Marian would be the one to decide when Roy would play the role of pleasurer, and she would be the one directing his pleasuring of her, Marian would still be playing her role of "active passivity."

Although relabeling activity as passivity and passivity as activity appears to be paradoxical, the intention of this relabeling is not to produce paradoxical effects. What is intended is to blur the distinction between these two terms in this couple's relationship, to have Roy and Marian begin to see that labels such as "active" and "passive" are relative and do not represent stable personality traits and characteristics, and to help them understand that "activity" and "passivity" draw their meaning from and have relevance only within a particular context.

Upon completion of this assignment, the couple was free to engage in sexual activities that were more satisfying to both partners. At this time, another evaluation session was scheduled with Roy and Marian to assess progress and to determine whether additional clinical work was necessary. Both Roy and Marian agreed that their relationship had improved considerably, but that there were still some "kinks" left in their marriage that they wanted to work out. They agreed to contact the therapist after their summer vacation to resume treatment.

11

Couples' Mythologies
in Marital Therapy—Part III:
Conclusions and Outcome Evaluation

W HEN MARIAN AND ROY reentered therapy in the fall, they focused their
attention on the two remaining areas of SIDCARB that required
resolution: children and friendships. They had been discussing the possibility of having another child, but both Roy and Marian had some reserva-
tions about doing so. Roy's hesitancy stemmed from his insecurities about
having responsibility for an additional person. Marian was less uncertain.
Time on her biological clock was "running out" and she did not want to be
bearing children into her late thirties. However, she appreciated the fact
that her relationship with Roy was still somewhat fragile and that adding
another child at this time might overtax their marriage.

Being aware of the personal themes of each spouse, especially Marian's theme 4 with its prohibition against sexual enjoyment and its belief
in procreation as the only acceptable reason for engaging in sexual intercourse, the therapist approached this issue cautiously. It would be naive
to assume that such deeply ingrained moral and superego prohibitions
against sexual enjoyment for its own sake could be totally eradicated and
replaced by a less stringent morality and a more permissive superego in
the short period of time that Marian was involved in individual treatment. Therefore, another technique, we refer to as "conjugal theme
exploration," was used.

CONJUGAL THEME EXPLORATION

Conjugal theme exploration is one of the few methods we use that
requires the spouses to become aware of how their unconscious personal
themes are joined together to form conjugal themes and unconscious,

quid pro quo, mutually protective contracts. Most of our editing of conjugal themes is done indirectly. In conjugal theme exploration, however,
the therapist identifies a thematic contract and brings it to the couple's
attention for discussion and modification. This strategy is similar to the
psychoanalytic interpretations used in individual work and discussed in
Chapter 4, in that it brings into conscious awareness the central conflicts
and the defenses used by the spouses to avoid experiencing the unpleasant affects associated with these conflicts.

This direct interpretation of unconsciously held agreements is called
for in two situations:

1. When the therapist believes that the manifest content of the couple's
   unresolvable conflict is not really the issue with which the couple is
   struggling and that the couple is actually fighting about a perceived
   violation of an unconsciously negotiated quid pro quo contract.
2. When the therapist believes that a consciously negotiated contract
   actually violates or has the potential for violating an existing unconsciously negotiated contract between the spouses.

This latter case was seen as being relevant for Roy and Marian. In using
this approach, the therapist simply outlined what he believed to be the
pairing of themes that constituted two closely related unconscious contractual agreements relevant to Roy's and Marian's deliberations concerning having a second child. These were:

1. Roy agrees not to make excessive sexual demands upon Marian if in exchange she agrees to take care of him and does not expect him to take
   charge of their relationship or to take care of her in times of illness.
2. Marian agrees to engage in sexual intercourse with Roy on a limited
   basis to fulfill her wifely duty, as long as their sexual experiences do
   not become too pleasurable for either of them. If, however, they
   begin to enjoy their sexual experiences, some type of pain or punishment must be introduced (e.g., physical illness, psychological
   distress, pregnancy) to distance the couple.

When the therapist outlines what is believed to be the contractual
relationship between and among various themes, he/she does not de-
bate the veracity of his/her speculations with the couple. He/she simply
states them as his/her way of understanding the couple's relationship.
The goal is not to convince the spouses but to help them consider the
possible effects of any decision that appears to make a substantial modification in this unverbalized contract.

In some cases, when the therapist wishes to suggest a possible solution to the couple's dilemma, he/she might tell the spouses a metaphorical story which appears to have nothing to do with their unconscious agreement but hints at a solution to the problem at hand. Using metaphors is often appropriate with couples who are not psychologically minded and insight oriented. When spouses have been involved in treatment for a considerable time and when they are introspective about the causes of their difficulties, conjugal theme exploration should be attempted before more indirect methods.

Roy and Marian responded well to the therapist's suggestion that they consider the existence of these two unconsciously negotiated contracts in their discussions concerning their decision to have another child. Using the Structured Guidelines, they discussed this issue at length and decided that they would begin their efforts to conceive a child with the understanding that this would be their last offspring. After the birth of this child, Roy would undergo a vasectomy to prevent any future unwanted pregnancies.

Marian became pregnant within six weeks, and her pregnancy caused some disruption in the marriage. Roy began to revert to his former way of handling frustration and disappointment. He withdrew and suffered from mild, periodic depressions. Marian also had a mild regression. She again experienced Roy's distancing as rejection. However, this time the couple's conflicts did not get out of hand, and both spouses were able to discuss their feelings about Marian's pregnancy and the changes in their life that the birth of their second child would bring. No backsliding was evident in the couple's dealings with Marian's family of origin and her mother's attempts to realign herself with her daughter. Roy and Marian's ability to maintain their marital coalition in the face of Marian's mother's maneuverings was reinforced by the therapist.

The couple was also pleasantly surprised to find that Marian's two older sisters responded appropriately to the news that Marian was again pregnant. In a stunning gesture of support, Marian's father took Marian to lunch in order to celebrate this happy event.

Introducing New Themes and Models, Exploring Their Potentials, and Encouraging their Development

In some instances we have come across individuals whose development and ability to change are severely curtailed because their personal myths are so restrictive that little or no room exists for modification.

Such restrictions may stem from a paucity of themes in one's personal mythology, a simplicity or narrowness of thematic plots, a lack of variation among themes, or the absence of a variety of characters which provide the person with different models for identification. This frequently happens when splitting is the major defense used by the person. Splitting often results in the polarization of themes and characters.

Under such circumstances, active encouragement of the person to seek out new characters and explore different themes can be used by the therapist to stimulate the development of alternative models and behavioral patterns. Such was the case with Roy and Marian. For Roy, the restrictiveness of his personal themes and the absence of a variety of character models was evident. Marian, on the other hand, posed a different problem. Character models from her personal life and Personal Myth Assessment were plentiful, but the theme that made up her Personal Myth Assessment was outmoded and no longer served its original purpose. "The Cosby Show" storyline was a dead end. Roy's main characters in his Personal Myth Assessment were also inappropriate for his current life circumstances and roles as husband and father. Therefore, the couple was encouraged to select new fairy tales, stories, novels, etc., whose themes and characters seemed to be more relevant to their current life experiences, stage of the family life cycle, and issues being considered by them (e.g., friendships).

Depending upon the nature of their relationship, spouses can be asked to select the same new fairy tale, story, novel, etc., to serve as a model for how they are to approach the problem at hand, or each spouse can be asked to choose his/her own new fairy tale, story, or novel. If increased cohesion is desired, the spouses might be asked to use the same story; if, on the other hand, the therapist believes that spousal autonomy, separateness, and differentness should be fostered or strengthened, then each spouse might be asked to select his/her own new fairy tale, story, movie, etc.

The reader will recall that differences concerning closeness and separateness (cohesion) were central issues identified on FACES III and that Roy and Marian spent some time negotiating interpersonal distance during the early stages of treatment. The couple's difficulties concerning friendships turned out to be another manifestation of the struggle to negotiate mutually acceptable rules governing separateness and connectedness (i.e., cohesion). For example, Marian wanted to cultivate friendships, as a couple, with other families having children their daughter's age. Roy, on the other hand, was uncomfortable with this idea, and he pushed for exploring independent separate friendships with members of the same sex. The reader can see how Marian's theme 1 (closeness = love) and Roy's theme 4 (retreat from, or submission to, male/father figures) are reflected in this conflict. Although Marian was disappointed that Roy did not share her desire to develop a close circle of mutual friends (as her parents had done), she did appreciate Roy's willingness to pursue friendships with other men as symbolizing a change in his feelings about himself and his adequacy. She acknowledged his growing sense of self-confidence as something new and very positive. Roy also did not close off the prospect of developing associations with other couples in the future. He explained to Marian that he preferred to move slowly, and at his own rate of speed, in this area of his life. He asked that Marian be patient and not rush him. Marian agreed not to pressure Roy.

With the couple's difficulties conceptualized in this way, the therapist decided to have each spouse select his/her own new story, so as not to disturb the couple's newly established equilibrium in the realm of interpersonal closeness and intimacy. Roy chose *The Hobbit* by J. R. R. Tolkien as his new story, and Marian selected a novel by Alice Munro entitled *Lives of Girls and Women*. Both novels seemed appropriate for the task at hand, because they both chronicled the protagonists' development as individuals and traced the evolution of intimate relationships between same-sex friends.

Once Roy and Marian had selected these two new stories, they were asked to reread them carefully and to highlight in some fashion any passages that had special significance or meaning for them. When this rereading assignment was completed by both spouses, Roy and Marian were asked to exchange books. Next they were directed to read their partner's book and to pay close attention to the underlined sections. When this task was finished, Roy and Marian were given the opportunity to discuss what they had read, to ask each other questions, to share insights, etc., using the Structured Guidelines. This exercise is used as a prelude to the next intervention strategy, which we call "Role Compromise." Unlike role playing and role taking, Role Compromise is used to help couples fashion a new conjugal theme and is not primarily designed to alter personal themes or a spouse's self-concepts. Once spouses have devised such a theme, the therapist might prescribe cognitive-behavioral rituals designed to foster the new theme's integration into the marital system and help secure its place within the couple's mythology. We assume that the new fairy tales, stories, novels, etc., chosen by the spouses contain the germs of additional themes, underdeveloped character traits, and heretofore unrecognized aspects of the self. These dormant themes, character traits, aspects of the self, etc., all have the potential for behavioral expression. The goal of "Role Compromise" is to help spouses share in the mutual shaping of new conjugal themes and interaction patterns in a specific area of their relationship. The intervention procedure is briefly outlined below.

ROLE COMPROMISE

Role Compromise was the final intervention strategy used with Roy and Marian. They were asked to discuss their respective novels using the 14 questions of the Personal Myth Assessment Interview as a guide. Roy chose the hero of *The Hobbit*, Bilbo Baggins, as the character with whom he identified. Roy described Bilbo as a mild-mannered, stay-at-home, peace-loving creature who gets caught up in the hair-raising adventures of a troop of boisterous dwarfs, elves and other assorted characters who are preparing to do battle with the horrific fire-breathing dragon, Smoog. Smoog had driven the dwarfs and their ancestors from their homeland and usurped the dwarfs' treasure. The novel tells of Bilbo's exploits as he accompanies the dwarfs and their comrade, Gandolf the wizard, on their quest to regain what is rightfully theirs. The lifelong friendships made by Bilbo throughout the novel are central to the story's main plot. Essentially, *The Hobbit* can be seen as a Jungian tale of the dawning of consciousness of the archetypal hero (Campbell, 1949; Neumann, 1954b). It is a story of transformation (Jung, 1956) and of the unfolding of the self (Jung, 1959). Its perennial themes of cosmic struggles between instinctual forces (good and evil), separation-individuation (the dragon fight), and the coming together of desperate aspects of the self (various and sundry characters in the novel) are the novel's main elements. They symbolized Roy's personal struggles and graphically outlined the unresolved developmental tasks with which he was then grappling.

Marian's identification with the main character in her story, Del Jordan, was obvious. This story is less complex and more straightforward than *The Hobbit*. It tells of the heroine's development from middle childhood through her early adult years. There are several aspects of this story that are of particular importance because of their relevance to Marian's personal journey through these same developmental eras. Unlike Marian, Del Jordan's relationship with her mother is not at all ambivalent. Del's mother is supportive of her growth, development, and attempts to separate and individuate. She speaks very frankly and openly about sexual matters and love relationships between men and women. However, Del's father is distant and aloof, much like Marian's own dad. Del is her parents' only child; therefore, the problems of sibling rivalry

and favoritism do not surface as issues in this novel. The central focus of
the story is Del's own developmental experiences, especially her sexual
experiences, which are shared with her childhood friend, who is her
confidant throughout much of the novel. The nonjudgmental and accepting attitudes of all the characters are a far cry from Marian's own
childhood experiences.

Not surprisingly, both these novels depict the current state of affairs for
both Roy and Marian. Marian's coming to grips with her own sexuality
and Roy's struggles with assertion and aggression are graphically outlined in these two stories. Similarly, both stories deal with what can be
considered the "chumship" (Sullivan, 1953) preadolescent era of interpersonal development, the formations of a personal identity during adolescence (Erikson, 1968; Sullivan, 1953), and the movement into adult
developmental tasks that were incompletely mastered by both spouses.

For their final assignment, Roy and Marian were asked to complete the
following exercise:

> You are to work together on a short story. The goal of this short story is to help
> the two main characters, Bilbo Baggins and Del Jordan, develop friendships
> and friendship networks that: (a) will be supportive of each character's
> unique personality, needs, style, behavioral patterns, etc., and (b) will not
> jeopardize the special type of relationship that exists between Bilbo and Del.
> Include, in your story, the time frame needed to bring this plot to a successful
> conclusion, and describe what the outcomes will look like in as behaviorally
> specific a manner as possible.
>
> Knowing what you know about the two main characters, you should take
> into consideration each character's past achievements, innate potentials, and
> future goals. Be as creative as you desire, considering the diverse nature of
> these two characters.

Roy and Marian were given as much time as they needed to complete
this final assignment. They called the therapist two weeks later saying
that they had done their homework and were ready for their next
session.

One thing that had become crystal clear for these spouses as they
worked on this assignment was that they both expected very different
things from their friendships with members of their own sex. Roy, who
had always avoided any type of conflict or competition with males, was
now ready for a relationship where some type of friendly competition
was involved. Marian, on the other hand, wanted to cultivate supportive
and noncompetitive relationships with women who had children her
daughter's age. Roy realized that it was important for him to gain a sense

of adequacy in his dealings with other men in a relationship that was separate from his relationship with Marian. Marian realized that she had a "need" to bring all those persons whom she knew together in order to have them "all become friends." This was what her mother had done. Traces of Marian's theme 1 can still be seen in this attitude.

Marian and Roy arrived at the following solution: They both would pursue relationships independently, but they would set aside time, with each other, to discuss these relationships. Marian would make no attempts to involve Roy in her friendships. In exchange for this, Roy would actively explore (in his relationships) the possibility of involving Marian in social situations with a male friend and his spouse. A year's time was considered long enough to accomplish this latter goal. With this agreement finalized, treatment was brought to a close. Both Roy and Marian said that they were satisfied with the therapy and its outcome. However, both indicated that they still had some unfinished personal conflicts related to their families of origin that required additional work. The therapist left this option open to them and said he would be available for both of them in the future, should the need arise.

IMMEDIATE POST TREATMENT EVALUATION

Pre-treatment and post-treatment scores of both spouses for all empirically derived measures are presented below. Our discussion and interpretation of these scores are offered in this section. Each instrument will be considered separately.

Results for IMAGES subscales are listed in Table 6. Total discrepancy score differences between pre-treatment and post-treatment for Roy and Marian were: 33/210=16% to 17/210=08% and 47/210=22% to 32/210=15%, respectively.

FACES III scores for Roy and Marian also demonstrated more congruence between ideal and perceived levels of cohesion (intimacy) for Roy but not for Marian. These scores and their corresponding conceptual dimensions are presented below in Table 7.

It appears that, as a result of therapy, Roy achieved his desired degree of cohesion but Marian did not. However, when one examines the range of raw scores for all four categories on this dimension of FACES III, one finds that the numerical difference between connected and enmeshed in Marian's case is only a magnitude of 1. This difference of one numerical point places Marian in a totally different and conceptually dysfunctional category of interpersonal closeness according to the normative categories developed by the FACES III authors. We believe that this enmeshed

TABLE 6 IMAGES

Roy	Pre-treatment Ideal/Perceived Discrepancies		Categories (factors)	Post-treatment Ideal/Perceived Discrepancies
	7/48 = 14%	I	Emotional gratification	0/48 = 0%
	5/36 = 14%	II	Sex role orientation and physical attraction	3/36 = 08%
	4/18 = 22%	III	Spousal satisfaction	2/18 = 11%
	1/24 = 04%	IV	Parent sibling identification	1/24 = 04%
	2/24 = 08%	V	Emotional maturity	1/24 = 04%
	4/18 = 22%	VI	Intelligence	3/18 = 17%
	10/42 = 23%	VII	Homogamy	7/42 = 17%

IMAGES

Marian	Pre-treatment Ideal/Perceived Discrepancies		Categories (factors)	Post-treatment Ideal/Perceived Discrepancies
	16/48 = 33%	I	Emotional gratification	9/48 = 19%
	7/36 = 19%	II	Sex role orientation and physical attraction	5/36 = 14%
	6/18 = 33%	III	Spousal satisfaction	4/18 = 22%
	2/24 = 08%	IV	Parent sibling identification	2/24 = 08%
	6/24 = 25%	V	Emotional maturity	5/24 = 21%
	0/18 = 0%	VI	Intelligence	0/18 = 0%
	10/42 = 23%	VII	Homogamy	7/42 = 17%

designation does not accurately reflect what Marian truly desired in her relationship with her husband. Therefore, we again asked her to draw her perceived/ideal levels of closeness as part of her post-treatment evaluation. Marian's pre-treatment drawings are compared with her post-treatment drawings in Figure 4.

Obviously, the post-treatment graphic depiction of perceived/ideal closeness does not portray enmeshment. *The assumption that digital and linear computations of interpersonal closeness and marital cohesion are sufficient representations of what is also a highly symbolic dimension of interpersonal*

TABLE 7 FACES III

	Pre-treatment		Post-treatment	
Roy	Perceived/Ideal		Perceived/Ideal	
	Separated/Connected		Connected/Connected	
Raw scores	(37)	(44)	(43)	(44)
	Pre-treatment		Post-treatment	
Marian	Perceived/Ideal		Perceived/Ideal	
	Separated/Enmeshed		Connected/Enmeshed	
Raw scores	(37)	(48)	(45)	(46)

relationships must be seriously questioned. Much of the marital and individual treatment with Marian addressed her struggles to separate and individuate from her mother, to define personal ego boundaries, and to erect subsystem boundaries in relation to her family of origin. Her success in doing this *is* reflected in all of her post-treatment scores on the PAFS. However, one does not get any sense of change if one simply compares pre-treatment and post-treatment scores for the Cohesion dimension of FACES III. This supports the value of using a variety of empirical instruments in one's clinical assessment, treatment, and outcome evaluations. These results also suggest that with some couples, a more symbolic method of assessing intergenerational relationships may be more valid. The age-old question concerning the relationship between statistical comparisons and meaningful clinical change surfaces in regard to FACES III.

We now turn to the comparison of pre-treatment and post-treatment scores for the Personal Authority in the Family System Questionnaire

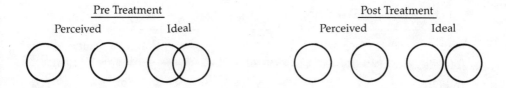

FIGURE 4 Marian's pre treatment and post treatment drawings of her perceived and ideal levels of interpersonal closeness.

(Table 8). As we said above, Marian's post-treatment scores certainly reflect changes on all four subscales used in this assessment.

Roy's scores also reflect changes; however, some of these changes are not in the expected direction. It will be recalled that there was some suspicion that Roy's responses to PAFS were defensive and did not actually represent the true status of his involvement with his family of origin. As he became more involved in therapy and as his trust in the therapist increased, Roy was better able to give less socially desirable responses to PAFS questions. Pre-treatment and post-treatment comparisons on this measure are shown in Table 9.

As a result of therapy, both individual and marital, Roy developed much more insight into the true nature of his relationship with both parents and his two older brothers. This understanding translated into a more accurate and less defensive appraisal of the unresolved conflicts in the area of separation-individuation. Here again we see how paper and pencil, self-report questionnaires may fail to accurately reflect positive changes. We can argue, quite convincingly we believe, that Roy's post-treatment scores on the PAFS questionnaire represent positive changes and improvement because they are less defensive and more accurately reflect his experiences in his family of origin. They also demonstrate a deeper personal understanding and insight into the nature of key intrapsychic difficulties that require additional psychotherapeutic work.

The final pre-treatment/post-treatment comparison of scores derived from empirically developed instruments deals with the spouses' responses to SIDCARB (Table 10).

An examination of pre-treatment/post-treatment scores for the first factor shows a considerable decrease in the amount of behavior change desired by Marian in her relationship with Roy. Similarly, her perception of exchange inequities in the marriage has also diminished appreciably. Essentially, her post-treatment score for the first factor is indicative of a

TABLE 8   Marian's PAFS Scores

Marian	Pre-treatment	Post-treatment	Low	Range of Scale Medium	High
INFUS	19	26	8	24	40
NFTRI	25	33	10	30	50
INTRI	20	34	11	33	55
INTIM	65	87	29	87	145

TABLE 9   Roy's PAFS Scores

Roy	Pre-treatment	Post-treatment	Low	Range of Scale Medium	High
INFUS	30	26	8	24	40
NFTRI	45	42	10	30	50
INTRI	50	52	11	33	55
INTIM	100	80	29	87	145

nondistressed relationship. The same trend is evident in Roy's responses on Factor I. Again, his post-treatment score is one that is found in a nondistressed, satisfactorily married spouse.

It is not surprising to see slight increases in factor II scores for both Roy and Marian. It is common to find internal-psychological barriers increasing with the addition of children to the family. With the advent of Marian's second pregnancy, one would expect both spouses to perceive an increase. Similarly, with the increased financial responsibility brought about by the addition of family members, one would expect to see a slight increase in factor III scores.

It is interesting to note that treatment has also changed the balance of power to where both spouses share power more equally. Before treatment, Marian held more power by virtue of her perceiving considerably fewer external circumstantial barriers to divorce and separation than did Roy.

TABLE 10   SIDCARB

	Pre-treatment Factors:		Post-treatment Factors:	
Marian	I	64	I	52
	II	55	II	59
	III	40	III	48
Roy	I	54	I	44
	II	52	II	57
	III	52	III	55

12

Levels of Change

A s we have noted earlier in this volume, personal myths are the organizing premises (cognitive schemata, symbolic reconstructions,
basic assumptions) by which a given individual's reality is maintained.
Environmental (in particular interpersonal) experiences serve as cues
that activate a particular theme, which in turn determines how the experience is processed, understood, and acted upon. In this way, personal
myths organize the individual's realities.

In addition, individuals, spouses, or family members may seek out
new acquaintances or attempt to influence current significant others to
enact complementary role patterns that maintain their personal themes
in a reciprocal manner. In this way, familiar, commonly shared interpersonal marital and family realities are stabilized and maintained.

In still other situations, individuals, couples or families may need to
modify or *change* a current theme in response to new or unfamiliar experiences or relationship styles. When new experiences are dissonant with
existing themes, the new information may be *distorted, denied,* or
assimilated to fit the current theme, or the theme may *accommodate* itself to
the new data. Thus, some themes may be overly rigid and unresponsive
to new input. Others, however, may be flexible enough to incorporate
new information into existing cognitive structures or they may be capable of modification so that they develop toward greater complexity and
become more harmonious with one's actual experience. When describing family systems and recurring interactional patterns, Watzlawick
(1978) refers to the assimilation of new information or behaviors into
currently existing rules as "first order change." He calls the shift to a
different organizational structure with different interactional rules (including those governing the symptomatic behavior) a "second order
change."

In our framework, the assimilation of new information into an existing theme is similar to Watzlawick's concept of first order change, while the modification of an existing theme to a more complex and environmentally congruent cognitive structure is similar to his concept of second order change. *According to our conceptualization of personal mythologies, first-order changes include changes in individuals' self-statements, internal dialogues, or specific behaviors without accompanying changes in the theme itself.* For instance, a woman whose personal theme includes the role of "loner" and a script of isolation and fear of emotional involvement may decide, after some ambivalence, that she is comfortable with this world view and lifestyle because this style allows her ample opportunity to develop her career as a writer. Another example of first-order theme change would be the incorporation of a new role into a currently existing role complex. For example, the addition of Alfred the Patient Listener into Mr. G.'s ALF role constellation (see Chapter 4) may not have been sufficient to alter his central theme of ambivalence concerning interpersonal closeness and distance and yet enabled him to derive more satisfaction from his interpersonal contacts.

At the conjugal or familial level, communication training or problem-solving skills may enable family members to function more effectively on a day-to-day basis without directly affecting the ideal images held of other family members and the accompanying, reciprocally maintained role relationships and central themes. In the treatment of Roy and Marian, for example, communication training, straightforward contingency contracts, and sensate focusing procedures for heightened awareness and communication of their sexual feelings were of this type. These skills training procedures built a foundation for increased trust between them and served to create positive expectancies for second order changes later in treatment.

Second order changes in one's personal mythology involve shifts in the character or structure of the individual's central themes or the relationships between central themes or components of themes (e.g., idealized images). For Roy and Marian, second order changes in personal themes were seen in those themes that dealt with Marian's loyalty to her family of origin (mother) and Roy's passivity in relationship to women and perceived inadequacy in meeting others' needs. As a result, Roy became better able to meet Marian's needs for emotional support, while Marian was able to establish her primary loyalty to her own family of procreation rather than to her family of origin. She relinquished her Cosby family personal myth script and adopted more developmentally appropriate scripts of Rapunzel and Del Jordan. Although both scripts still emphasized the theme of mother-daughter (family of origin) relationships, they did so in a way which offered new solutions and possible changes in the structure of these relationships.

Second order changes in conjugal or family mythologies involve shifts in the character or structure of shared themes or the relationships between several shared themes, and are most discernable as changes in the reciprocal role arrangements between spouses or other family members. Second-order changes were evident near the completion of treatment, when Roy and Marian worked to create a new conjugal script accommodating each's central themes and current developmental needs in the areas of interpersonal intimacy.

We have found however, that first and second order theme changes do not adequately account for all the reorganizations seen in treatment. For example, an entirely *new* personal theme may emerge when parts of an existing myth become outdated or when environmental input exceeds the myth's "accommodation capacity" (Piaget, 1977). In such cases, higher order cognitive structures are necessary (Feinstein, 1979). These higher order structures may incorporate elements from previously existing themes and yet have a qualitatively different structure. The example offered earlier, of the young woman who had experienced the role of "loner" and the accompanying theme of isolation can serve as an illustration. If this young woman no longer finds this "loner" view of the self and the self-in-relation-to-significant-others tolerable, she may develop a qualitatively different sense of self, which is accompanied by an entirely new affective and interactional script. For instance, a reorganized sense of self capable of engaging in intimate interpersonal relationships where one is valued and accepted could be said to reflect a *third order change.*

The emergence of a new individual theme is often preceded by an ambivalent personal struggle, which may include debilitating stress and symptom development. Behavior patterns associated with old themes are usually highly resistant to extinction and may persist in spite of one's conscious desire to relinquish them (Feinstein, 1979). Koestler (1978) has referred to the perception of a situation or event in two mutually exclusive associative contexts as "bisociation." The result of this bisociation can be an abrupt transformation of the train of consciousness to a different track, governed by a different logic. Koestler (1978) has convincingly argued that this mental process is the central ingredient in humor, wit and artistic creativity. Inability to make the leap to what has been referred to as a third order change (Berenson, 1987) or Learning III (Bateson, 1972) results in continued distress, confusion, ambivalence, and related psychological and behavioral symptoms. Success at completing a third order change can be accompanied by dramatic second order shifts in the individual's marital and family relationships.

References to such third order transformations are alluded to occasionally in psychotherapy (Bettelheim, 1976; Fromm, 1951; Jung, 1959) religious conversions (Coomaraswamy, 1916; Frazer, 1942; Watts, 1954) and in other contexts where there is a dramatic reorganization of the self. For instance, Morihei Uyeshiba, founder of the martial art Aikido, was driven by a personal theme of becoming powerful and strong. He vowed never again to be weak and helpless. As a child, he had seen his father beaten up by some neighborhood toughs, but was unable to do anything because he was too frail and sickly. Following that incident, he became obsessed with learning whatever he could about fighting and self-defense. After mastering a number of martial arts, and following his father's death, he went into seclusion for a period of seven years. During this period of mourning, he had time to study and to reflect upon his existence.

His transformation occurred after Uyeshiba had fought with a man who had come to visit him. Following this fight, standing alone under a tree wiping the perspiration from his face, he was overcome with a feeling which he had never experienced before. He could neither walk nor sit. He felt rooted to the ground. He recalled this experience:

> I felt that the universe suddenly quaked, and that a golden spirit sprang up from the ground, veiled my body, and changed my body into one of gold. At the same time, my mind and body became light. I was able to understand the whispering of the birds, and was clearly aware of the mind of God, the creator of this universe. At that moment, I was enlightened: the source of Budo (fighting arts) is God's love—the spirit of loving protection for all beings. Tears of joy streamed down my cheeks. Since that time, I have grown to feel that the whole earth is my house and the sun, the moon and the stars are all my own things. I had become free of all desire, not only for position, fame, and property, but also to be strong. I understood: Budo is not felling the opponent by our force; nor is it a tool to lead the world into destruction with arms. The true Budo is to accept the spirit of the universe, keep the peace of the world, correctly produce, protect and cultivate all beings in nature. I understood: The training of Budo is to take God's love, which correctly produces, protects and cultivates all things in Nature, and to assimilate and utilize it in our own mind and body. (Uyeshiba, 1958, p. 5)

A similar transformation to a qualitatively new personal mythology was described by Hermann Hesse (1951) in the novel *Siddhartha*. Siddhartha was in deep despair over his runaway son and his recollections of how he too, in a similar manner, had left his own father and never returned home again. Hesse wrote:

> Everything that was not suffered to the end and finally concluded, recurred, and the same sorrows were undergone. Siddhartha climbed into the boat again and rowed back to the hut, thinking of his father, thinking of his son, laughed at by the river, in conflict with himself, verging on despair, and no less inclined to laugh aloud at himself and the whole world. The wound still smarted; he still rebelled against his fate. There was still no serenity and conquest of his suffering. Yet he was hopeful and when he returned to the hut, he was filled with an unconquerable desire to confess to Vasudeva, to disclose everything, to tell everything to the man who knew the art of listening. (p. 132)

After having confessed to Vasudeva, Siddhartha returned to the river to contemplate. Hesse (1951) then describes Siddhartha's transformation:

> His wound was healing, his pain was dispersing; his self had merged into unity.
> From that hour Siddhartha ceased to fight against his destiny. There shone in his face the serenity of knowledge, of one who is no longer confronted with conflict of desires, who has found salvation, who is in harmony with the stream of events, with the stream of life, full of sympathy and compassion, surrendering himself to the stream, belonging to the unity of all things. (p. 136)

The initial pain and despair, followed by surrender to a greater power, the accompanying sense of awe and humility, and the dramatic alteration of one's basic premises about the self and the world reflected in these experiences are similar to the "bottoming out" experience reported by some members of Alcoholics Anonymous. For example, Bill W., cofounder of AA, after four hospitalizations for alcoholism and after receiving a hopeless prognosis from his physician, reported the following experience:

> My depression deepened unbearably and finally it seemed to me as though I were at the very bottom of the pit. I still gagged badly on the notion of a Power greater than myself, but finally, just for a moment, the last vestige of my proud obstinacy was crushed. All at once I found myself crying out, "If there is a God, let Him show Himself! I am ready to do anything, anything!"
> Suddenly the room lit up with a great white light. I was caught up into an ecstasy which there was no words to describe. It seemed to me, in the mind's eye, that I was on a mountain and that a wind not of air but of spirit was blowing. And it burst upon me that I was a free man. Slowly the ecstasy

subsided. I lay on the bed, but now for a time I was in another world, a new world of consciousness. All about me and through me there was a wonderful feeling of Presence, and I thought to myself, "So this is the God of the preachers!" A great peace stole over me and I thought, "No matter how wrong things seem to be, they are still all right. Things are all right with God and his world."

This experience produced a fundamental reorganization of Bill's character and world view that had a lasting impact on his life. Bill never drank again (Berenson, 1987). Bateson (1972) has noted how the transformations described above require revision of the most fundamental premises by which individuals operate. These premises, located in the deep levels of the unconscious, are "prelinguistic and the computation which goes on there is coded in primary process" (p. 327). They are "hard programmed" and difficult to change. Bateson (1972) noted that, "if a man achieves or suffers change in premises which are deeply embedded in his mind, he will surely find that the results of that change will ramify throughout his whole universe. Such changes we may call 'epistemological'" (p. 336). For the alcoholic, these premises are rooted in excessive pride and a symmetrical struggle against the self (and significant others) to prove that "I am the master of my own fate. I can control my drinking." The shift from a symmetrical premise to a complementary one in which the alcoholic acknowledges a power greater than himself (both a spiritual power and the power of the substance) allows him to revise the false dichotomy of self versus substance and to accept a unity between the self and the substance. This allows the alcoholic to develop a new identity and personal mythology which includes self-statements such as, "I am an alcoholic" and "Once an alcoholic, always an alcoholic".

Third order changes of the magnitude noted here are certainly not everyday occurrences in our clinical practice. As a rule of thumb, we start with more direct, straightforward cognitive and behavioral first order procedures before attempting to bring about second order changes in clients' personal, marital, or family mythologies. Third order changes are generally not planned, though an appreciation of clients' personal myths and the "fundamental themes" and "premises" which comprise them can facilitate these types of changes. It is our position that, while such third order changes can occur in marital and family therapy as well as in individual therapy, such changes are always deeply personal and individual in nature. However, this is not to say that such changes are not contextual or that significant others do not play a part in the individual's transformation. For instance, alcohol counselors often refer to making an "intervention" where significant others (spouses, children, employers, parents, friends, etc.) confront the alcoholic about his/her drinking and outline the interpersonal contingencies they will impose if the person continues to drink (spousal separation, loss of job, etc.). Such interventions can play a pivotal role in the alcoholic's experience of "bottoming out." Also, the proposition that such third order transformations are deeply personal does not imply that these changes cannot have profound effects on couple and family dynamics.

How an understanding of central mythological themes can facilitate third order change is illustrated in the case of a young married couple seeking treatment for the wife's depression. When each spouse's history and personal mythology were assessed, the following themes emerged as central:

In Mrs. M.'s family of origin, her mother was a powerful force. All the members of Mrs. M.'s family of origin (including herself, her father and two sisters) shared a similar orientation toward Mrs. M.'s mother. No one dared challenge her authority. As a result of this family structure and other factors, Mrs. M. developed a personal mythology which can be summarized as:

> I'm not as important, nor are my needs as important as the needs of others in my life. When disputes arise between my needs and the needs of significant others, I should withdraw, defer to them and not challenge the status quo. To challenge would mean risking the support of the important people in my life. I would then be alone, vulnerable and unable to defend myself against powerful others particularly women who have only their own selfish interests at heart.

In Mr. M.'s family of origin, a somewhat disengaged family structure prevailed. Mr. M. and his two brothers were free to come and go as they pleased. His parents had divorced during his school years and contact with his father was limited. While living with his sickly mother, he often had to fend for himself. Conflicts, when they arose in this family, were generally avoided. Mr. M.'s personal mythology included the following themes:

> Life is fine as long as I'm in control. When I can take responsibility without interference from others, work gets accomplished, I'm more relaxed, and I can be more responsive to others emotionally. At times, I feel tired and overextended. However, this would not be a problem if others would allow me to function without interference so I can still be in control. When conflicts arise, I can usually keep others at bay with my powerful temper. This temper is a

force to be feared. I almost killed someone once when I lost control and it erupted. If my threat fails, and because I dread using this weapon, I must withdraw from others to deal with my feelings and reactions alone. I must always leave myself a way to withdraw from interpersonal encounters. Otherwise, I might have to fight, lose control and really harm someone.

While this couple's conjugal mythology was far more complex than this example will illustrate, several elements of it are relevant here. Mrs. M. felt overpowered and defeated in her relationship with her husband in much the same way she had with her mother in her family of origin. In disagreements with either, it was she who "gave in," "sacrificed [her]self" for the sake of the other. Much of the beginning phases of therapy addressed this issue in an effort to bolster her self-esteem and to enable her to challenge her husband in more productive and direct ways than were available to her in her family of origin. Mr. M's style of unleashing intense anger, fearing his anger's destructive potential, and then distancing from conflict to deal with his feelings had always been effective and reinforced periodically in both his family of origin and in his present marriage. In each area of his life (work, family of origin, marriage) he experienced pressure to take responsibility for the well-being of others. He was often criticized because his efforts were unappreciated or misunderstood. His response was to retreat. This was accompanied by a desire to retain the interpersonal power and security this strategy provided.

Threaded throughout this couple's conjugal mythology were efforts to reenact unresolved personal themes by collusively arranging for each spouse to play the reciprocal roles required by the other. For Mrs. M., this involved an intense monitoring of her husband's behavior, checking how he was feeling toward her, and in numerous ways communicating to him that she did not want her needs to be ignored. For Mr. M., this involved feelings of being cornered by his wife. His typical response included the following:

You are trying to corner me and make me give up my independence (self) and the little freedom in my life that remains. If you keep pressuring me I will explode. I've exploded before and the consequences were nearly catastrophic. If I lose control, I fear that I will be left alone as you will not be strong enough to handle my rage and vulnerability. My relationship with you is the most important thing in my otherwise empty, disengaged life. Therefore it is safer to handle my feelings on my own rather than risk losing you. Leave me alone.

Initial therapeutic efforts included the development of a strong, trusting therapeutic relationship with the couple, some preliminary work on Mrs. M.'s family of origin (and her self-esteem), and some work on the couple's style of communication. Following this, the focus shifted to Mr. M. In the context of a strong therapeutic relationship, a firmly restated commitment of each spouse to their relationship, and their stated commitment to completing the therapy, it was possible for the therapist to align with Mrs. M. and to persistently "pick a fight" with Mr. M. With his customary style of retreating blocked, Mr. M. was placed in the position of having to face his worst fear: that he would explode, lose control, and likely lose his wife in the process.

The results were dramatic. Mr. M. became extremely anxious and confused. In the session his desire to flee was addressed and verbalized. He left the session still quite anxious and tense. The following week, with both Mr. and Mrs. M. present, Mr. M. related an experience he had had several days earlier. He had remained tense since the previous week's session. One morning, prior to both spouses' leaving for work, the couple had had a "fight." On this occasion, Mrs. M. did not "back down" as she previously had, and they both left for work extremely upset. At work, Mr. M. was unable to concentrate. As this continued, he became more and more angry, disoriented, confused, and frightened. He left work, went to Mrs. M.'s office, and the two of them went home, where Mr. M. proceeded to "break down" and cry. Throughout the episode, Mrs. M. was "strong, supportive, and amazingly calm." Later, Mr. M. reported that he had never before felt so "humbled," nor had he realized just how strong his wife really was.

This experience was a turning point in the therapy. The most dramatic and profound effect was experienced by Mr. M. His personal sense of self was transformed from one which included a symmetrical struggle between conflicting aspects (the controlled, responsible self versus the uncontrolled, angry self which was avoided and feared) to one which recognized a more complementary relationship between conscious and unconscious aspects of himself. This transformation was evidenced in Mr. M.'s increased sense of humility and his tremendous relief at being able to surrender to previously unacknowledged feelings of anger, helplessness, and vulnerability. It was equally obvious that the intervention produced alterations in certain conjugal themes. Following this experience, the couple's relationship changed from one of rigid complementarity to one of alternating complementarity, greater mutual respect, closeness, and the ability to tolerate separateness. Central themes in Mrs. M.'s personal mythology underwent changes as well. However, in her case it was less clear whether the "fight" with Mr. M. or her earlier work on her own family of origin was a more significant factor.

A final noteworthy observation occurred in a follow-up session held six weeks after the couple had terminated treatment. Mr. and Mrs. M. reported that, after many years of noninvolvement, they had begun to attend religious services regularly. Here we see the couple expanding the areas of their intimacy to include the spiritual dimension.

In each of the vignettes described in this chapter, a third order shift to a new and revised self organization in the individual's personal mythology was accompanied by a heightened sense of stress, confusion and urgency. *This was accompanied by the individual's relinquishment of a dearly held premise about the self and the self's relationship to significant others, a sense of surrender, a heightened sense of humility and greater tranquility* (i.e., reduced anxiety). As Fromm (1951) has noted, an understanding of the symbolic language of myths brings us in touch with one of our most significant sources of wisdom and reveals to us the deeper layers of our own personalities. It is during those instances of third order change that his comment is most easily appreciated.

Thus far, we have limited our conceptual framework and discussions to work with individuals and couples. In Chapters 13 through 16, we will broaden our emphasis to include the entire family system. In the final chapter, we will focus on issues related to training and supervision.

13

Family Mythologies:
Theoretical Formulations

E ARLIER WE SAID THAT family myths are comprised of a number of separate, yet interrelated, factors and components. The first two components, personal mythologies of all persons who are considered to be part
of the family unit and themes from parents' conjugal mythology, have
been discussed at length. Here we will discuss the three accompanying
components: (a) each parents' conscious and unconscious expectations
for his/her children as they manifest themselves in the form of cognitive
ideal children; (b) submyths, subthemes and fables that develop between
and among family members and serve to maintain various family coalitions, power alignments, structural configurations, procedural rules and
hierarchical arrangements; and (c) family group myths that evolve out of
the interactions and shared life experiences of all family members.

THE IDEAL CHILD

The birth of the first child represents a critical period in the family's
development requiring the mastery of a number of family developmental
tasks (Anderson, Russell, & Schumm, 1983; Duvall, 1977). Each spouse
brings to the marriage his/her ideal cognitive representation of each child
that is born into the family system. How each child is seen depends
upon a number of factors. For instance, the sex of the child, the child's
physical appearance, the child's position in the birth order, the parent's
hopes, dreams, aspirations, unresolved personal conflicts, etc., all play a
part in the construction of the parent's ideal for a particular child. In
addition, specific roles and script expectations accompany each ideal. All
children are expected to fulfill these roles and play out their unique
scripts in order to fit into each parent's model of the *ideal family*.

Like the *ideal spouse*, the *ideal child* and *ideal children* are cognitive images which have conscious as well as unconscious dimensions. Identification, projection, idealization, splitting, projective identification, and transference play a significant part in determining the qualities that are attributed to each *ideal child*. *As was true for the ideal spouse and the ideal marriage, the ideal child and the ideal family and their relation to the self become central themes in the family mythology as children are introduced into the system*. Family themes, like their personal and conjugal counterparts, tend to cluster around personal and family developmental tasks, unresolved interpersonal conflicts, and family milestones. Frequently, unresolved conflicts from the parents' own personal mythologies become reactivated when a child with whom the parent is strongly identified or with whom the parent is involved in a transferential relationship approaches and begins to confront those developmental tasks that the parent himself/herself has not successfully mastered or completely resolved.

For example, a wife who had incompletely separated and individuated from her own mother experienced severe anxiety attacks whenever she left her daughters with baby sitters. She continually projected her own separation fears onto her daughters, whom she nursed until they were well into their third year. Additionally, she was unable to put her preschool children to bed at night without spending hours with them at bedtime; frequently she fell asleep with them while putting them to bed. All this was rationalized as her fear that her daughters were afraid of being "abandoned" by her. The realization that she was actually attempting to deal with her own fears of separation and abandonment came about when her oldest daughter told her, "Mamma, you don't have to worry about us. We will still be here when you wake up tomorrow morning."

Essentially, a process similar to *mutual shaping toward the ideal spouse* takes place with each child who enters the family. Both parents attempt to make the child into a preordained ideal image. Obviously, it is highly unlikely that both parents will have constructed identical or very similar ideals for any child, and conflicts are inevitable. If the parents are unable to resolve their differences concerning their expectations for a child, the child finds himself/herself caught in the middle of a deadly power struggle. Under such conditions, the child may come to symbolize a number of things. The child may represent the battle ground where this civil (or not so civil) war is fought. He/she may become the prize that goes to the victorious parent, who then has the freedom to mold the child into his/her ideal. In many instances, the child becomes an ally of one parent by conforming to that parent's ideal. In exchange for this conformity, the child gains power and leverage in the family system. In other instances, the child becomes an arbitrator or pacifier in the parental struggles. Frequently, the child who attempts to conform to both parents' conflicting and contradictory expectations for him/her develops a psychiatric symptom. This symptom serves to maintain both intrapsychic and interpersonal equilibria. It also can be seen as a metaphor for the parents' conflicts and struggles.

As family therapists, we are concerned with how the conflicting expectations of parents for the same child affect that child's acquisition of a specific group of personality characteristics, behavioral traits, perceptions and world views critical for the development of a psychologically healthy and stable individual, one who is capable of forming successful and satisfying interpersonal relationships as an adult.

THE MERGING OF PARENTAL IDEALS

In healthy functioning families, each parent's consciously held ideals for a particular child are thought to be consistent with his/her unconsciously held ideal for that child. Similarly, in functional family systems, both parents are believed to share (more or less) very similar or congruent ideals and expectations for the same child. This consistent-congruent condition is schematically outlined in Figure 5 as an ideal type.

Although it is highly unlikely that any two parents will ever totally agree upon each and every personality factor, behavioral trait, perception, and world view for a given child, the conflicts that inevitably develop between parents are not necessarily dysfunctional for the family system. However, when the parents fail to resolve these interpersonal incongruities and/or intrapsychic inconsistencies, and the child becomes the focal point of the parents' struggle, the child may be unable to move out of his/her triangulated position in the family system. Figure 6 represents what we consider to be a "simple conflict condition." Here both parents consciously and overtly disagree, and the child does not become confused because their disagreement is straightforward, open, honest, and both parents' expectations are internally consistent.

Clinically, such overt parental disagreement and conflict can be dealt with in a very direct and behavioral manner if both parents are willing and able to negotiate their differences and to compromise their positions. The degree to which the targeted child, "the identified patient," is actively involved in these negotiation processes will depend upon the

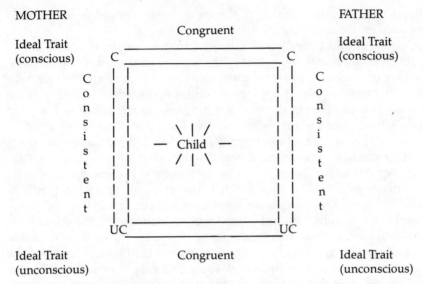

FIGURE 5   Optimal merging of parental ideals for child

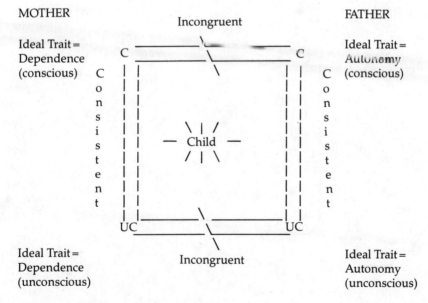

FIGURE 6   Simple conflict condition

child's age. The older the child, the more he/she should be included in the parents' discussions.

Open and direct conflicts of this type are not usually characteristic of families that present themselves for therapy. In clinical families, intrapsychic inconsistencies and interpersonal incongruities are the rule rather than the exception. For example, intrapsychic inconsistencies often manifest themselves in the parent's inconsistent treatment of the child coupled with ambivalent feelings toward that child. The parent's ambivalence may take a number of forms (e.g., double bind messages, mind reading attempts, disconfirmations, disqualifying communications, indirect requests and directives, vague and unclear statements, confusing and mystifying verbalizations). This condition, for one parent, is outlined in Figure 7 for two personality traits: autonomy and dependence.

Although the children in Figure 7 receive inconsistent messages from only one parent, they still cannot escape becoming the focal point of that parent's personal struggle concerning his/her conflicting ideals for the child. Whenever a child finds himself/herself caught in such a dilemma and he/she is unable to leave the field of interaction or to metacommunicate about the contradictory or double bind nature of the communications he/she receives, two options are available. The first is to develop a

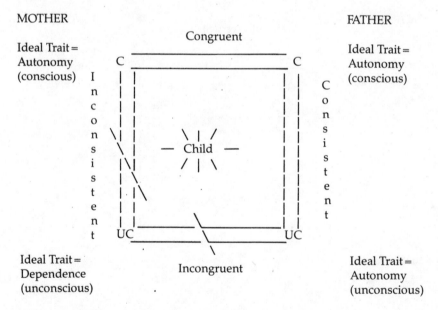

FIGURE 7   Intrapsychic conflict in one parent

psychiatric symptom (Bateson, Jackson, Haley, & Weakland, 1956). Symptomatic behavior is the only compromise that allows the child to behave in accordance with two incompatible, projected ideals with which he/she has become identified.

The second option is to behave in accordance with the ideal projected by the consistent parent and repudiate, as much as possible, identification with the inconsistent parent's conflicting projections. Frequently, when this condition occurs, an overt parent-child validation results between the child and the parent whose ideal the child has chosen to identify with and emulate. In extreme cases, marital skews and schisms may come to characterize the family's way of functioning (Lidz, Cornelison, Fleck, & Terry, 1957). However, the repudiated ideal is not extinguished. It is simply repressed and split off from the self. The activation of this denied, repressed, and repudiated part of the self always remains a possibility. Given the right circumstances, it may erupt as uncharacteristic behavior.

Figure 8 depicts the condition that results when parents make unconscious contractual agreements concerning a particular child. This family condition is frequently seen by family therapists.

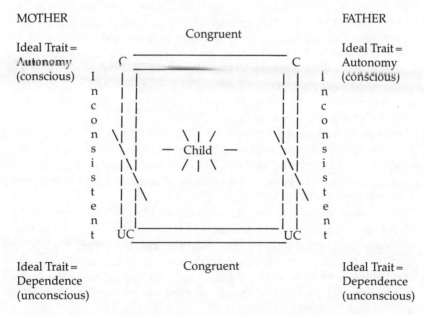

FIGURE 8   Unconscious contractual arrangement between parents

Both parents consciously acknowledge and agree that they would like the "identified patient" to develop the specific ideal trait or personality characteristic, but unconsciously they have agreed to shape (in this case) the opposite trait or characteristic. The type of family structure that develops under such conditions is similar to the pseudo mutual family systems described in the pioneering work of Wynne, Ryckoff, Day, and Hirsch (1958). A brief example of how such a condition comes about is given below.

Mr. and Mrs. Mann came in for consultation because their 12-year-old son was being disruptive at school, disobeying his teachers and misbehaving at home. Both Mr. and Mrs. Mann consciously agreed that they wanted their son, Randy, to behave at school and not to "back talk" to Mrs. Mann. Both parents were genuinely upset with Randy's disobedience at school and his misbehavior at home. Family Relationship Histories and Personal Myth Assessment Interviews were completed by all family members. Mr. and Mrs. Mann were also asked to complete Ideal Child Profiles for Randy. The Ideal Child Profiles created by Mr. and Mrs. Mann showed few inconsistencies. Consciously, these parents were in agreement. However, themes derived from Mr. and Mrs. Mann's Family Relationship Histories and Personal Myth Assessment Interviews told a different story. Two themes, one from Mr. Mann's personal mythology and one from Mrs. Mann's personal mythology, are pertinent.

First, Mr. Mann came from a home that was dominated by women. His maternal grandmother, his mother, and his maternal aunts were all powerful, strong-willed women who ran their husbands' lives. A central theme in Mr. Mann's personal mythology was "women will dominate men every chance they get to do so. Men must constantly fight to get out from under women's control."

Second, Mrs. Mann was the "baby" in her family of origin, which consisted of her parents, herself, and three brothers. Her father was very protective of her mother, and her brothers were very protective, if not possessive, of her. Mrs. Mann had grown up with the belief that men are the "senior partners" in marriage.

Mrs. Mann identified her son, Randy, with her youngest brother, whom she considered to be the closest and whom she liked the most. Although they often "argued over little things," they were the "best of friends." Mr. Mann, on the other hand, identified his son as his projected rebellious self who constantly fought, as a child, to free himself from female domination by deliberately disobeying his mother, his grandmother, and his maternal aunts.

The complementary meshing of these two personal themes resulted in childrearing practices that encouraged Randy to disobey his mother and to become disruptive in school, where he found it necessary to "stick up for his own rights" with teachers and other female school personnel.

In this example, both parents consciously desired a child who was well behaved and respectful of his elders. However, unconsciously Mr. and Mrs. Mann reinforced noncompliant and argumentative behavior in their son for reasons that became evident only through exploring both parents' personal mythologies and the ideals they held for the "identified patient." For Mrs. Mann, the implementation of clear, firm limits upon Randy's behavior at school and toward her would have jeopardized their "best of friends" relationship. For Mr. Mann, the implementation of clear, firm limits on Randy's behavior would have jeopardized his vicarious fight to free himself from female domination.

Figure 9 represents a more complex condition. Here we have a situation in which parents appear consciously and overtly to disagree about the character trait they wish their child to develop, yet unconsciously they are in agreement. This type of collusive arrangement is one that is also frequently presented by dysfunctional family systems.

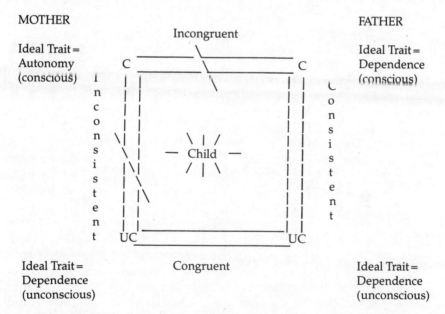

FIGURE 9 Conscious disagreement; unconscious agreement with intrapsychic conflict in one parent

In these types of families, parents frequently argue and disagree about the proper way to discipline, parent, interact with, etc., the identified patient in order to produce the consciously agreed upon behavioral trait or personality characteristic. However, the child responds only to the consistently shared nonverbal directives and expectations.

In conditions depicted in Figures 8 and 9, the child is involved in the unconscious collusive agreement with his/her parents. However, in the latter situation, he/she can side openly with one parent against the other, altering sides as serves the family's needs and his/her own purposes. In all three conditions, symptomatic and acting-out behaviors are acceptable as long as the child conforms to the unconscious expectations of the parents.

Figure 10 represents a family condition more complex and more difficult to assess than any of the conditions outlined thus far, because it requires the introduction of a third and different (as opposed to a polar opposite) unconsciously held expectation for a characteristic or behavioral trait. In this condition, the child also may side openly with one parent against the other. However, the ideal trait agreed upon by both parents

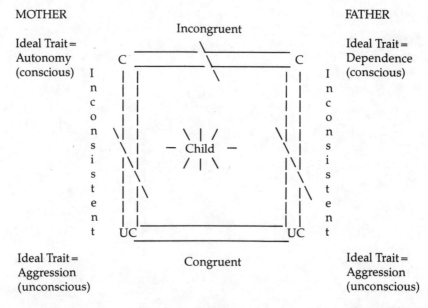

FIGURE 10 Conscious disagreement with intrapsychic conflict and unconscious agreement between the parents

(in their unconscious contract for the child) is not even part of the parents' open disagreements.

This condition proves to be very confusing and perplexing for the targeted child, and symptomatic behavior may be the only option available if the child is unable to decipher which character trait or behavior he/she is supposed to acquire. Confusion can be compounded even further under the conditions depicted in Figures 11, 12, and 13. Probably the most confusing and perplexing condition for the child is that shown in Figure 14. Here a fourth variable is introduced into an already complex situation.

IDEAL CHILDREN, IDEAL FAMILY SYSTEMS, AND THE DEVELOPMENT OF FAMILY SUBMYTHS

Associated with each cognitive representation of an ideal child is a role that he/she is expected to play in the parents' model of an *ideal family system*. Obviously, even in the most functional family systems, it is highly unlikely that parents will share identical ideals for their children or

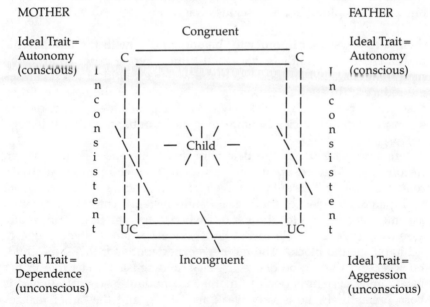

FIGURE 11 Conscious agreement between parents with both parents having intrapsychic conflict resulting in unconscious disagreement

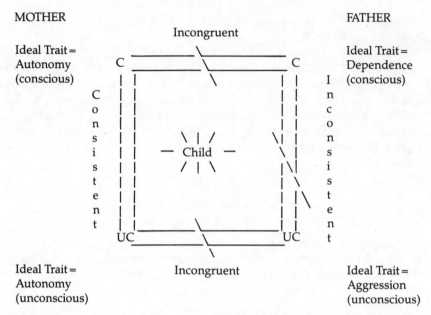

FIGURE 12 Conscious disagreement with intrapsychic inconsistency in one parent resulting in unconscious disagreement

their family systems. In order for parents to deal with the intrapsychic and interpersonal conflicts that result from differing expectations, they might: (a) change their ideals so that any perceived/ideal discrepancies are reduced; (b) attempt to change the behaviors of the target child so that he/she conforms more closely to each parent's ideal; or (c) defend against any discrepancies by employing any number of intrapsychic ego defenses.

A final way for parents to deal with their differences is to create an unconsciously agreed-upon submyth about each child and that child's role in the family. This submyth must be vague enough to accommodate both parents' models of their ideal family systems. For example, let us assume that a father's ideal son is one who is very athletic and physically assertive. This son's role in the father's ideal family system is one of "chip off the old block." The mother's expectations for this same child, however, are that he be docile, passive, and sensitive. His role in her ideal family system is one of "mother's confidant." When the child is born prematurely, he is very weak and sickly, and the father realizes immediately that his son will never become the assertive, self-confident athlete he desires. Mother, on the other hand, sees the possibility of this

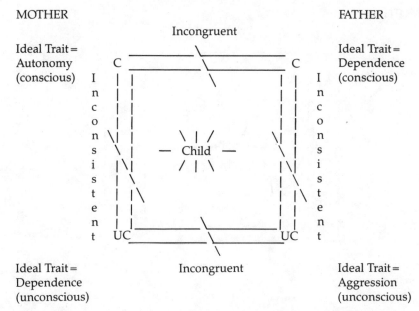

MOTHER   FATHER

Ideal Trait =   Ideal Trait =
Autonomy   Dependence
(conscious)   (conscious)

FIGURE 13   I. Pervasive incongruent—inconsistent parental expectations

Ideal Trait =   Incongruent   Ideal Trait =
Dependence   Aggression
(unconscious)   (unconscious)

child's becoming very much like her ideal. She also believes that he will fit very neatly into her model of the ideal family system. From the time she brings her son home from the hospital, mother pampers him and spends a considerable amount of time with him. As far as she can tell, she does not have to do very much to shape him into fitting her ideal. However, if father does not modify his cognitive ideals and change his expectations for his son, or if he attempts to force his child into becoming more like his ideal, serious power struggles and conflicts may ensue between him and his wife. Both parents realize this on an unconscious level. In order to avoid any confrontation, therefore, they create a sub-myth of the "sickly, but verbally assertive son" who can be mother's confidant as well as being sufficiently assertive to please his father. As the child grows older, if his behavior does not deviate too drastically from this "consensus role image" (Byng-Hall, 1973) that his parents have settled upon, family harmony and tranquility may prevail.[1] The "consen-

---

[1]"Consensus role image" is the term used by Byng-Hall (1973) to describe the role that all family members agree each individual family member should play.

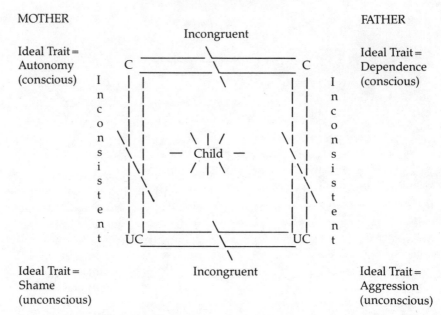

FIGURE 14   II. Pervasive incongruent—inconsistent parental expectations

sus role image" may never require revision, and it may remain functional and viable for the family and the child.

Submyths also come into being in order to maintain specific structural configurations between and among family members. For example, a wife who possesses relatively little power in her relationship with her husband may develop a coalition with one or more of her daughters, who side with her in her disagreements with her spouse. In order to solidify and justify this power alignment, mother and her daughters develop a belief system or submyth about men which they secretly share (e.g., "men cannot be trusted," "all men are out for what they can get"). This submyth usually has its roots in the mother's own personal mythology, which is disclosed, in part, to her daughters and becomes part of their personal mythologies and world views.

As each new child (or member) is added to the family, submyths come into being which allow for the smooth (or not so smooth) transition from one type of family configuration and family process to another. If this does not happen, the family cannot remain viable.

Some submyths also develop for the purpose of maintaining intergenerational alignments, allegiances, and coalitions. For example, in one family treated by the first author, all male children born to the couple become "property" of the husband's parents. The submyth devised to maintain this arrangement was that it was the male grandchildren's responsibility to carry on the family name, traditions, and business operations. The female children, on the other hand, became "property" of the mother's parents. The submyth used to maintain this intergenerational coalition was graphically stated by the children's maternal grandmother, who had always told her daughters and granddaughters: "mothers lose their sons to their wives, but the mother-daughter relationship can never be lost."

We believe that the roles and functions of children within a family system are always negotiated between the parents in the form of unconscious contracts. Frequently, these unconscious contracts about the children require that parents renegotiate and redefine the couple's primary relationship rules. The reader will recall that in Chapter 5 we outlined four primary areas of conjugal relationship rules:

1. Rules for interpersonal intimacy (closeness and separateness).
2. Rules for distributive justice and social exchange.
3. Rules for marital power sharing, influence, and leadership.
4. Rules for communicating love, value, and worth.

Some examples of how these relationship rules become renegotiated and redefined when children or new members enter the family are given below:

1. *Interpersonal intimacy (closeness and separateness).* Couples who have never been able to establish mutually satisfying levels of intimacy may draw up an unconscious contract which permits the spouse (e.g., the husband) who desires more closeness to have his intimacy needs fulfilled through his relationship with a child. In exchange for this, the husband no longer turns to his wife for closeness, and she then is able to achieve the degree of separateness that she desires without having to worry about her husband continually making demands on her for closeness.

2. *Distributive justice and social exchange.* Whenever spouses perceive inequitable or unfair exchange systems in their marriage, they can use their children (or their relationships with their children) as resource commodities. For example, if a husband controls the purse strings and thereby his wife's behavior, the wife may be granted sole dominion over all children who give their allegiance to her. Her children's loyalties are

given as compensation. Their loyalty also increases her power in other areas of the conjugal exchange system.

3. *Power sharing, influence, and leadership.* A spouse (e.g., the wife) who has been in the inferior, one-down, complementary power position with her husband can gain a more dominant position in decision-making by "speaking for" and "representing the best interests" of her children. As a result, the power, influence, and leadership once concentrated solely in the husband's hands are now shared more equally.

4. *Communicating, love, value, and worth.* In situations where there exists a noncorrespondence of rules between husband and wife, children can be trained to use both sets of rules in their relationships with their parents. For example, if the parents' noncorresponding rules for communicating love are as follows:

Husband/father = If you love me you will not call attention to any of my shortcomings, and I will not call attention to any of your shortcomings to show my love for you.

Wife/mother = If you love me you will give me constructive feedback about my mistakes, and I will try to improve myself. I will show my love for you by giving you constructive feedback whenever I think you can profit from it.

Children of such parents can learn to discriminate between these two conflicting rule systems. They also can learn to apply the appropriate rules with each parent and to differentiate their responses accordingly. As a result, both parents feel loved, understood and appreciated by their children. Conflicts having to do with the noncorrespondence of rules may erupt less frequently between the parents if the parents unconsciously contract to use their own rules for sending and receiving value messages only with their children and not with each other. Here again, submyths must be devised to preserve the newly erected structures and processes that result from these renegotiated contractual agreements and arrangements.

FAMILY GROUP MYTHS THAT EVOLVE OUT OF MUTUALLY SHARED FAMILY EXPERIENCES

Family group myths come into existence as a result of the shared experiences of all family members. Probably the first time such group myths crystallize is when the parents and their first child come to an understanding and unconscious agreement about that child's "consensus role image." Family homeostasis is maintained as long as the child's behavior is congruent with his/her parents' "consensus role image." When each family member behaves in accordance with his/her "consensus role image," the family comes close to approximating a vaguely defined *ideal family image* that all family members share to a greater or lesser degree. The loosely integrated group of "consensus role images" that constitute the members' shared ideal family image must undergo periodic revision and modification in response to the growth and development of family members. It must also change as the family proceeds through the various stages of the family life cycle. Finally, if the family is to remain viable, the ideal family image must accommodate to external demands, changing environmental contexts and existing realities.

Dysfunction occurs whenever the shared ideal family image cannot be modified to accommodate to changing needs and demands of family members, external systems, and environmental forces. Holding tenaciously to an outmoded, distorted, or dysfunctional *ideal family image* can reach delusional proportions in some severely distressed family systems. Frequently, family members who "go against" a distorted ideal family image by refusing to behave "as if" the rigidly held image were in fact a reality, become ostracized, scapegoated, believed bad, or treated as mad by those who cling to this distorted image.

The ideal family image is transmitted to each incoming member through overt and covert communication channels. Family members' (particularly parents') nonverbal messages carry with them approval or disapproval of one's behavior that is thought to be incongruent with one's "consensus role image." Behaviorally, the ideal family image is reinforced through daily routines and rituals; shared family mottos, jokes, humorous stories, reminiscences; family recreational activities, religious practices, ethnic customs, etc. Verbally, the ideal family image is communicated via specific values and rules of conduct. These are often couched in statements like: "This is the way we do things in our family," "We don't care what your friends' parents allow their children to do; in this family, we have different rules and standards," "In our home, we don't do such things," or "Good Christians (Catholics, Baptists, Methodists, Episcopalians, Jews, etc.) don't behave in such a manner."

We know from our clinical experience and from the original research done by Ferreira (1963, 1966) that the family's mutually agreed-upon ideal image of itself may differ considerably from the way in which outsiders view the family. We use the term ideal family image in place of Ferreira's term "family myth" because we believe it more accurately describes this phenomenon.

The reader will recall that husbands and wives unconsciously collude to play out reciprocal and complementary roles from their spouse's personal mythologies in order to help them rework and resolve intrapsychic conflicts. A similar process involving all family members is commonly seen in clinical practice. As was true for the development and maintenance of conjugal myths, projective identification and multiple transference reactions play a significant role in the family group process. The most frequently observed example of this phenomenon is family scapegoating. Systems theorists have emphasized the group homeostatic qualities of scapegoating in families, but they have failed to realize that scapegoating also maintains the intrapsychic homeostasis of all who participate in the scapegoating process.

A family that presented itself for treatment after the adolescent daughter had made a suicidal gesture demonstrates how this process works. She had attempted to "cut her wrists" while her parents and her younger brother were swimming in the family pool.

Family Relationships Histories and Personal Myth Assessment Interviews of all family members and Ideal Child Profiles of the parents for both children revealed a number of important thematic issues. For example, the Family Relationship Histories of both parents contained themes of parental rejection. Both parents were "cut off" from their families of origin when they decided to marry; neither set of parents approved of the couple's marriage. The "identified patient," who was conceived shortly after the couple married, became the repository for each parent's unacceptable personality traits. These were projected onto her by both parents, who frequently attacked her for possessing these undesirable characteristics. The reader will not be surprised to learn that these same characteristics were the ones that the parents had been punished for by their own parents.

The parents' Ideal Child Profiles for the "identified patient" were fairly congruent in that both parents consciously desired that she be "polite," "kind," and "not rebellious." However, they were distressed because she had turned out to be "just the opposite." Their Ideal Child Profiles for their son, however, appeared to be consistent and congruent at both levels of awareness. This child was "polite," "kind," "considerate," and "helpful." He did not have a "rebellious bone in his body."

Scapegoating allowed both parents and their son to attack the repudiated aspects of themselves that were projected onto the "identified patient," who colluded with them by playing out their consensus role image of her as the rebellious daughter. Intrapsychic equilibria were maintained for the parents and the son, who did not have to face these negative traits in themselves. "Cutting her wrists" was a symbol of both parents' personal themes of being "cut off" from their families of origin. This theme was in the process of being replayed in this family system, since both parents were seriously considering placement of their daughter in a residential treatment facility (i.e., she too would be cut off).

The Family Relationships History of the daughter was helpful in highlighting just how many people, outside the nuclear family, were participating in this scapegoating process. She identified her maternal grandmother and her paternal grandfather as the persons she "liked most" and "felt closest to." She "liked" her maternal grandmother because she understood her; and she "felt closest to" her paternal grandfather because he always "stuck up for her" with her parents. The reinforcement she received from her grandparents was enough to insure that she would continue to play the scapegoat role of the "rebellious child." It also insured that both sets of grandparents would continue to be actively involved with their own children over the fate of this granddaughter. This myth of the "rebellious child" can be seen as maintaining intrapsychic equilibrium as well as maintaining family group homeostasis.

This example also sheds light on two additional functions of shared family myths: (a) by incorporating themes from the parents' personal and conjugal mythologies, they maintain thematic continuity from one generation to the next and allow the parents additional opportunities to rework unresolved developmental conflicts through their relationships with their children; and (b) they serve to maintain intergenerational ties.

Experiences that all family members share as a cohesive group add to the crystallization of the family's *ideal image* of itself. The process by which crystallization takes place involves three steps: (a) the actual event or experience itself and the family's response to that event (e.g., encounters with systems external to itself, developmental transitions, crises); (b) each family member's individual appraisal of the family's success in mastering the event or experience; and (c) the family members' reconstructed view of the experience and their agreed-upon appraisal of their success as a family unit. This latter step requires that all family members reach a general consensus. Frequently, this means that some family members will have to modify, revise, or distort their original perceptions in order to conform to the agreed-upon group norm or consensus. Once this reconstructed experience is openly discussed and agreed upon, it becomes part of the *ideal family image*. It also becomes a guide for handling similar experiences in the future.

The reader will remember that in Chapter 1 we said that cultural myths are imaginative narratives dealing with significant acts and events in human history which have taken place at a particular time, and that these cultural myths have their source in the common life and experiences of a particular group or community. Furthermore, they tend to persist over generations and become part of the group's tradition. Finally, we said that these shared beliefs become prized and inseparable parts of the group's life. Here we see how myth and ritual become linked to the ideal family image. The ideal family image, much like the self, is a superordinate structural system having cognitive and affective components which operate at conscious and unconscious levels of family group awareness. Like the self, the ideal family image has definite rules of operation which members of the family must obey in order to retain membership in the family unit. Family group experiences are organized into some coherent whole by the members who use their unconsciously shared ideal family image as a referent. This shared image is used to organize group perceptions, to lend continuity to the group's past and present experiences, and to serve as a guide for group actions in the future.

14

Family Assessment Procedures

FAMILY ASSESSMENTS INCLUDE the following:

1. Family Relationships Histories for all family members.
2. Personal Myth Assessment Interviews for all family members.
3. Couple's Relationship History for the parents.
4. History of Presenting Problem taken with all family members present and including all members' inputs.
5. IMAGES for both parents.
6. SIDCARB for both parents.
7. Ideal Child Profiles of both parents for the identified patient.
8. Faces III for all family members old enough to complete the family version of this instrument.
9. Personal Authority in the Family Systems Questionnaire for all family members old enough to complete the instrument.
10. Behavioral observations of the entire family group engaged in a specific interaction task (e.g., problem-solving, conflict negotiation, planning something together as a family, setting goals) in order to get an appraisal of salient relational-communication control and dominance patterns and characteristic rules for communicating love, value and worth among family members.

The reader should be familiar with all these assessment tools except the *Ideal Child Profile*, which has not been discussed thus far. The Ideal Child Profile is a 26-item questionnaire that parents are asked to complete for the identified patient. Parents are asked not to consult with each other while completing this questionnaire. The Ideal Child Profile is reproduced in Table 11.

In addition to using these instruments and procedures, we also pay close attention to the following processes that signal the presence of

TABLE 11 Ideal Child Profile

Parent's Name _____ Child's Name _____ Date _____

Please answer the following questions about your son/daughter.

1. (Mother) How did you feel when you first realized that you were pregnant with this child?
2. (Father) How did you feel when you first learned that your wife was pregnant with this child?
3. Were you and your spouse married to each other at the time of conception?
4. Is this child an offspring from a previous marriage or relationship? Explain:
5. Was the pregnancy planned by both you and your spouse? If the answer is no, please explain:
6. Was the child wanted by you? Was the child wanted by your spouse?
7. Were there ever times when either you or your spouse gave serious consideration to terminating this pregnancy? Why was the option considered? Were any active steps taken to end this pregnancy that failed?
8. Was the child conceived in order to replace a deceased loved one (e.g., parent, sibling, another child) for either you or your mate? If yes, please explain:
9. Was the child conceived in order to improve an unhappy relationship between you and your spouse? If yes, please explain:
10. What was your reaction and your impression when you saw this child for the first time?
11. What was your mate's reaction and impression to seeing this child for the first time?
12. What were your parents' reactions and impressions to seeing this child for the first time?
13. What were your in-laws' reactions and impressions to seeing this child for the first time?
14. What reaction did the child's siblings have to seeing him/her for the first time?
15. How did you feel about this child's gender (sex) when he/she was born? How do you feel about his/her gender now?
16. How did your spouse feel about this child's gender (sex) when he/she was born? How does your spouse feel now about this child's gender?

TABLE 11 *(Continued)*

---

17. Who named this child and how was the child's name selected?
18. How do you expect this child to behave in order for him/her to be a productive member of this family? Explain:
19. How does this child *actually* behave? Do you consider him/her to be a productive member of this family? Explain:
20. What role do you expect this child to play in relation to you, your spouse, and his/her brothers and sisters in order to keep this family running smoothly? Explain:
21. What role does this child *actually* play in relation to you, your spouse, and his/her brothers and sisters? Does he/she contribute to the smooth operation of your family? Explain:
22. What attitudes, beliefs and values do you want this child to develop? Explain:
23. What attitudes, beliefs and values (for this child) do you consider to be unacceptable? Explain:
24. Below is a list of character traits and behaviors that may or may not be characteristic of this child. On the lefthand side of this sheet, please indicate, by circling one number, the degree to which the child possesses the particular character trait or behavior. On the righthand side of this sheet you will see that the same character trait or behavior appears again. Please indicate, by circling one number, the degree to which you would like this child to possess or acquire the particular character trait or behavior in question. For example:

	Perceived Very little Very much		Ideal Very little Very much
Trusts people	1 ②3 4 5 6 7 8 9	Trusts people	1 2 3 4 5 6 ⑦8 9

In this example, the parent perceives the child to trust people at a #2 (in the *very little* range). However, he would like his child to trust people at a level of #7 (in the *very much* range).

Please rate your child on the following character traits and behaviors:

	Perceived Very Very little much		Ideal Very Very little much
1. Trusts people	1 2 3 4 5 6 7 8 9	1. Trusts people	1 2 3 4 5 6 7 8 9
2. Self-assured	1 2 3 4 5 6 7 8 9	2. Self-assured	1 2 3 4 5 6 7 8 9
3. Stable personality	1 2 3 4 5 6 7 8 9	3. Stable personality	1 2 3 4 5 6 7 8 9

(continued)

TABLE 11 (*Continued*)

	Perceived Very Very little much		Ideal Very Very little much
4. Independent	1 2 3 4 5 6 7 8 9	4. Independent	1 2 3 4 5 6 7 8 9
5. Feels ashamed	1 2 3 4 5 6 7 8 9	5. Feels ashamed	1 2 3 4 5 6 7 8 9
6. Feels guilty	1 2 3 4 5 6 7 8 9	6. Feels guilty	1 2 3 4 5 6 7 8 9
7. Doubtful	1 2 3 4 5 6 7 8 9	7. Doubtful	1 2 3 4 5 6 7 8 9
8. Indecisive	1 2 3 4 5 6 7 8 9	8. Indecisive	1 2 3 4 5 6 7 8 9
9. Autonomous	1 2 3 4 5 6 7 8 9	9. Autonomous	1 2 3 4 5 6 7 8 9
10. Competent	1 2 3 4 5 6 7 8 9	10. Competent	1 2 3 4 5 6 7 8 9
11. Secure	1 2 3 4 5 6 7 8 9	11. Secure	1 2 3 4 5 6 7 8 9
12. Aggressive	1 2 3 4 5 6 7 8 9	12. Aggressive	1 2 3 4 5 6 7 8 9
13. Assertive	1 2 3 4 5 6 7 8 9	13. Assertive	1 2 3 4 5 6 7 8 9
14. Passive	1 2 3 4 5 6 7 8 9	14. Passive	1 2 3 4 5 6 7 8 9
15. Active	1 2 3 4 5 6 7 8 9	15. Active	1 2 3 4 5 6 7 8 9
16. Submissive	1 2 3 4 5 6 7 8 9	16. Submissive	1 2 3 4 5 6 7 8 9
17. Dominant	1 2 3 4 5 6 7 8 9	17. Dominant	1 2 3 4 5 6 7 8 9
18. Positive	1 2 3 4 5 6 7 8 9	18. Positive	1 2 3 4 5 6 7 8 9
19. Optimistic	1 2 3 4 5 6 7 8 9	19. Optimistic	1 2 3 4 5 6 7 8 9
20. Antisocial	1 2 3 4 5 6 7 8 9	20. Antisocial	1 2 3 4 5 6 7 8 9
21. Dependent	1 2 3 4 5 6 7 8 9	21. Dependent	1 2 3 4 5 6 7 8 9
22. Negative	1 2 3 4 5 6 7 8 9	22. Negative	1 2 3 4 5 6 7 8 9
23. Isolated	1 2 3 4 5 6 7 8 9	23. Isolated	1 2 3 4 5 6 7 8 9
24. Intimate	1 2 3 4 5 6 7 8 9	24. Intimate	1 2 3 4 5 6 7 8 9
25. Sexual	1 2 3 4 5 6 7 8 9	25. Sexual	1 2 3 4 5 6 7 8 9
26. Competitive	1 2 3 4 5 6 7 8 9	26. Competitive	1 2 3 4 5 6 7 8 9
27. Masculine	1 2 3 4 5 6 7 8 9	27. Masculine	1 2 3 4 5 6 7 8 9
28. Feminine	1 2 3 4 5 6 7 8 9	28. Feminine	1 2 3 4 5 6 7 8 9
29. Strong	1 2 3 4 5 6 7 8 9	29. Strong	1 2 3 4 5 6 7 8 9
30. Shy	1 2 3 4 5 6 7 8 9	30. Shy	1 2 3 4 5 6 7 8 9
31. Fearful	1 2 3 4 5 6 7 8 9	31. Fearful	1 2 3 4 5 6 7 8 9
32. Respectful	1 2 3 4 5 6 7 8 9	32. Respectful	1 2 3 4 5 6 7 8 9
33. Other _____	1 2 3 4 5 6 7 8 9	33. Other _____	1 2 3 4 5 6 7 8 9

25. Please describe, in a few short sentences, how this child fits into the family system:
26. What is it about this child that makes him/her unique in your family? Explain:

family group themes: (a) redundant interaction patterns; (b) recurrent topics of concern; (c) repeated resurfacing of affect-laden conflicts; and (d) the predominant feeling tone and atmosphere in the family system.

During our initial interview with the family, we attempt to identify the consensus role image of each family member. In order to do this, we ask each family member to describe what he/she does to maintain the family's smooth functioning (homeostatic balance). We also ask each family member what he/she does that encourages the family to grow and develop as a system (viability). Another method used to detect each family member's consensus role is identify any labels that are used to describe particular family members. Once these have been noted, we attempt to trace their origins in order to determine the specific behaviors, roles and scripts that these nicknames, pet names, derogatory names, epithets, etc., prescribe for the family member thus labeled.

Frequently, we have each family member describe the family system in analogical and/or metaphorical terms. For example, what does the "identified patient" actually mean when he describes his family's characteristic mode of functioning as "we are like marbles in a clothes dryer"? After each family member has offered his/her analogy or metaphor, we ask that person to describe his/her role in the analogy or metaphor and the roles of other family members. For example, the identified patient who characterized his family's operations as "marbles in a clothes dryer" saw himself and his siblings as "marbles." His mother represented the circular clothes dryer itself. His father, an alcoholic, was described as the "rotating inner drum" of the dryer which caused all the marbles to be thrown together in chaotic turmoil. We also ask all family members to try to agree upon an analogy or metaphor that describes the family's characteristic way of functioning. This helps us get a better understanding of how each family member's consensus role image fits into the shared ideal family image.

After the initial family interview, we attempt to draw a structural description of the family as it now appears. We use the guidelines and symbols suggested by Minuchin (1974) to highlight hierarchical arrangements; types of personal ego boundaries; coalitions; affiliations, overinvolvements; conflicts; triangles; and intergenerational relationships that appear to be significantly related to the presenting problem. We then attempt to understand the relationships between and among any submyths (conjugal or otherwise) and how these submyths maintain the various structural arrangements that have been observed.

Finally, we attempt to identify any family rituals, secrets, or symbols which might alert us to the presence of central family themes or submyths. The most obvious symbols appear in the form of psychiatric symptoms. We see the psychiatric symptoms as a symbolic attempt to maintain intrapersonal (intrapsychic) and interpersonal (dyadic and systemic) equilibria simultaneously. We think that it is extremely important to pinpoint in time precisely when a symptom first appears, because the circumstances surrounding the symptom's development provide valuable clues as to the nature of the conflicts which gave rise to it.

Occasionally, families come in for treatment who appear to have some understanding of a particular "theme" or "family myth" that has plagued the family for some time. For example, a father might say that he and his wife had always refrained from arguing and fighting in front of their children in order not to expose them to the same type of strife that he and his wife experienced in their families of origin. Both parents then report that their avoidance of conflict might be the cause for the identified patient's aggressive behavior at school. The parents then go on to explain that no one is permitted to express anger in their family, and that they have always attempted to create a happy and tranquil home life. They add that this also may be a contributing factor in their son's behavior problems. Such revelations may seem, at first, to be evidence of the parents' understanding of the importance of intergenerational themes in their current family life circumstances. The therapist may also take such disclosures, on the part of the parents, as indications of deep psychological "insight" into their unconscious contractual agreements. However, we have come to see such prepackaged understanding of family themes and family myths as family group defensive maneuvers designed to divert, to confuse, and to lead the therapist away from the actual themes and submyths which are used to maintain the family's homeostatic balance.

CONCEPTUALIZING THE PRESENTING PROBLEM

As was true for our work with individuals and couples, we begin our intervention with families by using a straightforward behavioral approach. Our initial premise is that the presenting problem is a result of faulty learning. The identified patient's behavior or the family's dysfunction is treated as if it were simply a problem requiring first-order change solutions. The presenting problem is translated into specific, observable behaviors that can be easily identified and monitored by all family members. The family is then asked to agree upon a specific behavioral outcome or goal that will be the focus of treatment. Dysfunctional behaviors are described in a way that will make them amenable to treatment.

Basically, modification is seen as increasing the frequency, duration, consistency, etc., of desirable behaviors; decreasing the frequency and/or duration of undesirable, punishing, noxious behaviors; eliminating, suppressing or extinguishing altogether specific undesirable behaviors; and acquiring new, more functional and desirable responses.

Providing Families with Feedback

In the initial feedback session with families, where we discuss our assessment findings, we explain our philosophical/theoretical/pragmatic premise concerning the presenting problem, i.e., that the family's problem stems from faulty learning. This disclosure usually puts the family, especially the parents and the identified patient, at ease, because it does not single out one individual as the cause of the family's distress. This having been done, we turn to a discussion of our assessment findings. We review the instruments and procedures that were used to arrive at our interpretations. We then focus upon those aspects of family structure and functioning that various family members have identified as problematic. We pay particular attention to areas of interpersonal conflicts, problems, ideal/perceived discrepancies, exchange inequities, rule differences, family-of-origin difficulties, etc., and offer our interpretations concerning how dysfunction in these areas of family life and family process appear to be contributing to and/or maintaining the family's presenting problem and/or the behavior of the identified patient.

Material gathered from the parents' Family Relationships Histories, Personal Myth Assessment Interviews, the Couple's Relationship History and the parents' Ideal Child Profile is discussed only if it has direct and obvious bearing upon the presenting problem or the behaviors of the identified patient. At the conclusion of our feedback session, we recommend a specific course of action which we believe will help the family achieve its stated behavioral goals. The type of behavioral program suggested will depend upon a number of factors. Some of the major considerations are: (a) the number of presenting problems and their complexity; (b) the age of the identified patient; (c) the number, severity and duration of the identified patient's symptoms; (d) the presence of more than one identified patient and the number, severity, and duration of these persons' symptoms; and (e) the family members' philosophies, beliefs and values concerning human nature, "mental illness," behavior change, behavior modification practices, insight, etc.

Before the conclusion of the feedback session, family members are prepared for what is to take place in treatment. An induction procedure, similar to the one used in marital therapy, has been developed which outlines the differences between individual therapy and family therapy, clarifies the roles of the therapist, and outlines expectations for the family members. As was true for orienting couples to marital therapy, family members are also told that their willingness to cooperate, collaborate, compromise, negotiate their differences, make specific behavioral changes, and complete homework assignments can be seen as concrete manifestations of their verbal commitment to resolving the presenting problem. Parents are told that if they are not prepared to follow through on these commitments then they should not expect to see any change in the presenting problem or the behavior of the identified patient. Again, the therapist tells the parents that their lack of commitment means that the family may not be ready for the changes that successful therapy might produce. Having been thus prepared, the parents are asked to consider whether they are willing to engage in family therapy. If either parent is uncertain, the family is given as much time as it needs to come to a decision. No further interviews are scheduled, however, and any future contact is left up to the family.

Early Treatment Strategies and Considerations

If the family decides to begin treatment, a contract for the modification of specific behaviors is negotiated. The first in-session task is to teach family members functional communication skills that they can use to negotiate differences, resolve conflicts, solve problems and set goals. Family members are given guidelines and asked to use them in their discussion of the presenting problem (Table 12).

Stanton (1981) has offered some procedural guidelines for the use of both structural and strategic techniques with families. Believing that it is possible to apply structural and strategic approaches separately, concurrently, and contrapuntally, because these two schools of therapy are compatible at both operational and pragmatic levels, he offers three procedural rules for guiding practice. These are:

1. *"Initially, deal with the family by using a straightforward structural (behavioral) approach."* The rationale given for this is that the structural-behavioral approach is more direct and parsimonious. In addition, the structural approach has been shown (through empirical research) to be effective with a variety of symptoms and presenting problems. Stanton also stresses that the structural approach is more comprehensible (especially for the inexperienced therapist), because the therapist can track and observe the family's reaction to in-session interventions more easily

TABLE 12 Rules for establishing functional communication in families

---

Speaker's Role

1. Speak directly to the person and look at the person to whom you are talking.
2. State what you think and feel clearly. Use short, concise sentences.
3. Don't attack, accuse, blame, or "put down" the person to whom you are talking or any other family member.
4. Don't interpret, mind read, or attribute hidden meanings to other family members' behaviors or statements. Take what he/she says literally.
5. When you have finished speaking to another family member, say that you have finished and ask that person if he/she has understood what you were trying to communicate.
6. Ask the person to whom you were speaking to paraphrase what you have just said so that you can know if he/she has heard you correctly.
7. Don't monopolize the conversation.

Listener's Role

1. Wait patiently while someone is speaking to you. Listen carefully to what he/she is saying, because he/she will ask you to paraphrase what was said to be sure you have understood correctly.
2. Look at the person who is speaking.
3. Don't interrupt when he/she is speaking. You will have your turn to reply when he/she is through.
4. As you listen, try to put yourself in the speaker's place. Try to understand how he/she feels, how he/she see things and how he/she experiences you.
5. If you are unclear or don't understand what the speaker means, ask him/her to repeat what was just said.
6. When the speaker is finished, repeat back to him/her what you have heard. This will help the speaker determine whether he/she has been understood by you.
7. When the speaker indicates that you have understood him/her, then it's your turn to reply.

---

than he/she can with strategic interventions designed to alter extra-session behavior.

Our use of skills training in functional family communication is seen in this way. The family's ability to carry out this simple task, to follow instructions, and to work as a team can be assessed by observing family members' attempts to complete this in-session task. Diagnostically, this simple assignment is telling, because it provides the therapist with data about the family's ability and willingness to modify dysfunctional communication patterns. Once the family demonstrates its ability to change its customary ways of communicating and interacting, it becomes difficult for family members to say that "communication is bad" or that "no one listens in the family," since the family has already shown its ability to use functional communication skills. Here family members are confronted with their own reluctance to use the skills that they have already mastered. "Poor communication" outside the therapist's office, therefore, can be seen as a conscious choice and decision on the part of each and every family member. Continued failure to use these skills outside the therapist's office, like repeated failure to complete homework assignments, indicates family group resistance. When this occurs, Stanton's second general rule applies.

2. *"Switch to a predominantly strategic approach when structural techniques do not appear to be working or when structural techniques are unlikely to succeed."* Since many of the strategic techniques were developed for work with severely dysfunctional (homeostatic) family systems, they are thought to be more effective for dealing with extremely rigid family systems. Empirical evidence to support this hypothesis is rather scanty. However, Stanton (1981) notes three family situations where strategic techniques appear to be called for:

1. (a) Families where a straightforward approach only seems to heighten the family's defensiveness, escalates conflict between and among family members or produces counterattacks against the therapist.
   (b) When tasks are never followed or are distorted to the disadvantage of the entire family, and the therapist begins to feel defeated.
   (c) The therapist makes a structural intervention which seems accurate, but nothing happens and there is no change in the family's characteristic interaction patterns.
2. The second situation in which a switch from a structural to a strategic approach appears to be warranted is when the therapist has certain pre-therapy information—for example, when a family has a

severely dysfunctional member or when a family has a lengthy history of unsuccessful treatment.

3. When the therapist becomes confused, is at a loss, cannot understand what is going on in the family or is unable to decide where to go with the treatment, he/she should consider switching to a strategic approach.[1]

In our work with families, it is at this juncture where we must decide whether to use a standard strategic approach, e.g., prescribing the symptom, restraining the family from changing, positioning ourselves on the side of "no change" rather than "change" or other clinical procedures based upon our understanding of the personal, conjugal and family mythologies of the family and its members.

The third, and final, general rule suggested by Stanton (1981) is straightforward and simple.

3. *"Following success with strategic methods, and given that a case is to continue in therapy, it may be advisable to revert once again to a structural approach"* (p. 433). It is not uncommon for us to switch back to a more structural-behavioral stance once we have been successful with a strategic intervention. If the strategic intervention has been successful in removing the "identified patient" from his/her pivotal role in the family, we may suggest that the parents consider devoting some time to clinical work on their own relationship. This is especially true when the strategic intervention has been effective in helping the identified patient leave home and establish a separate residence for himself/herself.

Often, we choose not to implement a standard strategic approach when a structural-behavioral approach is unwarranted. Instead, we opt for interventions which focus primarily on the family's symbolic system of meaning. In the next chapter, we will outline our clinical procedures based upon our understanding of the personal, conjugal, and family mythologies of the family and its members.

---

[1]As we shall see in Chapter 17, which deals with training and supervision, the therapist's confusion, loss of direction, or inability to clearly formulate a therapeutic goal may indicate that he/she has become "stuck" in the family's emotional process and is responding reactively to unresolved issues in his/her own personal mythology. In these instances, the therapist may need to become aware of his/her own contribution to the therapeutic impasse and be clear that the selected strategic intervention is not simply another way to reenact a counterproductive role, script, or interactional pattern in the family's mythological system.

15

Family Mythologies:
Intervention Strategies

I N THIS CHAPTER, we outline some of the clinical procedures used most frequently with families. When the straightforward behavioral approaches described in Chapter 14 are deemed inappropriate or ineffective, we turn to the data gathered from family members during the assessment process to gain a clearer understanding of how the parents' personal mythologies, conjugal themes, unconscious contracts, and ideal child images, as well as family members' consensus role images of the identified patient, ideal family images, submyths, subthemes, and family group myths, contribute to the genesis and maintenance of the presenting problem. We also speculate about how the identified patient's behavior serves not only to maintain his/her personal equilibrium but also to preserve the homeostatic balance of the entire family system.

CASE EXAMPLE: THE GEORGES

Mr. and Mrs. George came in for consultation regarding their five-and-one-half-year-old daughter's behavior. The presenting problem was Jessica's stubbornness; she was uncooperative, disrespectful, and defiant toward her mother and threw temper tantrums at home. Jessica's aggression toward Mrs. George had increased over the past several weeks. Both Mr. and Mrs. George found themselves unable to "handle her" or to bring her aggressive behavior "under control." The precipitating incident that brought the family into treatment was Jessica's assault upon her mother, who had recently given birth to the couple's second child, a son named Arthur. Jessica had been in the midst of throwing a "temper tantrum" and Mrs. George had attempted to "quiet her down." In defiant response to Mrs. George's requests that she "calm herself," Jessica kicked her mother in the abdomen. Mrs. George retaliated by spanking Jessica. Mrs. George then became overwrought with shame and guilt for having "beaten" her daughter.

When the family was seen for the first interview, Mr. George appeared anxious. Mrs. George was tearful and distraught. The couple had had an extremely difficult time getting Jessica to accompany them to meet "the doctor," because she was not "sick." The only way the couple was able to get Jessica to accompany them was to tell her that they were going to a "friend's house for a visit." When Jessica entered the therapist's office and was introduced to "the doctor," she refused to speak. She deliberately walked to the corner of the room and hid behind the therapist's desk, with her back facing her parents. She remained there for the remainder of the session. She refused to speak or to come to her parents when they called. She pretended not to hear or notice them. She did not respond to any overtures made by the therapist. After taking a thorough History of the Presenting Problem and gathering essential material about the marriage via a Couple's Relationship History, we taught Mr. and Mrs. George to identify and conceptualize "Jessica's problems" in behaviorally specific terms that would allow them to make behavioral observations, collect baseline data, identify discriminative stimuli that served as antecedent cues for the problem behaviors, and recognize what persons, events and consequences served to reinforce and maintain the behaviors under consideration.

When the therapist was sure that Mr. and Mrs. George had identified the specific behaviors that were to be the focus of intervention and understood his directions for collecting baseline data and making behavioral observations of Jessica, he gave them SIDCARB, FACES III, IMAGES, PAFS and two copies of the Ideal Child Profile to complete and return to him before the family's next scheduled interview.

Finally, Mr. and Mrs. George were asked to use Jessica's noncompliant behavior during the session as an opportunity to show the therapist how they usually dealt with her "stubbornness." The therapist then directed the couple to have Jessica leave her "hiding place" and accompany them on the sofa. Jessica responded by ignoring her mother's request. Mrs. George then ordered Jessica to come to her. Again, there was no acknowledgment of Mrs. George's command. Jessica continued to stare out of the window. Mr. George then intervened by attempting to coax Jessica, but she still did not comply. Mr. George then offered to buy her a "treat" if she listened to him. Still, there was no movement. At this juncture, Mr. and Mrs. George looked at the therapist, smiled faintly, shrugged their shoulders and proclaimed their helplessness. Mrs.

George appeared to become embarrassed, but then remarked to the therapist how much this scene reminded her of her own struggle with her mother when she was a child. To this, Mr. George added that his wife and his mother-in-law still had the same struggles "to this day."

It was time for the session to end, and the therapist began to escort Mr. and Mrs. George to the door. Again, parental requests, threats, and bribes did not move Jessica. Finally, Mr. George moved to take Jessica by the hand and lead her out of the room. She responded by throwing herself down on the floor and crying. Mr. George then picked her up and carried her, kicking and screaming, from the office. As they descended the stairs, Mr. and Mrs. George could be heard trying to soothe and comfort their daughter.

Mr. and Mrs. George returned to the next session without Jessica, who had refused to come with them. Although the couple had completed all assessment instruments given to them in the previous session and had mailed them to the therapist before returning for their second appointment, Mr. and Mrs. George had not been successful in completing their baseline observations of Jessica's problem behaviors. Mrs. George explained that she was "too harried" taking care of their new son, and Mr. George had worked overtime every evening until 8 or 9 p.m. the previous week. Mr. George's late hours had become a source of tension in the marriage, even though the couple needed the additional money that working overtime provided.

In order to determine what course to follow with Mr. and Mrs. George, the therapist drew upon the information already provided by the couple (i.e., History of the Presenting Problem, Couple's Relationship History, Ideal Child Profiles, the four assessment instruments, and the direct observations of Mr. and Mrs. George as they attempted to get Jessica to follow their directives and obey their commands). A summary of assessment findings is presented below:

ASSESSMENT FINDINGS

SIDCARB. Factor scores for the Georges were:

Factors	Mr. George	Mrs. George
I	60	68
II	65	70
III	68	76

Factor I scores reveal that both Mr. and Mrs. George perceived the couple's exchange system to be out of balance. Mrs. George perceived more inequities and was more dissatisfied with the marriage than her husband. Her major areas of concern, in order of their importance, were: children, sexual relations, and finances. Mr. George's were: finances, children, in-laws, and sexual relations. Both perceived fairly high barriers to separation and divorce. However, Mrs. George had less power in the marriage due to stronger dependence on the marriage, as seen by the strength of her barrier scores.

IMAGES. Scores for this couple did not show many ideal spouse/perceived spouse discrepancies. Overall percentage scores were low: Mr. George = 9% and Mrs. George = 12%. The major areas of discrepancies were Emotional Gratification and Maturity for Mr. George and Spousal Satisfaction and Parent-Sibling Identification for Mrs. George.

FACES III. Scores for perceived and ideal levels of cohesion for Mr. and Mrs. George were:

Mr. George		Mrs. George	
Perceived	*Ideal*	*Perceived*	*Ideal*
Separated	Connected	Disengaged	Enmeshed
(36)	(43)	(30)	(47)

FACES III scores reflect both spouses' desire to develop more intimacy in their marriage. However, Mrs. George's ideal level of cohesion falls in the enmeshed range. This score was interpreted as an overcorrection on Mrs. George's part, a response to the isolation she was feeling at the time. Such isolation is frequently experienced during the postpartum period.

PAFS. Scores showed Mr. and Mrs. George to have achieved median levels of individuation and low levels of both nuclear and intergenerational triangulation. However, both Mr. and Mrs. George showed high levels of intergenerational intimidation, indicating that there still existed some unresolved conflicts with both sets of parents.

Ideal Child Profiles. These data indicated that Jessica was a wanted and planned-for child who was born two years after the couple married. No unusual circumstances appeared to surround her conception, birth, or early rearing until the birth of the couple's second child. Mrs. George's parents, who had been indifferent to Jessica ever since she was born, now appeared to be all consumed with their grandson. Sibling rivalry was obvious, but neither parent knew how to handle Jessica's blatant jealousy and hostility toward her brother. Mrs. George's parents, however, had told Jessica that she was a "bad girl" for not loving her brother and that "God does not like little girls who don't like their brothers."

Jessica's name was chosen by Mr. and Mrs. George because they thought it was "a pretty name." Their son, however, was named after both his grandfathers. His full name was Arthur Percival George. Mrs. George's father, Percival, referred to his grandson as "Arthur P." Both Mr. and Mrs. George agreed that Jessica should be "ladylike" and a "big sister" to her brother and any other children that were to follow. They were very clear about the role of "big sister." A "big sister" did not have parental responsibilities for her younger siblings and was not expected to be a "surrogate" mother; however, she was expected to set an "example" and to "offer guidance" to her younger siblings.

There was little disagreement between Mr. and Mrs. George concerning their conscious perceptions of Jessica. They both saw her as "self-assured," "independent," "autonomous," "aggressive," "active," "negative," "antisocial," "competitive," and "assertive." Their conscious expectations for her also appeared to be congruent. They wanted her to maintain most of the above-mentioned traits and to become less "aggressive" and "antisocial," but there was some disagreement about her being "negative." Mrs. George saw Jessica's ability to say "no" and "to refuse to do what others wanted her to do" as a positive trait, a sign of autonomy and independence. Mr. George, on the other hand, interpreted this behavior as "stubbornness." Mrs. George also believed that a sense of "shame" and "guilt" were important qualities that Jessica should possess. Mr. George, however, believed that "shame" and "guilt" should not be "motivating forces in people's lives." It was assumed, therefore, that there was some degree of incongruence and conflict (at an unconscious level) concerning Mr. and Mrs. George's expectations regarding the role and importance of "shame" and "guilt" in their daughter's personality makeup. In addition, the therapist also speculated that "shame" and "guilt" might be recurrent themes in both Mr. and Mrs. George's personal mythologies, as well as playing a central role in their conjugal mythology.

The fact that one parent (in this case, Mrs. George) identifies major perceived/ideal discrepancies concerning one or more characteristics or traits in a child's Ideal Child Profile, and the other parent (Mr. George) does not see these discrepancies as important or as a cause for concern, but becomes angry or distressed when his/her spouse attempts to foster or shape that particular trait in their child, often indicates that there is unconscious incongruence and probably a power struggle between the parents concerning their ideals for the child. In this case, it appeared that

Mr. and Mrs. George were engaged in a "simple conflict condition," first diagrammed in Figure 6. In this case example, the "simple conflict condition" appeared as in Figure 15.

Whenever incongruities are detected, we assume that they are related to the presenting problem(s) in some way that is not readily apparent. Therefore, it was assumed that Jessica's temper outbursts and her stubborn, defiant, uncooperative, and aggressive behavior toward Mrs. George were related, in some symbolic way, to themes of "shame" and "guilt" in the parents' personal mythologies, as well as in the couple's conjugal mythology. Based upon this assumption and the information provided by the family, the therapist hypothesized that Mr. and Mrs. George's inability to follow through on their first homework assignment (i.e., collecting baseline data and making behavioral observations of Jessica's problem behaviors) might be related to an unverbalized, if not unconscious, struggle between them around these themes.

TESTING CLINICAL ASSUMPTIONS AND HYPOTHESES THROUGH TASK ASSIGNMENT

In order to determine whether Mr. and Mrs. George failed to complete their first assignment because of errors by the therapist in the prescription of the first task, or whether their failure to follow through was actually symptomatic of a deeper, more complex, unconscious conflict, the therapist reviewed the initial assignment with Mr. and Mrs. George. When the therapist was certain that the task had been completely understood and that he had not made any mistakes in prescribing their first homework assignment, the Georges were given the same task (observation and collection of baseline data) a second time. However, this time the therapist explained that if the couple had any difficulty carrying out the assignment a reevaluation of treatment goals and therapeutic procedures would have to take place in the subsequent session. In addition to this homework assignment, Mr. and Mrs. George were asked to complete Family Relationships Histories and Personal Myth Assessment Interviews and to return them to the therapist before their third session.

Once the therapist has gone over the assignment with the parents and is satisfied that all real obstacles to completion have been dealt with and removed, then failure to complete the assignment a second time is seen as "resistance." Before the end of the second session, an indirect approach is introduced. The spouses are asked to think of what situations, incidents, problems, etc., they might encounter that would prevent them from completing the homework assignment. When the couple has dis-

MRS. GEORGE   MR. GEORGE

Ideal Traits = Shame   Incongruent   Ideal Traits = Shameless
& Guilt   & Guiltless
(conscious)   (unconscious)

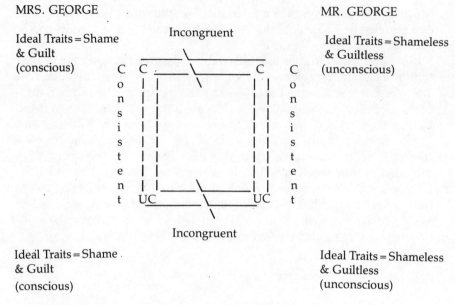

FIGURE 15   Georges' conflicting ideals for Jessica

cussed all possible issues (using the Structured Guidelines for Establishing Functional Communication in Marital Dyads), the second session is concluded.

Mr. and Mrs. George left the second session agreeing to put the behavioral child management plan into action. However, they returned the following week not having been able to follow through. Again, Mrs. George had become "overwhelmed" with taking care of their son, and Mr. George had worked overtime four out of five evenings. Therefore, a reevaluation of treatment goals and procedures was undertaken. The options presented to Mr. and Mrs. George, by the therapist were: (a) to discontinue treatment, (b) to accept referral to another therapist if they perceived a client × therapist, client × method or client × method × therapist mismatch,[1] (c) to explore some of the possible reasons for their inability to follow through with the homework assignments. Mr. and Mrs. George decided upon the latter alternative.

---

[1]Couples and family systems may be unable to progress in therapy for a number of reasons that cannot be attributed to therapist errors or incompetence or to client resistances. For example, therapy may get bogged down because of:

Exploring the "Ideal Child":
Projections, Identifications and Projective Identifications

We have developed a technique used in our initial effort to detriangulate the "identified patient" and to dislodge him/her from the scapegoat role. Essentially, this procedure has four foci. The first is to have both parents become aware of their projections so that they can begin to see their child in a more realistic manner. The second is to sensitize them to issues of transference and projective identification in their dealings with the identified patient. The third is to help both parents recognize when they are inducing the child to play out significant roles and scripts associated with specific themes from their personal and/or conjugal mythologies. Finally, when this technique is used with all family members present, its goal is the modification of the consensus role image allotted to the identified patient.

In using this intervention strategy, the therapist draws upon material gathered during assessment to guide and direct family discussions and influence family interaction processes. Family Relationships Histories and Family Myth Assessment Interviews from both parents are invaluable sources of information about the identified patient's possible role in his/her parents' personal and conjugal mythologies.

We begin exploration of the parents' expectations for the identified patient (i.e., perceived/ideal discrepancies) with a process similar to the one used to help couples discuss perceived/ideal discrepancies concerning their ideal spouses. Instead of using IMAGES, the parents are asked to follow the Structured Guidelines for Establishing Functional Communication in Marital Dyads to discuss ideal/perceived discrepancies reported on their Ideal Child Profiles. Initially, the therapist directs the parents to discuss Ideal Child Profile item discrepancies that appear to be directly related to the presenting problem behaviors. Next, the therapist helps the parents move to discussions of items that do not appear to be centrally associated with the child's problem behaviors, but represent consciously acknowledged differences and incongruities between the parents concerning specific personality characteristics, behavioral traits,

---

(a) Therapist × client system mismatch (incompatibilities).
(b) Clinical method × client system mismatch.
(c) Therapist × clinical method × client system mismatch.
(d) Therapist × family life cycle stage mismatch.
(e) Clinical method × family life cycle stage mismatch.
(f) Therapist × clinical method × family life cycle stage mismatch.
(g) Therapist × clinical method × family life cycle stage × client system mismatch.

attitudes, or affects. Finally, the therapist helps the parents become aware of those differences (incongruities) that are hypothesized to be the source of unconscious conflict between them. As each item is discussed by the parents, the therapist asks them to consider a number of questions. For example:

1. Why is this particular personality characteristic, behavioral trait, etc., so important to you?
2. What special (symbolic) meaning does this characteristic, trait, etc., hold for you?
3. Are there any persons in your family of origin who possess this trait or exhibit these behaviors?
4. To what extent do you possess this particular trait or exhibit these particular behaviors?
5. When your child exhibits (or fails to exhibit) these particular behaviors or personality characteristics, what memories or personal experiences are brought to mind?
6. When your child exhibits (or fails to exhibit) a particular behavior or characteristic what feelings does his/her behavior trigger in you?

With Mr. and Mrs. George, explorations of their "ideals" first began with discussions about Jessica's "stubborn," "uncooperative," "disrespectful," and "defiant" behavior. Early in these discussions, it became clear that Mrs. George had ambivalent feelings about Jessica's behavior and that this ambivalence had its roots in Mrs. George's own embattled relationship with her mother. Mrs. George became aware of her alternating and sometimes simultaneous identifications with Jessica in the role of "stubborn, uncooperative, disrespectful and defiant child" and with her own mother in the role of "domineering mother." She also became aware of projecting these ambivalently valanced qualities onto her daughter, with her inconsistent reactions to them depending upon her own identification (herself or her mother) at the time of the confrontation with Jessica.

When she identified with Jessica as a child herself, Jessica was permitted to "win" in her "struggle" with Mrs. George. Whenever Jessica "won," however, Mrs. George's identification with her own mother emerged and she felt "defeated" by her daughter. When Mrs. George identified predominantly with her own mother, Jessica was perceived as Mrs. George's own bad or negative self as a child. Jessica's "stubbornness," "defiance," etc., were then perceived as undesirable qualities that deserved to be punished. Here projective identification took over, and

Mrs. George would begin to treat Jessica as her own mother had often treated her (i.e., using physical punishment) during such confrontations. Once physical punishment was applied, however, Mrs. George would experience both identifications simultaneously. She would feel fear, shame, and intimidation (her daughter and herself as beaten children) and guilt and remorse (herself and her mother as child beaters). It is easy to understand why Mrs. George felt "overwhelmed" and frequently found herself immobilized.

Mr. George's insights into his handling of Jessica also proved to be enlightening. He, as a child and adolescent, "never" gave his parents "any trouble." He was the "perfect, overachieving, model son," his parents "only child." Three issues surfaced for Mr. George: (a) his unspoken admiration of Jessica's "stubbornness," even though it caused problems in the family; (b) his identification with Jessica as the "stubborn" child he had always wanted to be but did not have the "guts" to become; and (c) his belief that Mrs. George was overly harsh with Jessica, much like his mother had been with him. Essentially, Jessica was seen as acting out (in the true psychoanalytic sense of the term) Mr. George's unresolved conflicts with his mother.

The relationship between "stubbornness, defiance, disrespect, and uncooperativeness" and the parents' disagreement about "shame and guilt" in their daughter's personality makeup became clearer as the therapist helped the couple move through this process. Both Mr. and Mrs. George's parents had used (and were still using with their children and grandchildren) shaming and guilt-inducing techniques, in addition to physical punishment, to bring about conformity. Mr. George's vehement opposition to his wife's use of shame and guilt was seen, by the therapist, as having strong transferential components and some elements of projection of Mr. George's own superego onto his wife.

As an adolescent and young woman, Mrs. George experienced severe guilt reactions whenever she committed any sexual transgression. Her guilt was what "kept her a virgin" until she met Mr. George. As a matter of fact, it was the guilt that both she and Mr. George experienced in their premarital sexual relations that propelled the couple into marriage before either spouse had successfully separated and individuated from his/her family of origin.

Struggles to separate from a feared and domineering mother were central themes in the personal mythologies of Mr. and Mrs. George. "Guilt as a motivator of behavior" was also a theme shared by both spouses and had become a central theme in the couple's conjugal mythology.

Exploring each parent's "ideal" for Jessica, tracing the origins and meanings of specific traits and personality characteristics and unearthing the unresolved conflict themes associated with them was all that was needed to help Mr. and Mrs. George work cooperatively as a team to bring their daughter's problem behaviors under control through the use of behavioral management techniques. Once Jessica's problem behaviors were extinguished, Mr. and Mrs. George were asked if they would like to continue treatment to deal with any of the problem areas identified by SIDCARB, FACES III, IMAGES, and PAFS. They elected to postpone additional couple's work.

THE ROLE OF THE THERAPIST:
MODIFYING IDEALS AND EDITING THEMES

Throughout this exploration process, the therapist used a number of interventions previously described in this volume. For example, psychodynamic interpretations were applied to help Mr. and Mrs. George understand those identifications, projections, and transference distortions that were preventing them from setting limits with their daughter. Positive reframing was used to produce modifications in each parent's ideal child image, to reconstruct those personal relationship themes (between Mr. and Mrs. George and significant others) that they were trying to relive and rework through their dealings with Jessica, and to alter Mr. and Mrs. George's perceptions and interpretations of those current life situations and circumstances that were related to Jessica's presenting problems. In order to modify each spouse's perception of his/her own parents' actions (e.g., the use of physical punishment, shame and guilt as disciplinary techniques), reattribution of responsibility was employed.

TECHNIQUES FOR MODIFYING THE CONSENSUS ROLE IMAGE
WITH SCHOOL-AGED CHILDREN AND YOUNG ADULTS LEAVING HOME

Families with school-aged children, adolescents and young adults still living at home who are unable or unwilling to use behavioral contracting to resolve parent-child differences can be dealt with in several ways.

As was the case for Mr. and Mrs. George, parents can be asked to discuss their differences and incongruities identified through their responses to the Ideal Child Profiles in the presence of the identified patient and all family members who have come together for the consultation. Using the Rules for Establishing Functional Communication in

Families as a basic guideline for such discussion, the therapist encourages all participants present, especially the identified patient, to ask questions of the parents and other family members regarding any issue that comes up in the session. Here again, the therapist takes on the role of enabler and guides the parents' discussion by posing the six questions outlined earlier. These same questions (with appropriate modifications) are then presented to all family members for their consideration and exploration.

As the family discussions unfold, the various and frequently conflicting expectations, transference distortions, and projective identifications that have been heaped upon the "identified patient" become more and more apparent. It is at this juncture that the therapist draws upon what has been said by all family members to positively reframe the identified patient's behavior as his/her attempt to fulfill both parents' (and possibly some of the siblings') ideals and expectations. The therapist then adds that the "identified patient" believes that, if he/she is able to play out all roles and scripts assigned to him/her by all family members, the family unit will be preserved and everyone will be protected. The therapist also interjects that, since there can never be total agreement between parents and among all family members and since incongruities are inevitable in all families, the identified patient's behavior often appears "bizarre," "incomprehensible," "bad," or "mad" to family members as he/she attempts to play out these conflicting expectations, roles and scripts.

Next, the therapist adds that frequently when a person attempts to fulfill a number of conflicting expectations and roles, he/she begins to experience overwhelming anxiety and stress. He explains that the person who is caught up in such a dilemma may be "unable to cope" and may "give up." This giving up manifests itself as "symptomatic behavior."

Finally, the therapist explains that another outcome of such "role overload" is that the person may never have the opportunity to develop his/her own unique identity, because he/she has become too absorbed in "taking care of the family." When the person realizes that he/she has "sacrificed" his/her own identify for the sake of "maintaining family stability" he/she may attempt to discover his/her own identity by "experimenting" with new and different behaviors and roles that other family members do not recognize or understand. The therapist explains that these "new and experimental role behaviors" are often seen by the rest of the family as the person's problem behaviors.

The reader can see that the above interpretations and positive reframes offer the family members a variety of alternative explanations of the identified patient's behavior. The references to "role overload," stress, anxiety, family protection, and caretaking may be readily understood by many family members and thereby increase their ability and willingness to empathize with the identified patient. By presenting family members with a variety of interpretations from which to choose, the therapist makes it possible for each family member to select an explanation that fits within his/her personal mythology. The parental subsystem is also presented with a number of explanations from which to choose. Therefore, the identified patient's behavior can also be seen as fitting into any number of conjugal themes and unconsciously negotiated collusive parental contracts.

The therapist can also use his/her understanding of the parents' personal mythologies, conjugal themes, family submyths and family group themes to positively reframe the identified patient's behavior. It has been our experience to find that positive reframes that employ information gathered from the personal myths and themes of family members are rarely, if ever, met with resistance. Some brief examples of how this is done are presented below.

A family consisting of a mother, 37, a father, 39, and two children, 12 and 14, came in for treatment. The presenting problem was the 14-year-old daughter's obsessive ruminations about death and her compulsive door locking each evening before bedtime. Personal mythologies of both parents revealed themes of unresolved mourning. A central theme in this couple's conjugal mythology had to do with their unspoken fear (an unconscious desire) that their daughter might become pregnant, out of wedlock, and thereby recreate the circumstances leading up to their own marriage.

Positively reframing the daughter's obsessive thoughts about death as this child's attempt to help both her parents grieve for the loss of their own parents resulted in a gradual reduction of these obsessions.

By having both parents discuss their daughter's compulsive door locking (using the six questions outlined earlier to guide the discussion) and by encouraging both children to ask them questions they thought to be important, these parents finally divulged their "secret" of mother's out-of-wedlock pregnancy and the subsequent birth of the identified patient. Once the parents were able to talk about their fears that their daughter might become pregnant if she were to know about her mother's premarital pregnancy, the therapist interpreted the daughter's compulsive door locking as her way of "reassuring" her parents that she would "lock out any sexual advances by remaining a virgin until after she was married." With this interpretation and positive reframe, the daughter's compulsive door locking began to subside. The more she and her mother were able to discuss sexual matters, the less need there was for inappropriate door locking.

Another family presented itself for treatment because of the 16-year-old son's aggressive behavior at school and failing grades. This rural family was made up of a mother, 39, her two daughters, ages 21 and 19, and the identified patient. This was a close-knit family with strong kinship ties throughout the county. The mother's two older sisters were frequent visitors to her home and the mother's mother (the patient's maternal grandmother) lived not far from them. Both aunts and the grandmother had been overly involved in the boy's upbringing after "his father deserted the family" when he was three years old.

Family Relationships Histories and Personal Myth Assessments of the mother and her daughters revealed that they shared a number of themes about male-female relationships that constituted submyths binding the females together in a three-generation coalition consisting of grandmother, her three daughters, and their female children. They shared the belief that men were "weak and undependable" people who would say whatever they needed to say in order to get "into a girl's pants" and then leave her "with the problem." Another submyth which went hand in hand with the belief that all men were "undependable," was the "self-sufficiency of women."

The son's behavior at school and his poor academic performance were not considered to be major problems by his mother and grandmother. As a matter of fact, aggression and anti intellectualism are often thought to constitute desirable character traits for males living in small, isolated, rural mountain communities (Bagarozzi, 1982c). This boy and his mother had been referred to their local school district's psychoeducational facility for testing and evaluation because the teachers in his high school had been unable to manage his assaultive behavior. The family was seen by a two-women co-therapy team that was part of a larger training group of agency clinicians who were being supervised by the first author.

In the family's first assessment interview it became obvious that both his sisters and his mother depended heavily upon the son's financial contributions to the family and his physical protection. As a physically strong and emotionally dependable male, not an undependable weakling to be scorned by his mother, sisters, aunts and grandmother, he was the "exception to the rule." In this family system, his behavior was consistent with his "consensus role image." Psychological testing revealed that his I.Q. was considerably higher than average; actually, his scores placed him in the superior category.

A strategy used by the therapists to gain entrance into this family system was to disclose that they, too, had been divorced (deserted by men) and that they both had been able to complete their graduate degrees prior to remarrying (self-sufficiency). These disclosures permitted the therapists to gain immediate rapport, to build trust, and to foster identification with the mother, daughters, and key female figures in the mother's family of origin.

Once the system had been joined in this fashion, the therapists used their relationship with mother and daughters to begin the process of modifying the son's consensus role image. Pointing to his superior I.Q. as another example of his being an "exception to the rule," the therapists suggested that "cultivating his brains" might be beneficial to the family and someday to his own wife and children. The therapists explained that if he used his "brains" to get a good job, his family, and eventually his wife and children, would not suffer. In order to achieve these goals, however, he would have to succeed at school and some changes would have to be made in his aggressive behavior. The therapists mused about how such changes would really make him an "exception to the rule."

In this treatment strategy, the consensus role image is modified first and the identified patient's behavior is shaped to approximate the new consensus role image. Here we see that the essential submyth remains the same, but the identified patient's behavior, although modified, is still perceived as fitting into the role attributed to him/her.

In severely dysfunctional family systems, the identified patient becomes the focal point of both parents' unfulfilled expectations and unmet needs. As we said earlier, transference and projective identification play a major role in this process. Some of the most common, but by no means the only, dysfunctional expectations that fall upon the identified patient require him/her to: (a) fulfill one or both parents' unmet needs (e.g., nurturance, love, praise, admiration) that "should have" been satisfied by their own parents or significant others, (b) correct all wrongs and injustices that the parent or parents have suffered during their lives, (c) augment the parents' self-esteem or provide them with self-esteem by achieving for them what they could not achieve or were prevented from achieving by significant others, (d) become an extension of a parent who has poorly defined ego boundaries, a diffuse identity, or a fragmented self, or who experiences the child's attempts to separate and individuate as a threat of abandonment, (e) align with one parent against the other in marital conflicts and power disputes, and (f) take the place of a spouse who is physically absent or emotionally unavailable.

In the last example, we see how the identified patient's primary roles were those of fulfilling his mother's unmet needs for protection and security, correcting the wrongs done to his mother and sisters by his father, and taking the place of his father. Once mother and grandmother were convinced that the boy's nonaggressive behavior with peers and improved academic performance at school would crystallize and solidify their consensus role image of him even further and that these new behaviors would benefit them, as well as future generations, they began to encourage him to "quit cutting up at school and get an education so as not to be like your daddy." In a matter of weeks, his behavior improved. Follow-up, at the end of the academic year, showed that he had "settled down and was doing his schoolwork."

16

Using Ritual Prescriptions and Rites of Passage to Edit Family Themes and Submyths

O UR USE OF RITUAL prescription differs significantly from the work of most mainstream strategic therapists (e.g., Fisch, Weakland, & Segal, 1983; Keim, Lentine, Keim, & Madanes, 1987; Papp, 1983; Selvini Palazzoli, 1986; Selvini Palazzoli, Boscolo, Cecchin, & Prata, 1977, 1978; Selvini Palazzoli, Cirillo, Selvini, & Sorrentino, 1989) and is in keeping with our theoretical position. *We devise and prescribe rituals that are based upon material gathered from the personal, conjugal, and/or family group myths of our clients' own mythological themes and systems. The ritual prescribed must always make sense within the client's or family's own system of meaning. Giving invariant prescriptions to all families or assigning ritual tasks that are designed to change interaction sequences among family members, but which are not based upon the family's shared system of meaning, is not in keeping with our theoretical stance.* These methods may be used, however, in those situations where the therapist may have only one or two opportunities to see a family and practical considerations make it impossible to collect the information and conduct the empirical assessments needed to formulate prescriptions specific to the family's themes and myths.

THE FRANK FAMILY

Mr. Frank, a college professor, and his wife sought family therapy regarding the unacceptable behavior of their 17-year-old daughter, Christy. Christy had always been a "difficult child," but recently her behavior had become worse. She had been dating several boys, coming home after curfew, smoking cigarettes, and drinking. For the latter behavior, she had been "grounded" by her father. Her mother, on the other hand, believed that grounding Christy had been too harsh a punishment. The precipitating event that brought the family into therapy was Christy's most recent and most serious transgression. Two days before Mrs. Frank called for an appointment she had discovered that Christy had sneaked out of her room during the evening and spent the night with a group of friends. Mr. Frank became enraged when he found out about the incident and threatened to beat his daughter severely if the incident was ever repeated.

Christy, the only daughter and the oldest of three children, bore a striking resemblance to her mother. Mrs. Frank proudly admitted that they were frequently mistaken for sisters. Mrs. Frank, age 37, did not look her age. She appeared to be in her late twenties and dressed in the latest fashions to accentuate her youthful appearance. Christy, on the other hand, looked much older than her years. Anyone seeing mother and daughter together might think them both to be in their twenties. Mr. Frank, although only four years older than his wife, appeared to be in his mid to late forties. He was balding, overweight, and unkempt in his personal appearance. The couple's two sons accompanied the family on its first visit. Both boys, Peter, 14, and Paul, 9, appeared to be appropriate in their manner and dress. Neither son was considered to be a problem.

MR AND MRS. FRANK'S COUPLE'S
RELATIONSHIP HISTORY: SUMMARY

Mr. and Mrs. Frank met while they were both in college. Mrs. Frank initiated their dating. Mr. Frank, who had virtually no experience with women, was flattered by Mrs. Frank's attention. He could not believe that anyone so beautiful would even look at him. Mrs. Frank saw her husband-to-be as a way out of her previous existence. She came from an impoverished farm family where all children were expected to work in the fields. Education beyond grammar school was not encouraged. Mrs. Frank "rebelled" against her own father by going to high school and working in nearby towns in order to save enough money to afford one year of college. At 17, she left home for college, where she met Mr. Frank during the second semester of her freshman year. Mr. Frank, from a stable, moderately successful farm family, "fell in love at first sight" with his future wife. Although he knew that he was not attractive, he knew that he could "teach her things" and "provide well" for her and their children. The couple was married after dating for approximately three months. Christy was born the following year, while Mr. Frank was in graduate school.

Mr. and Mrs. Frank began having sexual intercourse on their first date. Mr. Frank was a virgin when the couple met. Mrs. Frank told her husband-to-be that she had had "some sexual experience" before she met him but did not go into any detail about her past. Mr. Frank was ecstatic after his first sexual encounter with Mrs. Frank. Mrs. Frank, conversely, was matter-of-fact about the incident. She knew that "putting out" was a good way to keep up Mr. Frank's interest. While she did not experience much pleasure or satisfaction in her sexual relationship with Mr. Frank, she "faked" enjoyment and interest.

Mrs. Frank's mother was pleased to hear of her plans to marry. Her father, who had not spoken to her since she left home to attend college, did not attend their wedding. Mr. Frank's parents were relieved, because they had been concerned that their son would never marry.

When Mrs. Frank was asked to describe any "legacy" that she might have brought into her marriage from her family of origin, she began to cry uncontrollably. In the privacy of an individual interview, she was able to reveal, for the first time in her life, that she had been an incest victim. Sexual intercourse with her father had begun when she was approximately eight years old and continued until she was a junior in high school. At that time, she moved out of her parents' home and took up residence with her maternal grandmother, ostensibly to care for the ailing woman.

The major themes in Mrs. Frank's personal mythology directly associated with the family's presenting problem were:

1. Men cannot be trusted; all men want is sex. They will lie and cheat and promise you anything just to get what they want from you. If you give them what they want, maybe they will leave you alone and maybe they will not. They may just keep coming back for more.
2. All men must pay for what my father did to me. I will use them every chance I get to get what I want. Men owe me my childhood and my adolescence, because my father took them from me.
3. I must make certain that my daughter is not robbed of her childhood and adolescence. It is my duty to protect her from her father. I will stand up for her like a sister, because none of my siblings (or my mother) ever stood up for me or protected me from my father.
4. Through my daughter, I can live vicariously. I can recapture my youth and have the fun and freedom denied to me by my father.

When Mr. Frank was born, his mother was 37, his father 42, and he had a 15-year-old-sister. Needless to say, conception was accidental. Born with congenital heart disease, Mr. Frank was closely watched and supervised by his mother and sister. His first memory of his family of origin was described as follows: "I am about three years old, and I am sitting in my playpen watching my mother get dressed. My sister is standing nearby, watching me. I remember how beautiful my mother looked. I feel safe and secure."

Mr. Frank was rarely, if ever, allowed to roughhouse or to play sports with boys his own age. He could not remember ever having a close male friend or chum while he was still a boy. Most of his free time during adolescence was spent reading and "cultivating" his mind. Intellectually superior to most of his classmates, he preferred the company of adults. Treated as special by his family and teachers because of his heart condition and intelligence, Mr. Frank missed out on much of the socialization that takes place within one's peer group. He did not learn how to "share things with others," had no opportunity to learn how to compete or to learn how to cooperate and collaborate with people his own age (Sullivan, 1953). He was socially inept and interpersonally incompetent. His mother and sister were still selecting his clothes for him when he entered college.

Mr. Frank sincerely believed that his mother and sister loved him dearly, even though he sometimes got angry at them for overprotecting him. He admitted, however, that when he was younger he relied very heavily upon them for protection from boys his own age who mocked him and called him "mamma's boy." He also believed that his father, who had been overjoyed at having a son after so many years, was very disappointed when he learned of his son's congenital heart problem and that his son would "never be normal." Mr. Frank said that "upon hearing this news from the doctors, my father abandoned me and left all the childrearing up to my mother and sister." Mr. Frank was named after his mother's brother, who had died of a heart attack several years before Mr. Frank was born. Mr. Frank could not determine what his father's hopes and desires had been for him as he was growing up. Their relationship was distant, at best. Mr. Frank knew that his mother wanted him to become a teacher so that he could further "cultivate" his mind and have financial security. Being a traveling salesman, like his father, was "out of the question."

Mr. Frank's role in his family was one that stayed with him throughout his life. He was "special" and "sickly" and shunned anyone or any group of people who did not treat him that way. Early in life, Mr. Frank learned that he could receive special treatment from his teachers, and pursuing an academic career allowed him to continue in his role as a "special one." Everyone in Mr. Frank's family of origin went out of the way to avoid upsetting Mr. Frank. Unpleasant events and occurrences were kept from him. The expression of strong emotions was taboo. The only family secret that Mr. Frank was able to identify was his suspicion that he might not be his father's child. He suspected, but had no "proof," that his mother might have been unfaithful to his father during his father's long absences on the road.

The major themes from Mr. Frank's personal mythology that seemed to have a direct bearing on the presenting problem were:

1. I am a very special person, because I am intelligent and sickly. My fragile health entitles me to special treatment from everyone. If you don't treat me as special, I will have nothing to do with you. Everyone's needs, no matter who that person is, are secondary to my own needs. People can do whatever they desire as long as they don't infringe upon my needs or expect me to go out of my way for them.

2. Women are strong, dominant, protective, and assertive. However, these qualities can also be used to control, dominate, and manipulate men. This is the price one pays for being dependent upon them.

3. I am totally inadequate as a man. I don't know how to relate to other men. I feel incompetent when I am around men. However, I long for a close, intimate relationship with a father figure. Sometimes this longing frightens me, because I think I may be homosexual.

4. The only time I felt adequate as a father was when my children were little. They looked up to me and thought I was someone special, especially my daughter. I was very important in her eyes. I was special to her like I was to my sister. Now she does not pay any attention to me. I am no longer special to her.

SIGNIFICANT CONJUGAL THEMES AND CENTRAL UNCONSCIOUS AGREEMENTS

Clinically, Mr. Frank manifests the dynamics of a narcissistic personality disorder and Mrs. Frank presents as having a borderline personality organization. When one compares the central themes from the personal mythologies of these two spouses, the majority appears to be either independent or complementary rather than competing or antagonistic. If one were to speculate about the mutually protective, unconscious, quid pro quo contractual agreements devised by Mr. and Mrs. Frank to permit full expression of both independent and complementary themes, the arrangements might take the following forms:

Mrs. Frank:

(theme #1): Men cannot be trusted; all men want is sex. If you give them what they want, maybe they will leave you alone or they just might keep coming back for more.

(theme #2): All men must pay for what my father did to me. Men owe me my childhood and adolescence.

Mr. Frank:

(theme #3): I am totally inadequate as a man. I don't know how to relate to other men and I feel incompetent when I am around them. However, I long for a close, intimate relationship with a father figure. Sometimes this longing frightens me, because I think I may be homosexual.

Unconscious Contract #1

Mrs. Frank: I agree to give you whatever you want sexually. You can be sexual with me anytime you wish. I know that this will make you feel competent as a man and special because I am so beautiful and you can have me all to yourself. I also agree to be sexually faithful to you. I will not cheat on you. I will not do what you think your mother did to your father, and you will not have to face your fears of homosexuality.

In exchange for this:

Mr. Frank: I will repay you for being sexual with me and bolstering my self-esteem and feelings of competence by giving you whatever you ask for, by allowing you to behave as an adolescent and sister to our daughter. This will give you the opportunity to relive your childhood and adolescence.

Mrs. Frank

(theme #4): Through my daughter, I can live vicariously, I can recapture my youth and have the fun and freedom denied to me by my father when I was growing up.

Mr. Frank

(*theme #4*): The only time I felt adequate and competent as a father was when my children were little. They looked up to me as someone special, especially my daughter. Now, she does not pay any attention to me. I am no longer special in her eyes (*theme #1*).

Unconscious Contract #2

Mrs. Frank: I agree to encourage our daughter to look up to you and see you as special. In this way, we will treat you as your mother and sister treated you.

In exchange for this:

Mr. Frank: I will allow you to try to recapture your youth by living vicariously through our daughter so long as you continue to encourage her to treat me as special and see me as a good father.

As often happens when a conjugal agreement has as its central focus a consensus role image for a particular child, the contract begins to break down and fall apart when the child is no longer willing to play out the assigned consensus role image.[1] It is at this point that families experience the crisis that brings them into therapy. This is what appears to have happened with Mr. and Mrs. Frank concerning their unconscious conjugal contract #2. The older Christy became, the less she was influenced by Mrs. Frank and the more she rebelled against the consensus role image that required her to treat her father as if he were special and her mother as if she were a sister. As this second contract began to unravel, two themes that had not been associated (Mr. Frank's theme #2 and Mrs. Frank's theme #3) came into direct, conscious conflict.

During assessment, both spouses' Ideal Child Profiles for Christy showed several major perceived/ideal discrepancies. Mr. Frank identified perceived/ideal discrepancies in the following areas: activity, assertion, dominance, and respect. He saw Christy as becoming too active, assertive, and domineering, and insufficiently respectful of her father (Mr. Frank's theme #2).

---

[1]Some aspects of "adolescent rebellion" in all families can be understood as the teenager's attempt to throw off parental projections and to free himself/herself from the confines of a static "consensus role image." This "rebellion" is considered to be an important part of identity formation.

Mrs. Frank, conversely, did not perceive Christy's activity and assertiveness as domineering, and she did not interpret her daughter's "speaking up for herself and saying what was on her mind" as disrespectful of Mr. Frank. As a matter of fact, Mrs. Frank had always encouraged her daughter to "stick up for herself" (Mrs. Frank's theme #3). Mrs. Frank identified only one perceived/ideal discrepancy that she found particularly distressing. This was directly related to her daughter's not treating her as if she were her sister. Mrs. Frank was very upset because Christy no longer "trusted" her, and she, in turn, was beginning not to "trust" her daughter. This breakdown in trust reached its peak when Christy sneaked out of the house without telling Mrs. Frank. It is important to note, however, that Mrs. Frank admitted that she would have given Christy permission to stay out most of the night if Christy had asked; in addition, she would have kept this incident hidden from Mr. Frank. The breach of trust between mother and daughter put an end to the submyth that maintained a long-standing mother-daughter coalition (i.e., women must protect each other, because men cannot be trusted).

Editing Dysfunctional Themes, Submyths and Portions of Family Group Myths through the Use of Theme/Myth-Specific Ritual Prescriptions

When one sets out to edit a family theme, submyth, or family group myth, one must decide whether to deal directly with the content material the family has presented, to make use of more symbolic and indirect means of editing, or to employ both strategies simultaneously. We agree with Seltzer (1989) and Van der Hart et al. (1989) that such editing should be designed to deal with both the concrete, behavioral, and interactional plane of family culture and the symbolic and ideational world of the family's experiences.

The first step in this process is to identify the theme, submyth, or family group myth that is contributing to the maintenance of the presenting problem and to understand how the identified problem is related both to the process and to family structure. Then, using our understanding of the personal themes of all family members, the conjugal themes and unconscious contracts of the spouses/parents, and the data collected throughout the family assessment process, we decide what information is most appropriate to use in designing a ritual prescription. Rituals can be constructed to edit family members' behaviors, roles, scripts, or entire themes, depending on the therapist's goals. Once the prescription has been formulated, a rationale (in the form of a psychodynamic interpretation, positive reframe, reattribution of responsibility, etc.) is devised that the therapist himself/herself accepts as valid and believes will be acceptable to the family. Each ritual prescription is presented to the family at the close of the session.

In the Frank family, several aspects of the family structure and process were identified as contributing to Christy's behavior. Two areas of structure and process in need of modification were:

1. A structural change was needed in the area of the parental subsystem because the husband-wife coalition had broken down and had been replaced by a cross-generational, mother-daughter coalition.
2. Closely related to this structural change was a process change that had to take place in the way that Mr. and Mrs. Frank functioned as a couple, once their parental coalition was reestablished. This modification in their behavior as a couple must insure that they were able to work cooperatively as a team and function effectively as an executive subsystem that could bring their daughter's behavior under control.

Once these two changes had been successfully implemented, intervention strategies would have to be introduced to strengthen the parental alliance and permit Christy to become more autonomous and independent (in a less destructive and more socially acceptable manner).

The structural change in the parental subsystem was brought about through the prescription of a ritual that made use of information gathered from the Family Relationships Histories of both Mr. and Mrs. Frank and their Ideal Child Profiles of Christy.

Treatment commenced with the symbolic separation of the generations and a reinforcement of the parental subsystem and husband-wife coalition. Christy and her two brothers were asked to wait outside the therapist's office while the therapist met separately with Mr. and Mrs. Frank. The therapist explained to the children that "mother and father have special and private aspects of their relationship that are not, and should not, be shared with their children." The children were then escorted into the waiting room by the therapist, who told them that he would return for them when a "family discussion was appropriate."

Next, the therapist met with Mr. and Mrs. Frank. Using the Structured Guidelines for Establishing Functional Communication in Marital Dyads and guided by the therapist, who helped them focus their discussion (using the six questions described in Chapter 15, p. 244), Mr. and Mrs.

Frank shared their thoughts and feelings about Christy's behavior, the perceived/ideal discrepancies identified by each spouse, and the incongruities noted for any behaviors that were associated with the presenting problem (i.e., activity, assertion, dominance, respect, and trust).

Shortly after their marriage, Mrs. Frank told her husband about the abuse she had experienced at the hands of her father, but the couple had avoided discussing these incidents in any detail or in any depth. They never considered that Christy's behavior might be related to Mrs. Frank's personal themes of mistrust of men, retribution against offending males, attempts to recapture her childhood and adolescence, and protection of her daughter. Similarly, they did not see how Mr. Frank's need to be a "special person" in his family's eyes, his self-image of inadequacy and poor health, and his dependence upon women whom he perceived as strong, dominant, and protective had been preventing him from taking an active part in family life and effectively disciplining his daughter.

Using information that surfaced during this discussion, the therapist reframed Mr. Frank's lack of assertion and involvement with Christy as his "nonverbal, unconscious message of assurance" to his wife that he would never "violate or abuse" his daughter as Mrs. Frank's father had done. His behavior, therefore, was a demonstration of his "love, caring and concern." His noninvolvement with his daughter was also reframed as "the inner strength of personal restraint." Mrs. Frank's confiding in her husband was used as "evidence" to show her "trust of Mr. Frank." Mrs. Frank trusted only one man throughout her whole life, her husband. The therapist remarked that this was certainly an indication that he was "special in her eyes."

After these positive reframes had taken hold, the therapist asked Mr. and Mrs. Frank to decide upon acceptable standards for Christy's behavior, to agree upon negative contingencies (punishments and sanctions) that would be instituted if she did not comply, and to decide upon a mutually acceptable procedure for setting limits with her. In order to strengthen the informational boundary that had been erected between the generations in this session, the therapist suggested that Mr. and Mrs. Frank continue to keep Mrs. Frank's experiences with her own father "secret" from Christy and their sons, since divulging this material at this time in Christy's life would serve no constructive purpose. In order to reinforce the structural modifications that were beginning to take place in the session, the children were called back into the therapist's office and told that their parents had decided upon a plan of action to deal with Christy's behavior. Mr. and Mrs. Frank were then asked to inform Christy about the decisions they had made concerning their expectations for her behavior. Negative consequences for noncompliance were explained and positive reinforcers for satisfactory performance were agreed upon.

The children were then informed that their parents would be attending the next few therapy sessions without them so that they could work on some issues that were important to their relationship as husband and wife—issues that were their parents' private concerns.

The therapist recommended that Mr. and Mrs. Frank attend the next few sessions without their children, unless they had difficulty following through on the agreed-upon assignments. The rationale given to Mr. and Mrs. Frank was that the therapist thought they should discuss a number of issues (identified on SIDCARB) that would be inappropriate to bring up in their children's presence. Again, this tactic was used to draw a line of demarcation between the parental and children subsystems.

At the next session, Mr. and Mrs. Frank had nothing significant to report about their daughter's behavior. Christy appeared to be complying with the contractual agreements without too much resistance. To this report, the therapist responded matter-of-factly and suggested that Christy's undesirable behavior might very well resurface in the near future. He added, "Sometimes it gets worse before it gets better."

This session and the next two meetings with the Franks were spent devising a series of ritual exercises and homework assignments which were designed to: (a) crystalize their parental coalition and strengthen the informational boundary surrounding the husband-wife subsystem, (b) edit portions of central themes in each spouse's personal mythology, and (c) introduce slight modifications and alterations in pivotal clauses of the couple's unconscious contractual agreements.

Mr. and Mrs. Frank were asked to set aside two one-and-a-half-hour time periods on two separate days of each week. They were to make sure that they could arrange for these time periods to be free from any distractions or interruptions from their children. These periods were to be strictly for Mr. and Mrs. Frank. Each time period was to be divided into three separate segments. These were: individual preparations time (segment I), couple sharing time (segment II), and parental appraisal time (segment III).

During individual preparation time, Mr. and Mrs. Frank were instructed to prepare for their couple meeting by spending time alone, in separate rooms of their home. During this time, Mr. and Mrs. Frank prepared for their couple meeting by engaging in progressive relaxation exercises. Audio cassette recordings of preprogrammed progressive relaxation instructions and procedures were used for this purpose. When each spouse felt that he/she had achieved complete relaxation, he/she would begin to recite, subvocally, a personal chant. This chant was made up of a series of statements about the self and the self-in-relationship to his/her spouse and his/her children. These statements had been developed specifically for each spouse during separate, individual sessions with the therapist.

The unique personal chant developed for each spouse actually represents a cognitive response chain designed to edit certain portions of personal themes and unconscious collusive agreements between the spouses.

The two personal chants developed for Mrs. Frank are reproduced below:

Chant I

- I can trust my husband to be honest with me.
- I can trust my husband because he is not like my father.
- It is unfair to hold my husband responsible for things he did not do.
- It is unfair to hold my husband responsible for things done to me by my father.
- My husband is not my father.

Chant II

- My husband loves me for who I am.
- My husband loves me for who I am, not for what I can give him.
- My husband loves me for who I am, not for what I can do for him.
- My husband loves me for who I am and I love me for who I am.
- My husband also loves my children for who they are.
- He shows his love by being strong with our children.
- He shows his love by being compassionate with our children.
- He shows his love by sharing with me the responsibilities of disciplining our children.
- Disciplining our children gives them a sense of security, predictability, stability, order, and trust in their parents.

Only one chant was developed for Mr. Frank. It was designed to effect changes in his perceptions of himself as being a weak male and inadequate father. It also was meant to have him begin to perceive himself as an equal participant and central figure in family life.

- My wife and I stand strong together,
- Like pillars of marble we uphold the family temple.
- My wife and I stand strong together,
- Like girders of steel, we support the family edifice.
- My wife and I stand strong together,
- Like cornerstone blocks, we are the family's foundation.
- As a marble pillar, my strength shines forth.
- As a girder of steel, I gleam in the sun.
- As a cornerstone block, I sparkle like granite.

During couple sharing time, Mr. and Mrs. Frank were asked to engage in the pleasurable sharing of the day's events. They were instructed to follow the procedures outlined in the Structured Guidelines for Establishing Functional Communications in Marital Dyads to share and exchange positive thoughts and feelings about each other and their relationship. Another part of couple sharing time was to have Mr. and Mrs. Frank plan a series of family events in which their children were to participate. They were to plan activities that would make it possible for them to take a "parental role as teacher" with their children. Later on, after the successful completion of these projects, they would be expected to plan activities that would make it possible to interact with Christy as a young adult woman/daughter.

The purpose of these exercises was threefold:

1. To highlight and strengthen generational boundaries.
2. To enable Mr. Frank to interact with his children in ways that would make it possible for them to express genuine admiration for some of his talents (e.g., Mr. Frank was a golfer, fisherman and gardener).
3. To provide Mrs. Frank with a number of different opportunities to develop a more age-appropriate adult-adult, mother-daughter relationship with Christy.

Parent appraisal time was included in this assignment to help Mr. and Mrs. Frank crystalize their dyadic role as parents, especially in terms of their relationship to Christy. They were encouraged to work as a "parent team" to resolve their difficulties with their children. Any "parental difficulties" that Mr. and Mrs. Frank could not resolve were to be brought in for discussion at the following therapy session for review, discussion and resolution.

The final task assigned to Mr. and Mrs. Frank in this series of rituals was designed to guard against any child's (especially Christy's) attempt to reactivate a parent-child cross-generational coalition. Using the expression "dysfunctional parent-child secret," the therapist explained that any secret kept between a parent and a child that excludes the other parent has the potential for destabilizing the parents' relationship and destroying the integrity of the marital unit. This expression was used because of its relevance to certain aspects of theme #3 in Mrs. Frank's personal mythology. The therapist stressed the importance of both parents' discouraging their children from trying to gain leverage in the family by sharing secrets with a more powerful parental figure. The therapist explained that, while giving the child inappropriate power, a secret also compromises the child by requiring him/her to betray the parent who is not party to the secret. It also creates in the child severe anxiety and guilt and may retard the child's personal growth and psychological independence. The point of this explanation was subtle but powerful. In essence the therapist intimated that Mrs. Frank's conscious attempts to protect her daughter from men and Mr. Frank and her efforts to help her daughter enjoy life and become an independent person may actually prevent Christy from achieving these goals.

Mr. and Mrs. Frank were asked to devise a procedure for discouraging their children from attempting to align with one parent against the other. They were also asked to think about developing a standardized, self-generated procedure (ritual) for discussing such attempts with the children involved.

Mr. and Mrs. Frank agreed upon two procedures to accomplish these goals. First, they called the children together and informed them that secrets between parents and children (that excluded other family members) would no longer be part of the family's way of functioning. Children, however, could continue to keep secrets among themselves, and parents were expected to discuss husband-wife and parental issues between themselves.

Mr. and Mrs. Frank then instituted weekly family council meetings where any problems or concerns could be shared, discussed, and resolved by all parties concerned. These council meetings were intended to resolve minor family conflicts before they evolved into major family issues or family crises. The Franks adopted the Structured Guidelines for Establishing Functional Communication in Families as a general procedure for speaking at family council meetings.

Once these rituals were in place, the therapist directed the couple to focus on SIDCARB areas of concern that appeared to represent overt manifestations of unconsciously held contractual arrangements, starting with the SIDCARB item, "Expressions of Love and Affection." Both spouses had indicated that they desired a moderate degree of change in this area.

The therapist's intent was to modify the Franks' unconscious contract 2, which appeared to be falling apart. The reader will recall the terms of this contract:

> Mrs. Frank: I agree to encourage our daughter to look up to you and see you as special. In this way, we will treat you as your mother and sister treated you.

In exchange for this:

> Mr. Frank: I will allow you to try to recapture your youth by living vicariously through our daughter so long as you continue to encourage her to treat me as special and see me as a good father.

The goal of this structured negotiation was to help Mr. and Mrs. Frank devise a new conjugal contract that did not require a child to fulfill a consensus role image where she was needed to bolster a parent's self-esteem, fulfill a parent's unmet needs, help a parent recapture his/her past, play an inappropriate role vis-à-vis a parent, make up for past wrongs and injustices done to a parent by others, etc. In order to achieve this end, the therapist prefaced the Franks' structured communication exercise with these comments:

> You both have indicated that expressions of love and affection constitute areas of your marriage where you desire some degree of change. In marriage, it is very important for spouses to feel *special* to each other and to experience *joy* together. Having a relationship with someone *special*, a person with whom you can *be yourself* and *express the child in you* is very satisfying. I see by your personal histories that neither of you had much opportunity to be a child. Although we can never go back and make up for our "lost childhood," we certainly can learn how to enjoy and indulge the *child in us* and the *child in our spouse*.
>
> In your discussions of expressing love and affection to each other, I would like you both to pay particular attention to what each of you would like the other to do that would make you feel *special* and *bring out the kid in you*.

This approach is used to help the spouses understand that their frustrations and disappointments with their mates derive at times from inappropriate expectations. It does not negate the fact that the spouse did not have one or more basic needs satisfied by his/her parents. However, it does bring home the reality that a developmental task that is not completed during a certain critical period of life can never be completely reworked and mastered at a later stage of the life cycle. Such an interpretation is not pessimistic because it suggests that the adult *derivatives* of these needs can be satisfied *to some extent* by one's spouse. It is important that the *spouse—not one's children—*be identified and recognized as the person to whom one should turn. Equally important in such an interpretation is the therapist's explanation that identifying one's *need derivatives*, communicating them to one's spouse, and asking one's spouse to behave in a way that will satisfy them is the responsibility of the person. One should not expect one's spouse to intuit these needs and expectations.

With these comments and directives as a context for negotiation, Mr. and Mrs. Frank began to explore various behaviors that they might exchange in order to make each other feel special. They also began to talk about ways of bringing out and nurturing the child within.

The final group of ritual tasks used with the Frank family was created to bring about a restructuring of the mother-daughter relationship. Two basic goals were identified: (a) to help Christy and Mrs. Frank replace their problematic cross-generational coalition with a more appropriate mother-daughter relationship, and (b) to help Christy achieve autonomy and independence from her family of origin in a less self-destructive and more socially acceptable manner. In order to begin work on these goals, the family was reconvened as a group. Material gathered from the Family Relationships Histories and the Family Myth Assessment Interviews of all children was used to construct the rituals. Information collected during the initial family interview was also used in ritual construction.

Christy had chosen the film "Clan of the Cave Bear" as her favorite story. Her responses to the questions in the Family Myth Assessment Interviews are summarized below:

> I identify with the main character of the story, Ayla, who is orphaned at an early age. The story is set in prehistoric times when humans still lived in small clans. Ayla is found and raised by a less human, less advanced tribe. She is very different from the tribe that adopts her. She has blond hair, fair skin and blue eyes. The people in the tribe that adopts her are dark and ape-like. Although Ayla is much more beautiful and intelligent than the others of the clan, she is treated as dumb and ugly, especially by the men. Brun, the chief's son, is the original male chauvinist pig. He wants to kill Ayla, because he is afraid of her intelligence and self-confidence. Ayla is protected by an old medicine woman. She won't let the men hurt her. When the old woman dies, Ayla becomes the medicine woman of the tribe. This role protects her from the envious men in the clan. Ayla earns the respect of the clan and learns how

to hunt better than the men, even though women are forbidden to use weapons. Later in the story, Brun gets to become chief of the clan when his father gets too old. When he again tries to kill Ayla, he is demoted back to his original rank of ordinary person. Although Ayla is very smart and powerful in the story, she suffers greatly, because she is so different. At the end of the story, Ayla leaves the clan and goes off into the sunset in search of other people like herself.

Christy's brothers, Peter and Paul, both selected the motion picture "Star Wars" as their favorite story. Peter identified with the older hero, Hans Solo, and Paul saw himself as the young Jedi knight apprentice Luke Skywalker. The selection of this film by the two boys is interesting for two reasons. First, nowhere in this epic saga does a mature maternal figure appear. Princess Lea represents the classic virginal anima archetype who offers hope and moral support to the hero, but she is not a mother figure. One can say that in Princess Lea the boys see both their sister and their adolescent mother who has not fully matured as a woman. Second, both boys expressed strong ambivalent feelings toward Darth Vader, feelings of love and hate, attraction and repulsion. The identification of Darth Vader with Mr. Frank was obvious.

When the children's favorite films are viewed against the backdrop of the Frank family, one can see how various themes from these films fit together to represent the Frank family's current organizational structures and life circumstances. For example:

1. Protection of the orphaned child, Ayla (Christy), from the men of the tribe (father and brothers) by the medicine woman (Mrs. Frank) and the powerful coalition that develops between these two women as Ayla (Christy) grows older.
2. The dissolution of the female coalition as Ayla (Christy) matures and the medicine woman dies. Then, Ayla's departure from the Clan of the Cave Bear and its developmentally inferior members (Mr. and Mrs. Frank) as she begins her search for "people of her own kind" (Christy's friends and peers).
3. The two young male heroes, Luke and Hans (Peter and Paul), who must confront their many developmental conflicts on their own without much support from their natural father, Darth Vader (Mr. Frank). They are helped, however, by a surrogate father, Obewon Canobe (various athletic coaches) and receive encouragement and moral support from Princess Lea (Christy and Mrs. Frank).

Several techniques were used to achieve the designated goals, including recasting the roles of family members, behaving and thinking as if one were the character, and the family role play. These interventions should only be attempted when the parents are willing to participate fully in the process.

The procedure begins with the therapist's asking the identified patient to create a role and sketch out a general script for each family member. The role assigned to each family member is to be based upon one of the characters in the individual's favorite story, film, novel, etc. However, he/she is told that none of the created roles or scripts is to be "negative," "bad," "evil," etc. The character that the identified patient dislikes, fears, etc., is to be "transformed" into a "likable" and "positive" individual. The goal of the exercise is explained as enabling family members to experiment with new ways of behaving that might help them resolve the problems that caused them to enter therapy.

Christy designed a role for her mother as the medicine woman from the "Clan of the Cave Bear." Mrs. Frank was asked to play the wise old woman who taught Ayla how to become "self-sufficient" and "independent" and to "deal with men." Christy added that the only change she would make in the story and the role ascribed to her mother was that the "medicine woman does not die, but sends Ayla on her way with love and hope." The role assigned to Mr. Frank as "chief" of the Frank clan was that of protector. Like the "chief" in the film, he had power to "demote" his sons if they treated Ayla (Christy) unfairly or badly. Christy's two brothers were given roles as men of the tribe who admired and respected Ayla.

Once these roles and scripts had been outlined, Christy and her mother were asked to spend some time, before the next session, talking about ways that Mrs. Frank could "use her wisdom as a grown woman and mother of three" to help her daughter "make it in the world of men." In addition, Mrs. Frank was asked to give some consideration to how she could "prepare Christy for moving out, going to college and living on her own."

The first part of the next session was spent reviewing these roles with all family members. The remainder of the interview was devoted to going through the same process with Peter and Paul, who were asked to cast Mr. and Mrs. Frank and Christy into roles taken from "Star Wars."

Peter and Paul cast Mr. Frank in the role of Obewon Canobe, Luke Skywalker's surrogate father, teacher, friend, and guide. Mr. Frank was flattered by this part and remarked that it was certainly not "type casting." From the look on his face, we could tell that this honor made him feel special in his children's eyes. A similar gleam was observed in his eyes when Christy assigned him the role of "chief" and "protector." The requests from Peter and Paul for changes in their father's behavior toward them did not require drastic modifications in father-son relationships. They simply asked for more time with him (this was also reflected in their FACES III scores), to go fishing and camping with him more often, and to be allowed to shoot his 22-caliber rifle under his supervision. They had no specific roles created for Mrs. Frank and Christy. They simply wanted them to be less "fussy" about their cleaning their rooms, and requested that Mrs. Frank show more interest in their athletic activities.

Depending upon the family, the presenting problem, and the appropriateness of the new roles and scripts developed by the identified patient, the therapist might ask some family members to try to think as their particular characters might think and to behave as if they actually were these characters for a short period of time. More or less structure can be used, depending upon the needs of the family. Self-instructed performance models can also be developed and cognitive-behavioral response chains and internal dialogues can also become part of the process. The reader must keep in mind that these editing strategies are not ends in themselves. They are simply techniques designed to change interaction patterns, rearrange problematic family structures, and modify the internal cognitive ideals of family members.

Within a period of weeks, the Frank family was stabilized. Christy no longer gave her parents trouble. She found a steady boyfriend of whom her parents approved. Peter and Paul did manage to get Mr. Frank to spend more time with them and Mrs. Frank "eased up" on the boys "a little." Mr. and Mrs. Frank then requested marital therapy to resolve some of their difficulties as a couple.

DESIGNING RITES OF PASSAGE WITH
FAMILIES OF ADOLESCENTS

Ancient cultures and primitive societies developed rites of passage to help individuals move from one stage of the life cycle to the next. We have found such rites of passage especially helpful in our work with families where the identified patient is an adolescent.

Adolescence offers young people in our contemporary Western society the developmental task of establishing and consolidating a unique personal identity, as well as a second chance to rework whatever developmental tasks remain unresolved from previous developmental eras (Erikson, 1968). The more triangulated the child is between conflicting parental projections and expectations, the more difficult it will be for him/her to establish autonomy in early childhood and to develop a clear, separate identity during adolescence. Adolescents who are trapped in such an impasse will often resort to drastic and desperate measures to separate from their families of origin, to rid themselves of parental projections, to develop their own set of values and moral principles and to consolidate their own unique personal identities. Acting-out behavior, substance abuse, sexual promiscuity, psychiatric disturbance, or suicidal attempts all can be seen as the adolescent's dramatic attempt to free himself/herself from such an intolerable position.

Scholars have identified three stages through which all rites of passage proceed: separation, transition, and incorporation (van Gennep, 1960). Initiation ceremonies are predominantly rites of transition which help the initiate progress from one stage of life (childhood) to the next stage (adulthood) in a smooth, orderly, and predictable fashion. In primitive societies, initiation usually takes place in same-sex groups. During such ritual practices, the initiates are removed from their families of origin. Males are usually subjected to ordeals and trials of endurance by their elders. These trials might include physical beating, hazing, humiliation, homosexual submission, and mutilation (e.g., circumcision, subincision, scarring, tattooing, removal of teeth, etc.). In addition, males are instructed in tribal lore, myths, male secrets, and traditions. A central theme of male initiation ceremonies is the ritual slaying of the initiate, his subsequent death, and his joyful resurrection as a changed person. All initiation rites take place under the watchful eyes of the elders and tribal gods.

Female initiation rites, though less common in primitive societies, usually consist of the recognition that menstruation has begun and that the young initiate has now begun the reproductive phase of her life. She, too, is taught tribal lore, myths, women's secrets, and traditions. Female initiation usually takes place in stages, i.e., dealing with menstruation, pregnancy and childbirth. Female initiations have as their central theme "the mystery of giving birth." The young woman learns that she is "creative upon the plane of life" (Eliade, 1960; p. 216). This revelation is a religious experience that has no masculine counterpart.

Unfortunately, in Western society there are few organized and culturally prescribed rites of passage to enable the teenager to make a relatively smooth passage into adulthood. In most instances, the adolescent experiences his/her rites of passage via a same-sex peer group unsupervised

by adults. For males and females attending college, fraternities and so-
rorities come closest to primitive societies in providing the major ingredi-
ents associated with tribal rites of passage. The military also serves this
function for many men, and now some women. In the first author's
work with fighting gangs that roamed the streets of the southeast Bronx,
Harlem and Spanish Harlem during the late 1960s, it was not unusual to
find many of the practices characteristic of tribal initiation ceremonies
present in gang inductions.

Same-sex peer groups, for better or worse, take the place of the tribal
group of elders for the majority of adolescents in our culture. Teenagers
who have not had the benefit of forming a close interpersonal "chum"
relationship (Sullivan, 1953) with a member of the same sex during
preadolescence can recoup their losses, to a large degree, if they can
become part of a same-sex adolescent peer group.

In our work with families where the identified patient is an adolescent,
we frequently find that he/she has been unable to find a peer group that
is able to support his/her attempts at separation-individuation from his/
her family of origin. The more isolated the youngster is from friends his/
her own age, the poorer the prognosis. The peer group is extremely
helpful, because it encourages the youngster to divest himself/herself of
parental projections and expectations and provides a supportive environment where he/she can try out various roles, experiment with interpersonal relationships, and begin the process of identity formation. In
such cases, we attempt to design intervention strategies (based upon our
understanding of each family member's personal mythology, the parent's conjugal mythology, and the family group myth) that simulate rites
of passage and facilitate the adolescent's entry into an appropriate peer
group.

We do this by helping families develop a number of carefully designed,
symbolic, ritual contracts that serve as rites of passage for the identified
patient. For example, permitting the identified patient to get a job that
will enable him/her to earn spending money, allowing the identified
patient to date members of the opposite sex, extending his/her curfew on
weekends, permitting the identified patient to use the family car in
exchange for improving school grades, or completing chores around the
house can be the first step in the emancipation process. As each contract
is negotiated, the identified patient is reminded of the increased responsibility that comes with "becoming a man" or "becoming a woman."

Parents are helped to discuss their ambivalence about their child's
newfound freedom. At times we have held sessions with parents on
Friday evenings when the identified patient was out on a date or using

the family car. During these sessions, we redirect parents to issues in their own relationship, help them negotiate new marital contracts that strengthen the parental coalition, and reinforce subsystem boundaries.

Ritual prescriptions that make use of central family themes can be devised to simulate death and rebirth of the identified patient or to celebrate the transition to womanhood for females in the family. Ceremonies where parents give their children treasured heirlooms or personal belongings and reveal family secrets are another way of introducing rites of passage into the family therapy session. Depending upon the family's sociocultural, ethnic and religious background, specific activities can be prescribed that represent initiation rituals into adulthood. For example, fathers can teach their sons how to hunt, fish, drive, play a particular sport, or follow the stock market. Mothers can teach their daughters how to cook, drive, put on makeup, say "no" to boys, or be assertive and compete on equal footing with males.

The reader is by now familiar with the various theoretical formulations, therapeutic models, and intervention strategies which comprise our method of intervening in individuals', couples', and families' mythological systems. When clinicians are sensitive to how these formulations and intervention strategies can be incorporated into their work, a variety of rituals can be designed to suit the needs of particular families.

17

Training and Supervision in Marital and Family Therapy

O**UR EXPERIENCE IN** training and supervising marital and family therapists comes from working with clinicians in a variety of settings, including university graduate training programs, mental health clinics, inpatient residential treatment facilities, and private practice. This diverse sample has sensitized us to the need for paying close attention to the trainee's/supervisee's level of therapeutic experience when attempting to teach our mythological approach. We have found it useful to employ a developmental perspective when considering work with any given trainee. We assume that beginning therapists must develop some basic clinical skills and experience some initial therapeutic successes before they can incorporate a mythological perspective into their work.

It is essential for therapists to learn how to think in terms of the "process" as well as the "content" (opinions, feelings, historical data, etc.) that clients report (Anderson & Russell, 1982). In the case of couple and family systems, this means being able to recognize redundant interactional patterns. In therapy with individuals, it requires that attention be given to transference, countertransference, and primary process phenomena. Trainees/supervisees must feel comfortable with themselves and their own creative playfulness and be aware of their own personal mythologies, since the therapeutic myths they create with clients will inevitably reflect their own underlying assumptions about the world, their definitions of family health and functioning, and their assumptions about how individuals and family systems change, grow, and develop over time. In this chapter, we will: (a) review the basic skills we believe to be essential for clinicians using myths in their work; (b) describe how a mythological perspective is used to broaden clinicians' perspective beyond the confines of their own theoretical orientation; and

(c) show how the mythological perspective can be used in case consultations and supervision with experienced clinicians.

The model of training we advocate takes into account the following factors: (a) interpersonal helping is a developmental, dynamic process of mutual influence; (b) the clinical and supervisory processes are effected by factors external to and inherent in the developing client-therapist-supervisor-training program system; (c) therapeutic skills can be broken down into three distinct groups: relationship skills, conceptual-theoretical skills, and intervention or executive-technological skills; (d) within each group of skills, at least two levels of expertise can be identified: primary and advanced; (e) advanced levels of therapeutic skills are generally required to implement our approach; (f) therapists' personal awareness plays an essential part in both the therapeutic and the training experience; and (g) evaluation/assessment skills are also essential to the therapeutic process. Each of these points will be addressed in this chapter.

DEVELOPMENT OF PRIMARY THERAPIST SKILLS

Relationship Skills

As noted in Chapter 4, we believe that the ability to establish and reestablish trust at various junctures throughout the therapy process is critical to therapeutic success. The ability to respond empathically to clients is at the core of a trusting relationship. In the clinical literature, relationship skills such as empathy, warmth, and genuineness have been found to be related to positive individual and family therapy outcomes (cf. Gurman & Kniskern, 1978; Rogers, 1957) and to keeping families in therapy (Shapiro, 1974; Shapiro & Budman, 1973; Waxenberg, 1973). Similarly, such relationship skills as affect-behavior integration, humor, and warmth have been associated with positive outcomes in family therapy (Alexander, Barton, Schiavo, & Parsons, 1976; Burton & Kaplan, 1968; Mezydlo, Wauck, & Foley, 1973; Thomlinson, 1974). Relationship skills also involve the ability to accommodate one's own style of communicating to variations in clients' styles of communicating (Beck et al., 1979; Minuchin, 1974).

In our approach to training and supervision, one of the most important indicators of the trainee's ability to establish a therapeutic relationship with clients is the quality of the involvement between supervisor and therapist trainee. Involvement here refers to the capacity to join, establish trust, tolerate intense affect, and exhibit spontaneity and humor in the supervisory relationship. This relationship may evolve in the context of live observation, reviewing videotapes of specific therapy sessions, exploring the trainee's family of origin, or examining transference-countertransference issues. In our experience, the most important consideration is that *the involvement between supervisor and therapist parallels the degree of involvement between therapist and client* (Gavazzi & Anderson, 1987). These parallel levels of involvement have been discussed by Liddle, Breunlin, Schwartz, & Constantine (1984) as the isomorphism inherent to any training system. Isomorphism implies that pattern, content, affect, and the bases for change tend to be replicated at different levels of the training system. Thus, any part of the therapeutic system (e.g., the client subsystem, the client-therapist subsystem, the therapist-supervisor subsystem) can be utilized to discuss qualities shared by all of its parts.

While the quality of the *supervisor-therapist relationship* has not been examined empirically in terms of therapeutic outcome for clients, the quality of the *therapist-client relationship* (e.g., therapists' relationship skills), as noted above, has consistently been associated with positive client outcomes (cf. Gurman & Kniskern, 1978; Rogers, 1957). Alexander et al. (1976) found that therapist relationship skills accounted for 44.6% of the outcome variance, while structuring skills (directness, clarity, self-confidence, information gathering, and stimulating interactions) accounted for an additional 15.4% of the outcome variance. If one accepts the premise that pattern, content, and affect tend to be isomorphically replicated at various levels of the training system, the quality of the relationship between supervisor and therapist becomes especially important in the development of a therapeutic relationship between therapist and client.

Conceptual Skills

A vast majority of practitioners and educators of marital and family therapists agrees that the ability to translate clinical observations into meaningful language is an essential skill (Barton & Alexander, 1977; Breunlin, Schwartz, Krause, & Selby, 1983; Cleghorn & Levin, 1973; Constantine, 1976; Falicov, Constantine, & Breunlin, 1981; Garfield, 1979; Garrigan & Bambrick, 1977). In our training model, conceptual skills include specific theoretical/conceptual knowledge *and* cognitive/perceptual skills.

The manner in which information is perceived, processed, organized, and stored for use by the therapist is determined by his or her conceptual model of interpersonal behavior and behavior change. Our mythological approach requires that trainees have a thorough conceptual understanding of family systems, ego psychological, object relations, and cognitive-behavioral theories. They must be familiar with structural, strategic, and intergenerational models of family therapy and proficient in the application of behavioral marital therapy techniques and child management strategies. However, in actual practice knowledge and skill do not always translate easily into smoothly integrated clinical strategies. Such an integrated gestalt requires a considerable amount of time, practice, and supervision.

It has been our experience to find that less experienced practitioners learn only one or two of the above theoretical/conceptual models. Therefore, we stress learning structural and intergenerational theoretical models initially. The structural school, with its clearly articulated emphasis on hierarchies, subsystems and boundaries (e.g. Minuchin 1974), and intergenerational approaches, with strategies for mapping family dynamics over time, offer trainees relatively straightforward ways of recognizing recurring interactional patterns and dysfunctional hierarchical arrangements. This makes the formulation of therapeutic goals manageable for the beginning therapist. The danger here is that students may attempt to copy or model themselves after the "masters" of these schools. This may inhibit the development of their own unique styles. Others may attempt to integrate techniques from many schools. A possible negative consequence here can be a confused "cookbook" approach to therapy that is devoid of any coherent theoretical understanding upon which to base clinical decisions. Students at this stage of training are usually not yet ready to incorporate a mythological approach into their practice. At this point in training, we prepare trainees to use straightforward behavioral techniques and structural approaches when working with couples and families.

We also consider the development of several perceptual skills as essential to the ability to translate clinical information into meaningful language (Bagarozzi, 1983c). One such skill is *concreteness*. Concreteness includes the ability to systematically collect relevant clinical data through direct behavioral observation or by asking appropriate questions when direct observation is not possible (Carkhuff, 1969). The focus of the therapist's observations and the specific content of his or her questions will be determined by the therapist's theoretical orientation. However, the abilities (a) to stay focused on the presenting problem, relevant themes, or clinical issues without being distracted, (b) to separate essen-

tial from nonessential bits of information, and (c) to take the time necessary to form a clear impression and to formulate hypotheses consistent
with a given theoretical framework are central to concreteness.

Another essential perceptual skill is the ability to *decenter*. Decentering is
the ability to reverse perspective and to take the role of another. This skill
enables the trainee to step back, to observe, and to cognitively process his
or her own involvement in and contributions to the system-therapist relationship. The ability to decenter also enables the therapist to metacommunicate (Watzlawick, Beavin, & Jackson, 1967) about the process and to
share observations, feelings, perceptions, and experiences with the client
system. The sharing of such material with clients in a nonthreatening,
nonaccusing manner also has been described as *immediacy* (Carkhuff,
1969; Gazda, Asbury, Balzer, Childers, & Walters, 1977).

Intervention Skills

The active posture we typically take in relation to our clients means
that the therapist must master a variety of intervention strategies. In the
family therapy field, the development of intervention skills which enable
trainees to disrupt dysfunctional family patterns is widely supported
(Barton & Alexander, 1977; Breunlin et al., 1983; Cleghorn & Levin, 1973;
Falicov et al., 1981; Garrigan & Bambrick, 1977; Haley, 1976; Lapierre,
1979; Minuchin, 1974; Piercy, Laird, & Mohammed, 1983). These intervention skills have been labeled "executive skills" (Cleghorn & Levin,
1973), "structuring skills" (Alexander et al., 1976), or "therapeutic skills"
(Breunlin et al., 1983; Falicov et al., 1981; Garrigan & Bambrick, 1977)
and typically include such therapeutic behaviors as taking charge of the
session, developing an initial therapeutic contract, stimulating interactions, gathering or probing for information, clarifying communications,
and assigning tasks. The importance of such intervention skills has been
demonstrated by Alexander et al. (1976), who found "structuring skills"
(directiveness, clarity, self-confidence, information gathering, and stimulating interaction) to be associated with positive outcomes for families
in therapy. Active interventions, such as firming up appropriate subsystem boundaries, restructuring dysfunctional subsystem boundaries, and
advice giving, have been found to be related to positive outcomes and
reduced dropout rates among families in therapy (Anderson, Atilano,
Paff-Bergen, Russell, & Jurich, 1985; Russell, Atilano, Anderson, Jurich,
& Paff-Bergen, 1984). While beginning therapists are not expected to
have mastered a wide variety of intervention skills, they are expected to
be able to assume an active role with clients and to demonstrate the
above basic skills.

Personal Awareness

As noted throughout this volume, the self and one's conception of the self-in-relation to significant others play a central role in our understanding of an individual's personal mythology. In turn, the individual's personal mythology is intimately linked to the conjugal and family myths that the individual co-creates with significant others. For this reason, a therapist trained in a mythological perspective must have a basic understanding of his/her own myths and their associated unresolved conflicts and symbolic-affective themes.

Conceptualizing an individual's, couple's or family's myths is a subjective process which is as much dependent upon therapists' own mythology as it is upon understanding the myths of their clients. Thus, in our approach, we are attentive to the reenactment of the therapist's own personal themes with clients and within the supervisory relationship. For instance, the presence of themes centering on ambivalence with regard to interpersonal closeness and distance may inhibit therapists' ability to establish basic trust or to be responsive to the most painful revelations of their clients. The presence of themes related to conflicts having to do with the expression of assertive as opposed to passive behaviors may restrain the therapist from taking charge of sessions, structuring communication, stimulating interactional patterns, probing for necessary but difficult information, or teaching specific skills.

The identification of the therapist's own mythological themes and understanding how these themes express themselves in the therapy to impede therapeutic progress is an important aspect of the supervisory/ training experience. Whenever a therapist appears to have difficulty with a particular relationship, conceptual, or intervention skill, we look for the personal theme(s) related to this difficulty. In this way, the development of clinical skills goes hand-in-hand with the personal development of the therapist.

The association between the therapist's own personal mythological themes and his/her ability to implement specific clinical skills is illustrated in the training experiences of Leslie. Leslie was an intelligent, young woman in her early twenties whose parents were both highly regarded university professors. Not surprisingly, Leslie's personal mythology included themes related to achievement. She felt pressure to be "excellent both academically and professionally" and was anxious about "being adequate or simply competent rather than outstanding" as a family therapist. Her choice of a career was also important, because, in addition to excelling professionally, members of Leslie's family had "always been

socially minded and concerned about helping others." Thus, it was important not only to succeed in her training program, but to be "better
than average" and "not just another trainee who didn't know what he or
she was doing." To fail would have meant she was not worthy of carrying
on the family tradition of helping others. To be simply competent rather
than exceptional would have meant falling short of the family standard.

Leslie's themes were evident in her approach to training and supervision. She was not satisfied with restricting herself to learning one or two
therapy models initially. She wanted to be well versed in *all* of the contemporary models of marriage and family therapy. Secondly, Leslie was
not interested in becoming a follower of any particular school or model.
Instead she wanted to develop her own personal model of therapy from
the outset.

With clients she often became confused and unsure of herself because
she could not restrict herself to one problem or goal at a time and instead
wanted to resolve *all* of their difficulties right away. Her own confusion
about which strategy to follow or her frustration with clients for not
moving as fast as she would have liked often left her anxious and fearful
that she would fail with them or that her supervisor would question her
competence.

As the connections between Leslie's personal themes and her clinical
behavior were addressed, she became more aware of the sources of her
own anxiety. She was able to use the supervision to formulate selected
goals with each client and to focus initially on helping clients to be less
anxious, less scattered, and more concrete about establishing clearly
defined goals for selected changes. She became more comfortable with
the idea of allowing her own style of therapy to emerge in a more deliberate and reasoned manner.

A central theme in Leslie's supervision was her willingness to accept
her current strengths and shortcomings and to be comfortable with her
own imperfections as a person and therapist. This theme was also evident in her work with clients, where she emphasized a style of "being
with" clients and accepting their vulnerabilities and shortcomings.

We assume that therapists interested in their own personal growth will
have the capacity for self-awareness and will be able to use their knowledge of their own personal mythologies as a primary source of information about clients' experiences in therapy. For instance, Leslie's increased
awareness of her own anxiety about succeeding and her pressure to excel
allowed her to be more sensitive to clients' anxieties about finding the
quick fix for their own problems and their reluctance, at times, to accept
their own shortcomings and limitations. As noted in Chapter 4, we use

our own feelings in order to spotlight the predominant affective themes of couples or families and assume that the affective tone between therapist and individual clients often mirrors significant themes in the client's personal mythology.

In addition, we are attentive to trainees' willingness to take risks, to tolerate ambiguity, and to be playful (as well as serious) in the therapeutic encounter. We assume that taking risks with clients will generally involve the therapist's willingness to face potential threats to his or her own self-definition. For instance, to push an adolescent to reveal previously denied or repressed feelings toward a parent may require that the therapist be faced with the dilemma of having to deal with the symbolic reenactment of his/her own unresolved relationship with a parent. Comfort with ambiguity is especially important when the therapeutic approach pays such attention to unconscious, primary process, and symbolic phenomena which are not readily grasped in a logical, concrete, left-hemispheric manner. Finally, attention to the multiple levels of meaning inherent in each client statement, behavior or gesture requires trainees to develop a willingness to play with words, objects, or dearly held values and points of view. Such playfulness is especially useful when therapists use metaphoric objects, ritual prescriptions, and other analogical forms of communication in their clinical work.

Assessment/Evaluation Skills

In keeping with our general approach to therapy, we view evaluation as an ongoing, collaborative process that takes place throughout the course of treatment. However, there are also several critical junctures over the course of treatment where assessment plays a pivotal role. Our model postulates that in the initial stages of the therapeutic relationship goals are behaviorally defined by the therapist and client. Once these goals have been agreed upon, a contract is negotiated between the therapist and client system which specifies procedural rules and guidelines that will be used to achieve the desired ends. However, during the course of treatment problems may arise which prevent the therapist and client system from achieving these agreed-upon goals. For example, clients may experience new crises which relegate the initial problem to secondary importance or clients may introduce new information which dramatically alters the therapeutic focus (e.g., a spouse acknowledges an extramarital affair or admits to having aborted a child without the husband's knowledge). When this happens, a number of problem-solving strategies can be used to facilitate therapeutic progress. New goals may

be set, contracts may be renegotiated, or termination (sometimes premature) may occur. If these unforeseen obstacles are overcome, the client(s)
and therapist can continue their efforts to resolve the clients' initial
difficulties.

As demonstrated throughout this volume, clients and therapists are
continually evaluating the effectiveness of their endeavors and each
must assess whether the exchange has been fair and equitable and
whether desired changes have taken place. A joint decision to terminate
treatment or to set new goals is made after each goal is achieved. This
view of the therapeutic process is in keeping with most contemporary
conceptions concerning the nature of living social systems, which stress
that in order for systems to remain viable, they must be able to: (a) set
goals, (b) develop mechanisms, rules, and procedures to reach these
goals, (c) evolve problem-solving strategies and make structural changes
in response to environmental inputs, (d) evaluate progress and goal
attainment, and (e) set new, more complex goals which further individual and system development (Bagarozzi, 1983c; Buckley, 1967).

From our perspective, there are several perceptual/conceptual and executive technological skills that are required for the evaluation of therapeutic progress and outcomes. The perceptual skill most germane to
clinical evaluation is scientific objectivity. We are aware of, and agree
with, the position taken by many systems therapists that pure objectivity
is itself a myth (cf. Hoffman, 1985; Keeney, 1982). These authors correctly point out that it is impossible for the therapist to stand outside of the
system he or she is observing while simultaneously participating in that
system's process. However, the skill to which we are referring is that of
objective evaluation. In using this skill, the therapist places outcome
efficacy above personal interest (Bagarozzi, 1983c). It assumes that the
instruments and procedures used to measure outcome effectiveness are
theoretically relevant, reliable, and valid.

The conceptual skills required for evaluation are those related to the
scientific method of inquiry. In addition, sound theoretical reasoning
provides the therapist with explanations for observable client behaviors
and suggests predictions about what one can expect as a result of specific
interventions. If desired outcomes are achieved, support is generated for
the underlying theory and accompanying interventions. Failure to
achieve the desired outcomes calls into question the theory, the therapeutic intervention, the method of assessing outcomes, the therapist's
errors in theory construction or choice of intervention (e.g. intervention
was not powerful enough, too global, too specific, poorly timed or not
appropriate for a given client), or all of the above.

The executive technological skills required for successful clinical assessment are those which permit the clinician to implement appropriate research designs and to collect and analyze data with some level of confidence. This includes the ability to assess the validity and reliability of empirical instruments (e.g., self-report questionnaires, rating scales, and observer coding schemes), to identity the units of assessment (e.g., specific affects, cognitions, attitudes, behaviors) relevant to one's theoretical model, and to determine the appropriate level of inference for evaluating one's treatment outcomes.[1]

It is obvious from this discussion that evaluation is a complex process requiring perceptual, conceptual, and executive technological skills which are different from those needed to engage in competent therapeutic practice. Evaluation requires that the therapist analyze not only whether treatment goals have been achieved but also why desired treatment outcomes have not been attained.

Advanced Skills

We expect the more advanced trainees and supervisees to have developed the following skills and abilities:

1. The ability to develop empathic and trusting relationships with clients and supervisors.
2. The ability to integrate one's own conceptual model of therapy into one's clinical practice. That is, the trainee/supervisee has developed a uniquely personal conceptual framework and is neither imitating others' models of therapy nor still loosely experimenting with numerous models of therapy. Secondly, the trainee's/supervisee's conceptual model is congruent with a broadly based and well-defined set of executive technological skills.
3. The ability to integrate cognitive and experiential knowledge of therapeutic "process" (e.g., interactional patterns, triangulation, transference/countertransference) as well as an appreciation that numerous "contents" (client complaints, interpersonal conflicts, problems) can be manifest in the same process. For some clinicians,

---

[1]Gurman and Kniskern (1978) have identified six levels of inference and the most appropriate sources available for making judgments at these levels. These range from simple behavior counts of frequencies tabulated by machines or trained observers at Level I to highly inferential, subjective judgments, such as Rorschach interpretations, made by expert judges at Level VI.

this understanding of process is accompanied by increased interest in therapeutic metaphors, symbolization, and analogical versus digital forms of communication. Such clinicians are especially suited to a mythological perspective.

4. Fluidity and creativity in the choice of intervention strategies. With the development of a personal conceptual model of therapy, a repertoire of executive technological skills and an understanding of therapeutic process, trainees/supervisees are less confused or overwhelmed by the unexpected. They can respond with confidence and be more open to novelty, ambiguity, and experimentation rather than being rigid and anxious.

5. The ability of trainees/supervisees to use their own sense of self as a primary vehicle for therapeutic change. This shift is often evidenced in less of a tendency to "do things to and for clients" or to "give clients an intervention" and more of an emphasis on "being with clients" or "responding" to clients with greater genuineness, honesty, openness and courage. This characteristic is also evidenced in the trainee's/supervisee's own degree of interest in personal growth, wholeness and integration. Here we often see trainees/supervisees initiating their own process of introspection with regard to the meaning of their clinical behaviors and earnestly seeking personal feedback from supervisors and peers. Clinicians invested in expanding the limits of their own self-awareness are especially suited to our approach because our mythological perspective assumes that therapists will replicate their own personal mythologies in their clinical practice. Therefore trainees/supervisees must be able to recognize when their own personal mythology inhibits rather than facilitates therapeutic progress.

6. The ability to select appropriate assessment instruments and evaluation procedures and to use them appropriately to evaluate the efficacy of their therapeutic endeavors.

To fully appreciate the complexities of the clinical process, one must understand its paradoxical nature. Whether clients desire changes in problem behaviors, attitudes, cognitions, affects or some combination thereof, they all hope to benefit from the experience while incurring as little cost as possible from the therapeutic exchange process. As treatment progresses, however, the client system may begin to perceive that the changes required to bring about more effective functioning may cost more than anticipated. When this occurs, the therapist may be experienced as an adversary or enemy and the cooperative alliance will be threatened. It is at this point in therapy that the paradox becomes most evident. The therapist finds that his/her attempts to offer assistance and to fulfill his/her end of the therapeutic contract are met with reluctance, ambivalence or "resistance." This is a crucial time in therapy, because reciprocal negative exchanges may ensue if the therapist attempts to force change or if he/she responds to the client's hostility in kind. The continuation of escalating, negative exchanges could ultimately lead to a homeostatic deadlock or premature termination. Therefore, it is important for the therapist to recognize what is taking place and to reverse this downward spiraling progression.

In order to understand the inherent therapeutic paradox and to interrupt spiraling, negative exchanges, the therapist must possess and be able to integrate a number of therapeutic skills. Conceptually, the therapist must be able to recognize: (a) that change is perceived as more costly to the system than the potential rewards; (b) that therapist and client(s) may have developed an interaction pattern that actually prevents them from achieving the therapeutic goal; (c) that the therapist may have become part of the homeostatic process by playing out a central role in the client(s)' personal, conjugal or family mythology; (d) that the effectiveness and appropriateness of the interventions being employed need to be reevaluated; and (e) that possible alternative intervention strategies must be explored.

Many of these skills have already been discussed. For instance, in order to recognize that clients may be perceiving more costs than rewards at certain junctures in the therapy, the therapist must be empathic and able to decenter (take the role of the other). To recognize a counterproductive interaction pattern between client systems and therapist, the therapist must be objective and honest. The ability to recognize having been inducted into a primary role in clients' personal, marital, or family mythologies requires self-awareness (awareness of one's own personal myths). To reassess the effectiveness on one's therapeutic interventions, a therapist must have developed specific assessment skills. The ability to explore and implement alternative intervention strategies requires flexibility and knowledge of a variety of intervention skills. However, what is most important is the therapist's ability *to draw on these numerous skills and to use them in a coherent and integrated manner when the emotional intensity of the therapeutic encounter has increased to the point where the threat of change and the possible painful outcomes that may result from these changes have become obvious and threatening to the client system.*

THE SUPERVISORY/TRAINING PROCESS

In our view, any model of supervision and training must incorporate the types of personal, conceptual, and technical skills outlined in the previous section. However, beyond the acquisition of skills lies the important, yet hard to measure, elements of the therapeutic experience. Few interpersonal encounters outside of our own familial and most personal relationships have the potential to consistently unleash such powerful affects and spontaneous personal responses as therapeutic or supervisory experiences. The supervisor/trainer, therapist, and client(s) make up a dynamic interpersonal system comprised of multiple personal mythologies. Clients' conjugal and family mythological themes have the remarkable, uncanny ability to mirror the therapist's own central mythological themes. Furthermore, the therapist's interpretations of and responses to clients' mythological themes generally bear a striking resemblance to the relationship themes that emerge between therapist and supervisor. We could broaden this script further to include the predominant themes that emerge in a given agency setting within which the therapy and training are occurring (cf. Gavazzi & Anderson, 1987). Ultimately, the prevailing cultural and societal myths also color the fabric of the therapy/training experience (cf. Goldner, 1988). Awareness of these issues offers the client/therapist/trainer system the option of either perpetuating currently existing themes or modifying these unconscious themes to more flexibly adapt to the current interpersonal context.

To address these unconscious, isomorphic qualities of the training system we attend to the following sources of information: (a) clients' personal mythology; (b) therapists' own personal mythology; (c) the supervisors' own personal mythology; (d) the interface between therapists' and supervisors' mythological themes; and (e) the interface between therapists' and clients' mythological themes.

Clients' Personal Mythology

The assessment of clients' mythological themes has been described throughout this book and will not be reviewed here. Our central concern in this chapter is the supervisory process. In addition to helping the therapist assess clients' mythological themes, we help supervisees/trainees select appropriate interventions designed to edit central themes in the client's mythology. The more pragmatic aspects of selecting therapeutic interventions to edit mythological themes have been discussed in earlier chapters. Therefore, we will not review them here. Other factors related to the selection of interventions have to do with the role the therapist is playing in the client system and the broader therapeutic system. We are especially attuned to whether the interventions chosen by the therapist perpetuate clients' dysfunctional mythological themes or modify them in a manner that offers new opportunities for growth and development. To understand whether the therapist's behavior with clients is introducing new potentials for change or maintaining a homeostatic impasse, we examine the therapist's own personal mythology.

The Therapist's Personal Mythology

In our approach to clinical supervision and training, the therapist's own personal origins, mythologies, and associated complexes of symbolic and affectively laden themes play a critical role in the development of the therapeutic system. We assume that therapists will perceive, define, and respond to others (clients, supervisors, colleagues, etc.) in ways that are congruent with their own preconceived cognitive schemata, attributions, values, beliefs, etc., and will attempt to reenact their own familiar scripts, roles, and personal themes in the therapeutic system. For this reason, we believe it is essential to understand the therapist's *view of himself/herself, the functioning of that self-in-relation* to other significant selves (e.g., members of the family of origin, spouses, children, the supervisor), and the *internalized ideals* the therapist has regarding significant others. These central elements of the therapist's personal mythology alert us to potential unresolved conflicts within the self or in relationships with significant others which may resurface in the therapist's/supervisee's personal encounters with clients. In addition to the internalized ideals of significant intimates, we are also interested in the therapist's idealized version of a "therapist." This is often easily derived from the individual's choice of those "master therapists" they most admire. Contained within such admirations are the rough blueprints the individual trainee has chosen to follow in his/her personal development as a therapist.

The therapist's/trainee's idealized version of a "therapist" can also manifest itself in an idealized view of his/her supervisor. In these instances, we consider the question: who does the master therapist or idealized supervisor represent in the therapist's/trainee's own personal mythology? For instance, one of the authors once trained a woman who thought the author could do no wrong. He was "always right." Her father could do "nothing right"; he was "totally incompetent." The author knew he was being set up for a fall. One day, in supervision, he took off his shoes and pointed to his "feet of clay." This opened up the woman's awareness to her own personal theme of "men are not really what they seem, and even if they appear competent, they are not and cannot be trusted." In marital and couples therapy, this supervisee always perceived men as "incompetent" and tended to discount any competence evidenced by her male clients.

We believe that our initial interactions with a therapist/supervisee/trainee mirror our initial efforts with clients. The development of an open, trusting, empathic relationship with the supervisee/trainee is essential to what is to follow in training and supervision. And, as with clients, this trust may have to be periodically reestablished between supervisor/trainer and supervisee/trainee over the course of the training/supervision experience. Central themes in the trainee's/supervisee's own personal mythology are identified by the supervisor through discussions of the supervisee's Family Relationships History and Personal Myths Assessment guidelines, the content of their verbal reports about client contacts, their interpretation of clinical interactions with clients which have been observed by the supervisor, their actual responses to clients, and their interactions and exchanges with the supervisor. Therapist-supervisor discussions center around transferential distortions in the form of projections, projective identifications, misperceptions, irrational beliefs, or faulty attributions. These distortions are noted both in terms of the therapist's interactions with clients and in the interactions between the therapist and his/her supervisor/trainer.

The type of information gathered with respect to central themes in the supervisee's personal mythology are illustrated in the training experiences of Jennifer. Jennifer was a single, white, protestant, 25-year-old woman from the midwest. She was currently in her second and final year of a marriage and family therapy masters degree program. Jennifer's family background was characterized by loss and intense conflict, often manifest in direct, angry verbal battles and occasional violence between her father and her two older brothers. Jennifer was often present during these physical outbursts. However, she was never the direct recipient of her father's anger. Jennifer thought her father's behavior represented unresolved grief and stemmed from his inability to get over his wife's (Jennifer's mother's) death. She had died when Jennifer was 10 years old. Jennifer's typical response to father's violent outbursts was to:

> initially withdraw to a safe distance, stay out of the line of fire, don't draw any unnecessary attention onto myself, and hope that the whole thing would blow over. However, if the outburst became potentially dangerous, I would intervene to stop it before someone either got killed or was forced to leave.

Once the outburst had ended, I would then help each person to recover by offering support and reassurance.

The predominant feeling that Jennifer experienced during these episodes was fear. She was afraid that one of her brothers would be hurt. She also believed that her father was too vulnerable because of his grief to be confronted with his part in initiating and perpetuating these violent arguments.

In her clinical work, Jennifer was especially adept at establishing rapport, supporting clients' movements toward growth, and helping them take more personal responsibility for themselves and their behaviors. From an "objective" standpoint, Jennifer was quite competent in attending to the therapeutic process and clearly conceptualizing the essential individual, couple, or family themes. However, she would avoid heated and direct emotional exchanges between clients. When conflict erupted between spouses or among family members, she could effectively block its escalation and support each member. However, she had difficulties in situations where conflict or unresolved negative feelings remained submerged and unexpressed. In these situations, Jennifer's own anxiety became heightened. She found it difficult to enable family members or spouses to discuss and address these unresolved conflicts openly.

Efforts to address this stumbling block in supervision took the form of open and frank discussions about how Jennifer's own personal themes were interfering with her clinical work. The supervisor pointed out how significant personal themes became operative with different individuals and client systems. These discussions led to insight concerning her behavior and she began to make conscious efforts to modify her in-therapy behavior.

Later in her training, the relationship between the supervisor and Jennifer was also analyzed. The therapist-supervisor relationship themes appeared to parallel those evident in Jennifer's relationship with her more affectively constrained clients. Here again, themes of personal rapport, conceptual clarity, and distance prevailed. Conscious identification of these themes in the supervisory relationship heightened both the supervisor's and Jennifer's anxiety and the intensity of their relationship. Throughout her training, the supervisor continued to highlight unresolved thematic issues of anger avoidance as they surfaced in Jennifer's work.

Near the completion of Jennifer's training, the degree of affective involvement between Jennifer and the supervisor increased substantially. However, the constraints on her emotional expressiveness had been reduced, and she found herself able to discuss her own negative and angry feelings toward her supervisor openly and honestly with him, without fear of reprisal or negative consequences. Jennifer's termination experiences with clients evidenced a similar progression, as they were permitted expression and resolution of their own anger.

Two obvious points with regard to the above training vignette are noteworthy. First, as the need became evident, Jennifer sought personal therapy to deal with some of these issues during the training experience. Second, the supervisor's own personal mythology dovetailed with some of Jennifer's in the supervisory relationship. This issue is addressed in the next section.

The Supervisor's Personal Mythology

The reader is by now familiar with our basic assumption that self-awareness, insight into the self and its relation to significant others, and personal understanding of one's ideal images are important to therapists' personal growth and development and to their therapeutic effectiveness. We view a firm theoretical/conceptual grounding and personal awareness of one's own mythological themes as essential to the therapist's ability to determine if she or he is enacting a homeostatic role in the client's mythological system or offering new and potentially more adaptive revisions to it. Thus, whatever role in the therapeutic system the practitioner is enacting (e.g., therapist, supervisor, supervisor's supervisor), two interdependent responsibilities prevail. One is to help *others* in the therapeutic system to become aware of (a) the themes (roles, scripts) they are enacting in the therapy drama and/or (b) to help these *others* revise those themes which are interfering with adaptation and growth in the therapeutic system.[2] The other is to be aware of *one's own part* in facilitating or interfering with the potentials for growth and adaptation in the therapeutic system. We believe it is the supervisor's responsibility to take whatever steps necessary—personal therapy, clinical su-

---

[2]As we have noted in earlier chapters, with some clients a more pragmatic or indirect approach may be preferred by the therapist so that revisions in central themes may occur out of conscious awareness. Basic communication skills, problem-solving and conflict negotiation skills training, or analogical, symbolic, metaphorical or ritualized interventions may all be utilized when clients demonstrate little affinity for personal awareness. However, at other levels of the therapeutic system, therapists, supervisors, etc., must be willing to develop this personal awareness in order to benefit from our model of training and supervision.

pervision, supervision of one's supervision, etc.—to understand the themes in his/her own personal mythology.

In the remainder of this section we will outline the central themes present in Jennifer's supervisor's personal mythology (noted above). Then, in the next section, we will examine the links between Jennifer's and her supervisor's mythological themes.

A central theme in S's (the supervisor's) personal mythology involved "Deaths and losses as pivotal transitional experiences." In S's background, deaths and losses were equated with personal turning points and periods of philosophical questioning. Deaths or losses were evidence of having strayed from the path of right living. They were also seen as warnings to get back on track. "Right living" demanded personal loyalty, commitment, hard work, and perseverance. One of S's earliest losses was the loss of his father to alcoholism and divorce during his high school years. The realization that his father would not be available (either physically or emotionally) for support precipitated a period of mourning, introspection, and reevaluation. During this period, S became a student of Eastern religions. He became intrigued with the search for "enlightenment" and "completeness." This was followed by a resurgence of personal resolve to become a more self-reliant and independent person.

Later, after completing college, the fatal accident of a friend accompanying S on a cross-country trip precipitated a similar experience of profound shock, grief, introspection and newfound resolve. This time his ambivalence had to do with being drafted to fight in the Vietnam War. Rather than avoiding the draft by moving to Canada as his deceased friend had planned, he opted to challenge his draft board by applying for conscientious objector status. The other alternative was imprisonment. His conscientious objector status was approved. This strengthened the theme of loss as a personal turning point and as an omen to get back on the track of right living.

A third major loss had occurred at about the time S began to supervise Jennifer. S's spouse lost her oldest brother as a result of a heart attack. He was 37 years old at the time of his death. His death sent profound shock waves through the entire extended family. The disequilibrium created by this untimely death created stress and increased conflict between S and his wife. Called into question were many of S's and his wife's previously unacknowledged value conflicts, which stemmed from their very different religious backgrounds. Here, returning to the track of "right living" meant "working hard" to resolve these issues and to find new appreciation and affirmation of his spouse and marriage.

A second theme in S's personal mythology had to do with "directly challenging, rather than retreating, from confrontations, danger or risks." In S's family of origin, he was often verbally assailed, criticized, and threatened by his alcoholic father. S's response to these threats was to become frightened. Nevertheless, he would rush to meet this confrontation head on using a counterphobic defense. He would "not back down." To "back down" was to risk losing integrity and self-esteem. The same theme of challenge versus retreat that characterized S's encounter with his draft board and his wife were echoed in any threatening encounters with clients in therapy or with his own clinical supervisor (in supervision of supervision). These "risky" encounters had to be faced "head on" rather than avoided. To avoid them was to "stray from the path of right living."

The reader may have already begun to speculate about possible links between S's personal themes, Jennifer's, the supervisory encounters that took place between them, and the common themes that were replicated in the client-therapist subsystem. In the next section we outline our interpretation of how all of these themes merged to form their own supervisor-therapist-client mythological system.

Interface Between Therapist's and Supervisor's Mythological Themes

At the outset of Jennifer's training, S was preoccupied with the recent death of his brother-in-law and the subsequent crisis in his own marriage. This was a time when he felt less able and willing to press Jennifer emotionally and more comfortable maintaining a safe distance. Jennifer's emotionally disengaged style did not directly challenge or confront S at a time when he was emotionally vulnerable. The theme of not confronting emotionally vulnerable men was a familiar one in Jennifer's personal mythology. At the same time, S's behavior as supervisor reinforced rather than challenged Jennifer's preferred style of minimizing emotional expressiveness and confrontation with men who were too vulnerable. This, in turn, placed less pressure on Jennifer to deal more demonstratively with those clients who were unable or unwilling to express and explore their own angry emotional conflicts.

In supervision, Jennifer's behavior with conflict-avoiding clients was objectively discussed. Attention was given to the links between her own personal themes and her difficulty confronting these clients. Discussions about intervention strategies emphasized how she might use structural techniques to revise conflict-detouring interactional patterns. The emphasis was on strategies Jennifer could use to engage clients more personally to increase the emotional intensity in sessions. However, these discussions were themselves low in personal involvement and emotional intensity.

Initially, direct analysis of the supervisory relationship and its similarities to Jennifer's interactions with clients intensified both Jennifer's and S's anxiety, and was avoided. However, as S became more resolved about his own marriage, he was able to examine with his supervisor his own role in constraining the emotional intensity in the therapeutic system. As the links between his own behavior and Jennifer's personal themes were clarified, this information was introduced into the therapist-supervisor relationship. S was able to increase his personal involvement and encourage Jennifer to express her anxiety, anger, frustration, etc., as these feelings developed toward clients or himself.

We believe that in training and supervision, much as in the therapist-client encounter, the absence of a sufficient level of trust, relationship development, and personal involvement limits the potential for learning, growth, and development. It may be possible to teach trainees specific conceptual skills and intervention skills in the absence of this personal component. However, we believe that the development of relationship skills and the trainee's own personal growth are best facilitated in an environment of personal disclosure. The potential for trainees to accommodate their central themes to new information or to reorganize their central themes is enhanced when they experience the personal safety afforded by an accepting and open supervisory relationship.

As the training year came to a close, Jennifer was confronted with issues of termination. The supervisor-trainee relationship took center stage. Central themes in both S's and Jennifer's personal mythology became activated. For Jennifer, this involved two major issues. One was her unresolved feelings about the loss of her mother. The second was her freedom to challenge and confront male authorities who would be able to withstand her attack (she had perceived her father to be too weak ever since the loss of his wife).

For S, the themes of "termination (losses, endings) as personal turning points and chances to get back on track" (theme 1) and "direct challenge rather than retreat in the face of confrontation, danger or risk" (theme 2) became activated. Thus, it became "necessary" for S to deal directly with his own and Jennifer's feelings of loss rather than back away from them. To back down would have meant a loss of integrity, self-esteem, and a straying again from the track of right living. Thus, the termination became a opportunity for growth for both supervisor and therapist. It provided S with a chance to stay on track and an opportunity to rework past losses. Jennifer was able to directly challenge, confront, and experience a male authority who would accept her more intense feelings without collapse.

The changes in the supervisory relationship were replicated at the level of therapist-client subsystem. Here Jennifer was able to more effectively challenge and confront her clients and to tolerate their challenges and confrontations (both towards her and among themselves). The greater flexibility in the therapeutic system for accepting loss and expressing intense, negative affects enabled clients to experience a sense of closure in their termination or their transfer to a new therapist trainee.

Interface Between Therapists' and Clients' Mythological Themes

Understanding the relationship dynamics which come about as a result of the meshing of the therapists' and clients' mythological themes is an especially important component of our training and supervision of students and supervisees. The impasses which emerge because of such meshing of themes have been referred to as countertransference, therapist triangulation in the family system, or "being stuck in the system." The focal point in many of these formulations is the therapist's own contribution to maintaining the system's homeostasis. This is thought to be brought about by the therapist's own emotional "blind spots" and unresolved personal conflicts, which interfere with clients' therapeutic progress. While we are quite concerned about helping therapists to understand what may be *inhibiting* them or their clients from reaching their therapeutic goals, our mythological perspective also attends to the *positive potentials* presented by the interface between therapists' and clients' mythological themes.

The positive merging of therapist and client themes is illustrated in the case of a single-parent mother with two teenage daughters, aged 15 and 17. This woman (who had been sexually assaulted by her father when she was an adolescent) had organized much of her interpersonal style of life around themes of betrayal, isolation, and loss. When she finally got the courage to tell her mother of her father's abuse, she was accused of lying by both parents. She also perceived her two brothers as siding against her because they were unwilling to confront their father even though they knew he was lying. Years later, when her mother died in an automobile accident, she again felt betrayed and isolated because she had never been able to reestablish a relationship with her.

Themes of betrayal, isolation and loss were prevalent in her relationships with men. She had been abandoned by her husband shortly after the birth of her second daughter. Prior to beginning therapy, she had become engaged to a man with whom she had been living for several years. Just following his proposal of marriage, he unexpectedly decided to break off the relationship and moved out of her home.

When she came into treatment, the presenting problems were the younger daughter's sexual promiscuity and running away from home. The older daughter also had had frequent conflicts with the mother (e.g., staying out beyond curfew, disobedience at home, declining school grades). The problem behaviors of both daughters were viewed as efforts to protect mother (and themselves) from the pain and anxiety of the recent loss of mother's fiancé who had become an integral member of their household. For mother, this loss reactivated themes of loss, mistrust, and betrayal. The theme of loss was further compounded by the older daughter's impending graduation from high school and her plans to move out of the home.

The course of therapy with this family had been extremely stormy. The therapist had been involved in numerous crises involving both daughters' running away. The mother had, on a number of occasions, filed missing person reports on her younger daughter. These had resulted in the therapist's being called by the police when she was located. Eventually, mother filed charges against her daughter for theft of several of her possessions, and the therapist was asked to appear in court to give recommendations for the disposition of the case.

Throughout treatment, the therapist concentrated on themes of loss, past and impending. Much of the younger daughter's problem behavior was interpreted as being designed to bring attention to herself, thus allowing the older daughter to begin the process of leaving home. In fact, as the younger daughter's behavior worsened, the older daughter's behavior (relationship with mother, school grades, involvement in school activities) improved. However, the intensity of recurrent family crises necessitated putting this central theme aside while attending to the smaller "brush fires."

Over time, the therapist became more ambivalent about continuing his work with this family. He began to question whether any progress was being made and whether his life would be easier without these late night calls, emergency trips to the police station, visits to the school, and continued high level of tension in the family system.[3] When the daugh-

---

[3]In fact, over the course of therapy the mother had become more aware of the connections between her current grieving and her past unresolved losses, had reinstituted contact with her brothers after many years of being emotionally cutoff, found new activities outside of the home to engage in for her own pleasure, and begun to be more clear and firm in establishing and following through on limits for her daughters' behavior.

ter was tried for the theft of her mother's possessions, out-of-the-home placement was recommended by court personnel. However, the therapist argued for the continuation of outpatient treatment with legal sanctions for any further misbehavior. Even though residential placement would have allowed the therapist to disengage from the family, he continued to work with them on an outpatient basis. His decision to "hang in" with this family mirrored a central theme in his own personal mythology:

> It is important to persevere, to accept all challenges and requests for help without attention to personal limits or depleted resources. To refuse is to betray my family's expectation that I represent and live out their deeply held religious values. To refuse would also jeopardize my own sense of self as competent.

In fact, the therapist's parents (his mother in particular) had strongly urged him to become a minister. Although he had deviated somewhat from this consensus role image, his choice of a helping profession allowed him to fulfill a number of family role expectations. For this therapist, however, deviation from the consensus role image of "selfless giver" was equated with imperfection, incompetence, and failure.

In this instance, the meshing of the therapist's own personal theme and that of the mother produced growth for both of them. The mother was confronted with a male who did not play out a complementary role in the theme of "men who are unreliable and who are likely to leave or disappoint women when they are most needed." This new relationship experience offered the mother an opportunity to revise her view of significant men, and she began to develop a more open, trusting, and disclosing relationship with the therapist. This enabled her to explore her past disappointments and to understand her current family crises in terms of these unresolved themes of loss, separation, abandonment, and betrayal. The therapist gained insight into his own personal mythology and learned how to identify the parallels between his own personal themes and the presenting problems of his clients. He learned firsthand how this knowledge could facilitate the development of therapeutic relationships and serve as a catalyst for positive change.

The role of the supervisor throughout the treatment was to identify the parallel themes between the therapist's beliefs and his client's presenting problems and to sensitize the therapist as to how his own personal themes were affecting the treatment process. The supervisor remained alert to how the therapist may have been invoked into reenacting his own themes with clients and how this may have interfered with therapeutic progress. In addition, the supervisor served as a consultant and sounding board helping the therapist to select intervention strategies which could achieve the therapeutic goals. This involved specific strategies for dealing with the various "brush fires" that developed, supporting mother's efforts to establish firm and clear limits for her daughters' behavior, helping the older daughter begin to separate from home, and helping each family member to address the unresolved themes of loss, separation, and abandonment.

The above example also illustrates some growth-inhibiting potential when therapist and client themes merge. Another theme closely related to the therapist's theme of "hanging in and not letting go" involved the perceived *consequences* of letting go:

> If I complete something I undertake, I will be forced to "let go" of it and to evaluate my success or failure. Therefore, it is better to leave tasks, goals, etc., incomplete. This protects me from having to face failure, imperfection, or incompetence for not living up to others' and my own expectations.

This theme was especially evident in this therapist's graduate school training. He had completed nearly all degree requirements but still had several courses listed as incomplete. Prior to making up these incompletes, he took on a full-time job in order to meet family commitments. These all made completion of his courses more difficult. On a symbolic level, completing his masters degree meant acknowledging his departure from the ministry and his repudiation of his family's "consensus role image" for him. His "day of reckoning" would come, however, if he were accepted into a doctoral program. By not completing his course work, he was able to avoid the confrontation with family members that a firm commitment to an alternative career would produce.

In the above case example, if the therapist pushed for resolution of the conflicts that existed between himself and this mother, he risked becoming a failure in this mother's (and his own) eyes. Therefore, it was better to "hang in there" with her, remain available to the family in times of crisis, but not to address her feelings toward men (him). To do so would leave him vulnerable to his own fears of failing (the family could drop out of therapy, unleash a barrage of accusations, or express disappointment with him). Such outcomes would force him to evaluate his competence and degree of success or failure. He would then have to confront potential feelings of incompetence and imperfection, because he would not have given enough of himself to make a difference in this woman's life.

Inherent in the therapeutic process are the potentials for positive change for both the therapist and the client. However, there is also the potential for clinical and personal stasis. The interlocking themes of therapist and client systems (i.e., the mother, each mother-daughter subsystem, and the broader client family system) form their own mythological system. The complementary, reciprocal playing out of denied, projected elements of each participant's personal themes described earlier in our discussions of conjugal and family mythologies are also in operation here. We assume that the supervisor's ability to identify these relevant themes and to sensitize the therapist to his/her own contribution to the collusive therapist-client pact can help tip the balance in the direction of progress and growth as opposed to stagnation for both client and therapist. Of course, the supervisor's own personal themes also become involved in the process. These further elaborate the form and content of the therapeutic system.

References

Adler, A. (1968). *The practice and theory of individual psychology.* Totowa, NJ: Littlefield Adams.

Alexander, J. F., Barton, C., Schiavo, R., & Parsons, B. (1976). Systems-behavioral intervention with families of delinquents: Therapist characteristics, family behavior and outcome. *Journal of Consulting and Clinical Psychology, 44,* 656–664.

Alexander, F., & French, T. M. (1946). *Psychoanalytic therapy.* New York: Ronald Press.

Allman, G., & Toler, D. (1980). *The Allman Band: Reach for the sky.* (Cassette recording no. 9535). New York: Arista Records and Tapes.

Andersen, T. (1987). The reflecting team: Dialogue and metadialogue in clinical work. *Family Process, 26,* 415–428.

Anderson, S. A. (1986). Cohesion, adaptability and communication: A test of an Olson circumplex model hypothesis. *Family Relations, 35,* 289–293.

Anderson, S. A., Atilano, R. B., Paff-Bergen, L., Russell, C. S., & Jurich, A. P. (1985). Intervention strategies, spouses' perceptions and dropping out of marital and family therapy. *American Journal of Family Therapy, 13,* 39–54.

Anderson, S. A., & Bagarozzi, D. A. (1983). The use of family myths as an aid to strategic therapy. *Journal of Family Therapy, 5,* 145–154.

Anderson, S. A., & Bagarozzi, D. A. (1989). Family myths: An introduction. *Journal of Psychotherapy and the Family, 4,* 3–16.

Anderson, S. A., Bagarozzi, D. A., & Giddings, C. W. (1986). IMAGES: Preliminary scale construction. *American Journal of Family Therapy, 14,* 357–363.

Anderson, S. A., & Fleming, W. M. (1986a). Late adolescents' home-leaving strategies: Predicting ego identity and college adjustment. *Adolescence, 21,* 453–459.

Anderson, S. A., & Fleming, W. M. (1986b). Late adolescents' identity formation: Individuation from the family of origin. *Adolescence, 21,* 785–796.

Anderson, S. A., & Russell, C. S. (1982). Utilizing process and content in designing paradoxical interventions. *American Journal of Family Therapy, 10,* 48–60.

Anderson, S. A., Russell, C. S., & Schumm, W. R. (1983). Perceived marital quality and family life-cycle categories: A further analysis. *Journal of Marriage and the Family, 45,* 127–139.

Ashby, R. W. (1954). The application of cybernetics to psychology. *Journal of Mental Science, 100,* 114–124.

Bagarozzi, D. A. (1981). The symbolic meaning of behaviors exchanged in marital therapy. In A. S. Gurman (Ed.), *Practical problems in family therapy.* New York: Brunner/Mazel.

Bagarozzi, D. A. (1982a). The symbolic meaning of behaviors exchanged in marital therapy. In A. S. Gurman (Ed.), *Questions and answers in the practice of family therapy.* New York: Brunner/Mazel.

Personal, Marital, and Family Myths

Bagarozzi, D. A. (1982b). Family therapy with violent families. *American Journal of Family Therapy, 10,* 69–72.

Bagarozzi, D. A. (1982c). The family therapist's role in treating families in rural areas. *Journal of Marital and Family Therapy, 8,* 51–58.

Bagarozzi, D. A. (1983a). Contingency contracting for structural and process changes in family systems. In L. A. Wolberg & M. L. Aronson (Eds.), *Group and family therapy 1982: An overview.* New York: Brunner/Mazel.

Bagarozzi, D. A. (1983b). Methodological developments in measuring social exchange perceptions in marital dyads (SIDCARB): A new tool for clinical interventions. In D. A. Bagarozzi, A. P. Jurich, & R. W. Jackson (Eds.), *Marital and family therapy: New perspectives in theory, research and practice.* New York: Human Sciences Press.

Bagarozzi, D. A. (1983c). A cognitive-sociobehavioral model of clinical social work practice and evaluation. *Clinical Social Work Journal, 11,* 164–177.

Bagarozzi, D. A. (1985). Implications of social skills training for social and interpersonal competence. In L. L'Abate and M. Milan (Eds.), *Handbook of social skills training and research.* New York: Wiley.

Bagarozzi, D. A. (1986). Premarital therapy. In F. P. Piercy & D. Sprenkle (Eds.), *Family therapy sourcebook.* New York: Guilford.

Bagarozzi, D. A. (1987). Marital/family developmental theory as a context for understanding and treating inhibited sexual desire. *Journal of Sex and Marital Therapy, 13,* 276–285.

Bagarozzi, D. A. (1988). Family myths: Some diagnostic guidelines. *Family Therapy Today, 4,* 1–5.

Bagarozzi, D. A. (in press). Spousal inventory of desired changes and relationship barriers (SIDCARB). In B. Perlmutter, M. Straus, & J. Touliatos (Eds.), *Handbook of family measurement techniques.* New York: Sage.

Bagarozzi, D. A., & Anderson, S. (1982). The evolution of family mythological systems: Considerations for meaning, clinical assessment, and treatment. *Journal of Psychoanalytic Anthropology, 5,* 71–90.

Bagarozzi, D. A., & Anderson, S. A. (1989). Personal, conjugal and family myths: Theoretical, empirical and clinical developments. *Journal of Psychotherapy and the Family, 4,* 167–194.

Bagarozzi, D. A., & Atilano, R. B. (1982). SIDCARB: A clinical tool for rapid assessment of social exchange inequities and relationship barriers. *Journal of Sex and Marital Therapy, 8,* 325–334.

Bagarozzi, D. A., & Bagarozzi, J. I. (1982). A theoretically derived model of premarital intervention: The making of a family system. *Clinical Social Work Journal, 10,* 52–56.

Bagarozzi, D. A., Bagarozzi, J. I., Anderson, S. A., & Pollane, L. (1984). Premarital education and training sequence (PETS): A 3-year follow-up of an experimental study. *Journal of Counseling and Development, 63,* 91–100.

Bagarozzi, D. A., & Giddings, C. W. (1982). A conceptual model for understanding and treating marital violence. *Arete, 7,* 49–59.

Bagarozzi, D. A., & Giddings, C. W. (1983a). Conjugal violence: A critical review of current research and clinical practices. *American Journal of Family Therapy, 11,* 3–15.

Bagarozzi, D. A., & Giddings, C. W. (1983b). The role of cognitive constructs and attributional processes in family therapy: Integrating intrapersonal, interpersonal and systems dynamics. In L. A. Wolberg & M. L. Aronson (Eds.), *Group and Family Therapy 1983: An Overview.* New York: Brunner/Mazel.

Bagarozzi, D. A., & Pollane, L. (1983). A replication and validation of the Spousal Inventory of Desired Changes and Relationship Barriers (SIDCARB): Elaborations on diagnostic and clinical utilization. *Journal of Sex and Marital Therapy, 9,* 303–315.

Bagarozzi, D. A., & Rauen, P. (1981). Premarital counseling: Appraisal and status. *American Journal of Family Therapy, 9,* 13–30.

Bagarozzi, D. A., & Wodarski, J. S. (1977). A social exchange typology of conjugal relationships and conflict development. *Journal of Marriage and Family Counseling, 3,* 53–60.

Bagarozzi, D. A., & Wodarski, J. S. (1978). Behavioral treatment of marital discord. *Clinical Social Work Journal, 6*, 135–154.

Bandura, A. (1977). Self-efficacy: Toward a unifying theory of behavioral change. *Psychological Review, 84*, 191–215.

Barton, C., & Alexander, J. F. (1977). Therapists' skills as determinants of effective systems-behavioral family therapy. *International Journal of Family Counseling, 5*, 11–20.

Bateson, G. (1935). Culture, contact and schismogenesis. *Man, 35*, 148–183.

Bateson, G. (1936). *Naven*. Cambridge: Cambridge University Press.

Bateson, G. (1949). Bali: The value system of a steady state. In M. Fortes (Ed.), *Social structure: Studies presented to A. R. Radcliffe-Brown*. Oxford: Clarendon Press.

Bateson, G. (1961). The biosocial integration of behavior in the schizophrenic family. In N. W. Ackerman, F. C. Beatman, & S. N. Sherman (Eds.), *Exploring the base for family therapy*. New York: Family Service Association.

Bateson, G. (1972). *Steps to an ecology of mind*. New York: Ballantine Books.

Bateson, G., Jackson, D. D., Haley, J., & Weakland, J. (1956). Toward a theory of schizophrenia. *Behavioral Science, 1*, 251–264.

Beavers, W. R., & Voeller, M. N. (1983). Comparing and contrasting the Olson circumplex model with the Beavers' system model. *Family Process, 22*, 85–97.

Beck, A. T. (1987). Cognitive therapy. In J. K. Zeig (Ed.), *The evolution of psychotherapy*. New York: Brunner/Mazel.

Beck, A. T., Rush, A. J., Shaw, B. F., & Emery, G. (1979). *Cognitive Therapy of Depression*. New York: Guilford Press.

Berenson, D. (1987). Alcoholics anonymous: From surrender to transformation. *Family Therapy Networker, 11*, 24–31.

Bergin, A. E., & Garfield, S. L. (1971). *Handbook of psychotherapy and behavior change*. New York: John Wiley.

Bertalanffy, L. von (1968). *General systems theory*. New York: George Braziller.

Bettelheim, B. (1976). *The uses of enchantment: The meaning and importance of fairy tales*. New York: Knopf.

Bienvennu, M. J. (1978). *A counselor's guide to accompany a marital communication inventory*. Saluda: Family Life.

Birdwhistell, R. L. (1970). The idealized model of the American family. *Social Casework*, April, 195–198.

Blos, P. (1962). The second individuation process of adolescence. *The Psychoanalytic Study of the Child, 25*, 162–185.

Boszormenyi-Nagy, I., & Sparks, G. M. (1973). *Invisible loyalties*. New York: Harper & Row.

Bowen, M. (1978). *Family therapy in clinical practice*. New York: Jason Aronson.

Bray, J., Williamson, D., & Malone, P. (1984). Personal authority in the family system: Development of a questionnaire to measure personal authority in intergenerational family processes. *Journal of Marital and Family Therapy, 10*, 167–178.

Breunlin, D. C., Schwartz, R. C., Krause, M. S., & Selby, L. M. (1983). Evaluating family therapy training: The development of an instrument. *Journal of Marital and Family Therapy, 9*, 37–47.

Brock, G. W. (1986). Beavers-Timverlawn Family Evaluation Scale. *American Journal of Family Therapy, 14*, 271–273.

Broverman, I. K., Vogel, S. R., & Broverman, D. M. (1972). Sex-role stereotypes: A current appraisal. *Journal of Social Issues, 28*, 59–78.

Buckley, W. (1967). *Sociology and modern systems theory*. Englewood Cliffs, NJ: Prentice Hall.

Buckley, W. (1968). *Modern systems research for the behavioral scientist*. Chicago: Aldine.

Burgess, A. W., & Holstrom, L. L. (1974). *Rape: Victims and crisis*. Bowie, MD: Robert J. Brady.

Burgess, E. W., & Locke, H. H. (1945). *The family: From institution to companionship*. New York: American Book.

Burton, G., & Kaplan, H. (1968). Group counseling in conflicted marriages where alcoholism is present: Clients' evaluation of effectiveness. *Journal of Marriage and the Family, 30,* 74–79.

Byng-Hall, J. (1973). Family myths used as defense in conjoint family therapy. *British Journal of Medical Psychology, 46,* 239–250.

Campbell, J. (1949). *The hero with a thousand faces.* New York: Pantheon Books.

Carkhuff, R. R. (1969). *Helping and human relations: A primer for lay and professional helpers (Vol. I): Selection and training.* New York: Holt, Rinehart & Winston.

Chodorow, N. (1978). *The reproduction of mothering.* Berkeley: University of California Press.

Church, C. D. (1975). Myth and history as complementary modes of consciousness. In L. W. Gibbs & W. T. Stevenson (Eds.), *Myth and the crisis of historical consciousness.* Missoula, MT: Scholars Press.

Cleghorn, J., & Levin, S. (1973). Training family therapists by setting learning objectives. *American Journal of Orthopsychiatry, 43,* 439–446.

Constantine, L. (1976). Designed experience: A multiple goal-directed training program in family therapy. *Family Process, 15,* 373–396.

Coomaraswamy, A. K. (1916). *Buddha and the gospel of Buddhism.* New York: G. P. Putnam's Sons.

Corrales, R. G., Kostoryz, J., Rotrock, L., & Smith, B. (1983). Family therapy with developmentally delayed children: An ecosystemic approach. In D. A. Bagarozzi, A. P. Jurich & R. Jackson (Eds.), *Marital and family therapy: New perspectives in theory, research and practice.* New York: Human Sciences Press.

Dicks, H. V. (1967). *Marital tensions: Clinical studies toward a psychological theory of interaction.* London: Routledge and Kegan Paul.

Dimond, S. J. (1972). *The double brain.* New York: Churchill-Livingstone.

Duval, E. M. (1977). *Marriage and family development.* Philadelphia: J. B. Lippincott.

Eccles, J. C. (1973). *The understanding of the brain.* New York: McGraw-Hill.

Edcoa Productions, Inc. (1976). *Sensate focus I, II, III, IV.* San Francisco, CA.

Eliade, M. (1960). *Myths, dreams and mysteries.* Harvill Press.

Ellis, A. (1962). *Reason and emotion in psychotherapy.* New York: Lyle Stuart.

Ellis, A. (1970). *The essence of rational psychotherapy: A comprehensive approach to treatment.* New York: Institute for Rational Living.

Ellis, A. (1973). *Humanistic psychotherapy: The rational-emotive approach.* New York: Julian Press.

Ellis, A. (1987). The evolution of rational-emotive therapy (RET) and cognitive behavior therapy (CBT). In J. K. Zeig (Ed.), *The evolution of psychotherapy.* New York: Brunner/Mazel.

Ellis, A., & Grieger, R. (1977). *Handbook of rational-emotive therapy.* New York: Springer.

Epstein, H. B., Bishop, D. S., & Levin, S. (1978). The McMaster model of family functioning. *Journal of Marriage and Family Counseling, 4,* 19–31.

Ericson, P. M., & Rogers, L. W. (1973). New procedures for analyzing relational communication. *Family Process, 12,* 245–267.

Erikson, E. (1950). *Childhood and society.* New York: Norton.

Erikson, E. (1959). *Identity and the life cycle.* New York: International Universities Press.

Erikson, E. (1968). *Identity: Youth and crisis.* New York: Norton.

Erikson, E. (1974). *Dimensions of a new identity.* New York: Norton.

Falicov, C., Constantine, J., & Breunlin, D. C. (1981). Teaching family therapy: A program based on training objectives. *Journal of Marital and Family Therapy, 7,* 497–506.

Feinstein, A. D. (1979). Personal mythology as a paradigm for a holistic public psychology. *American Journal of Orthopsychiatry, 49,* 198–217.

Ferreira, A. (1963). Family myth and homeostasis. *Archives of General Psychiatry, 9,* 457–463.

Ferreira, A. J. (1966). Family myths. *Psychiatric Research Reports of the American Psychiatric Association, 20,* 85–90.

Finkelhor, D. (1978). Psychological, cultural and family factors in incest and family sexual abuse. *Journal of Marriage and Family Counseling, 4*, 41–50.

Finkelhor, D. (1984). *Child sexual abuse: New theory and research*. New York: Free Press.

Fisch, R., Weakland, J. H., & Segal, L. (1983). *The tactics of change*. San Francisco: Jossey-Bass.

Flavell, J. H. (1963). *The developmental psychology of Jean Piaget*. Princeton, NJ: Van Nostrand.

Flavell, J. H. (1985). *Cognitive development* (2nd Ed.). Englewood Cliffs, NJ: Prentice-Hall.

Fleming, W. M., & Anderson, S. A. (1986). Individuation from the family of origin and personal adjustment in late adolescence. *Journal of Marital and Family Therapy, 12*, 311–315.

Fogarty, T. F. (1976). Systems concepts and the dimensions of self. In P. Guerin (Ed.), *Family therapy: Theory and practice*. New York: Gardner Press.

Fontenrose, J. (1966). *The ritual theory of myth*. Berkeley: University of California Press.

Ford, D. H., & Urban, H. B. (1963). *Systems of psychotherapy: A comparative study*. New York: John Wiley.

Forgus, R., & Shulman, B. (1979). *Personality: A cognitive view*. Englewood Cliffs, NJ: Prentice-Hall.

Frank, E., Anderson, C., & Rubinstein, D. (1980). Marital role ideals and perceptions of marital role behavior in distressed and nondistressed couples. *Journal of Marital and Family Therapy, 6*, 55–63.

Frazer, J. G. (1942). *The golden bough: A study in magic and religion*. New York: MacMillan.

Freud, S. (1913). *The interpretation of dreams*. New York: Macmillan.

Freud, S. (1927). *The ego and the id*. London: Institute of Psychoanalysis and Hogarth Press.

Freud, S. (1963a). Obsessive acts and religious practices. In P. Rieff (Ed. and Trans.), *The collected papers of Sigmund Freud* (Vol. 9, pp. 17–26). New York: Collier Books (original work published 1907).

Freud, S. (1963b). The unconscious. In P. Rieff (Ed. and Trans.), *The collected papers of Sigmund Freud* (Vol. 6, pp. 116–150). New York: Collier Books (original work published 1915).

Fromm, E. (1951). *The forgotten language: An introduction to the understanding of dreams, fairy tales and myths*. New York: Grove Press.

Garfield, R. (1979). An integrative training model for family therapists: The Hahnemann master of family therapy program. *Journal of Marital and Family Therapy, 5*, 15–22.

Garrigan, J., & Bambrick, A. (1977). Introducing novice therapists to "go-between" techniques of family therapy. *Family Process, 16*, 237–246.

Gavazzi, S. M., & Anderson, S. A. (1987). The role of "translator" in the case transfer process. *American Journal of Family Therapy, 15*, 145–157.

Gazda, G. M., Asbury, F. R., Balzer, F. J., Childers, W. C., & Walters, R. P. (1977). *Human relations development: A manual for educators*. Boston: Allyn & Bacon.

Gennep, A. van. (1960). *The rites of passage*. London: Routledge and Kegan Paul.

Goldner, V. (1988). Generation and gender: Normative and covert hierarchies. *Family Process, 27*, 17–31.

Goode, W. J. (1962). Marital satisfaction and instability: A crosscultural comparison of divorce rates. *International Social Science Journal, 14*, 507–526.

Graves, R. (1955a). *The Greek myths* (vol. 1). Baltimore: Penguin.

Graves, R. (1955b). *The Greek myths* (vol. 2). Baltimore: Penguin.

Grotstein, J. (1981). *Splitting and projective identification*. New York: Aronson.

Guerin, P. J., & Guerin, K. B. (1976). Theoretical aspects and clinical relevance of the multigenerational model of family therapy. In P. Guerin (Ed.), *Family therapy: Theory and practice*. New York: Gardner Press.

Guerin, P. J., & Pendagast, E. G. (1976). Evaluation of family system and genogram. In P. Guerin (Ed.), *Family Therapy: Theory and practice*. New York: Gardner Press.

Gunderson, J. G., & Singer, M. T. (1975). Defining borderline patients: An overview. *American Journal of Psychiatry, 132*, 1–9.

Gurman, A. S., & Kniskern, D. P. (1978). Research on marital and family therapy: Progress, perspective and prospect. In S. Garfield & A. Bergin (Eds.), *Handbook of psychotherapy and behavior change*. New York: Wiley.

Gurman, A. S., & Kniskern, D. P. (1981). Family therapy outcome research: Knowns and unknowns. In A. S. Gurman and D. P. Kniskern (Eds.), *Handbook of family therapy*. New York: Brunner/Mazel.

Haley, J. (1963). *Strategies of psychotherapy*. New York: Grune & Stratton.

Haley, J. (1964). Research on family patterns: An instrument measurement. *Family Process, 3*, 41–65.

Haley, J. (1973). *Uncommon therapy*. New York: Norton.

Haley, J. (1976). *Problem solving therapy*. San Francisco: Jossey-Bass.

Haley, J. (1980). *Leaving home*. New York: McGraw-Hill.

Haley, J. (1985). *Ordeal therapy*. San Francisco: Jossey-Bass.

Hart, O. van der, Witzum, E., & De Voogt, A. (1989). Myths and rituals: Anthropological views and their application in strategic family therapy. *Journal of Psychotherapy and the Family, 4*, 57–80.

Hawkins, J. L., & Johnsen, K. (1969). Perception of behavioral conformity, imputation of consensus and marital satisfaction. *Journal of Marriage and the Family, 31*, 507–511.

Hesse, H. (1951). *Siddhartha*. New York: New Directions.

Hess, R. D., & Handel, G. (1959). *Family worlds: A psychosocial approach to family life*. Chicago: University of Chicago Press.

Hoffman, L. (1981). *Foundations of family therapy*. New York: Basic Books.

Hoffman, L. (1985). Beyond power and control: Toward a "second order" family systems therapy. *Family Systems Medicine, 3*, 381–396.

Inhelder, B., & Piaget, J. (1958). *The growth of logical thinking from childhood to adolescence* (A. Parsons & S. Seagrin, trans.). New York: Basic Books.

Jackson, D. D. (1959). Family interaction, family homeostasis, and some implications for conjoint family psychotherapy. In J. Masserman (Ed.), *Individual and familial dynamics*. New York: Grune & Stratton.

Jackson, D. D. (1965). The study of the family. *Family Process, 4*, 1–20.

Jacobson, E. (1964). *The self and the object world*. New York: International Universities Press.

Jacobson, N. S., & Margolin, G. (1979). *Marital therapy: Strategies based on social learning and behavior exchange principles*. New York: Brunner/Mazel.

Jung, C. G. (1940). *The integration of the personality*. London: Kegan Paul.

Jung, C. G. (1951). Aion: Researches into the phenomenology of the self. In H. Read, M. Fordham, & G. Adler (Eds.), *The collected works of C. G. Jung* (Vol. 9). London: Routledge and Kegan Paul.

Jung, C. G. (1953). Two essays on analytical psychology. In H. Read, M. Fordham & G. Adler (Eds.), *The collected works of C. G. Jung* (Vol. 7). London: Routledge and Kegan Paul.

Jung, C. G. (1954). The development of personality. In H. Read, M. Fordham & G. Adler (Eds.), *The collected works of C. G. Jung* (Vol. 17). London: Routledge and Kegan Paul.

Jung, C. G. (1956). Symbols of transformation. In H. Read, M. Fordham & G. Adler (Eds.), *The collected works of C. G. Jung* (Vol. 5). London: Routledge and Kegan Paul.

Jung, C. G. (1959). The archetypes of the collective unconscious. In H. Read, M. Fordham & G. Adler (Eds.), *The collected works of C. G. Jung* (Vol. 9). London: Routledge and Kegan Paul.

Jung, C. G. (1960). The structure and dynamics of the psyche. In H. Read, M. Fordham & G. Adler (Eds.), *The collected works of C. G. Jung* (Vol. 8). London: Routledge and Kegan Paul.

Jung, C. G. (1961). Freud and psychoanalysis. In H. Read, M. Fordham & G. Adler (Eds.), *The collected works of C. G. Jung* (Vol. 4). London: Routledge and Kegan Paul.

Jung, C. G. (1973). Experimental research. In H. Read, M. Fordham & G. Adler (Eds.), *The collected works of C. G. Jung* (Vol. 2). London: Routledge and Kegan Paul.

Jung, C., & Kerenyi, C. (1950). Essays on a science of mythology: The myth of the divine child and the mysteries of Elessis. In H. Read, M. Fordham & G. Adler (Eds.), *The collected works of C. G. Jung* (Vol. 9). London: Routledge and Kegan Paul.

Kaplan, L. (1980). *Rapproachment and oedipal organization: Effects on borderline phenomena in rapproachment.* New York: Jason Aronson.

Keeney, B. P. (1982). What is an epistemology of family therapy? *Family Process, 21,* 153–168.

Keim, I., Lentine, G., Keim, J., & Madanes, C. (1987). Strategies for the past. *Journal of Strategic and Systemic Therapies, 6,* 2–17.

Kelly, G. A. (1955). *A theory of personality: The psychology of personal constructs.* New York: Norton.

Kernberg, O. (1967). Borderline personality organization. *Journal of the American Psychoanalytic Association, 15,* 641–685.

Kernberg, O. (1968). The treatment of patients with borderline personality organization. *International Journal of Psychoanalysis, 49,* 600–619.

Kernberg, O. (1970). A psychoanalytic classification of character pathology. *Journal of the American Psychoanalytic Association, 18,* 800–822.

Kernberg, O. (1974a). Contrasting viewpoints regarding the nature and psychoanalytic treatment of narcissistic personalities: A preliminary communication. *Journal of the American Psychoanalytic Association, 22,* 255–267.

Kernberg, O. (1974b). Further considerations of the treatment of narcissistic personalities. *International Journal of Psychoanalysis, 55,* 215–240.

Kernberg, O. (1975). *Borderline conditions and pathological narcissism.* New York: Jason Aronson.

Kernberg, O. (1978). Contrasting approaches to the psychotherapy of borderline conditions. In J. Masterson (Ed.), *New perspectives in the psychotherapy of the borderline adult.* New York: Brunner/Mazel.

Kernberg, O. (1980). *Rapproachment.* New York: Jason Aronson.

Klein, M. (1932). *The psychoanalysis of children.* London: Hogarth.

Klein, M. (1975). *Envy and gratitude and other works 1946–1963.* New York: Delacorte Press.

Knox, J. (1904). *Myth and truth.* Charlottesville: University of Virginia.

Kobak, R. R., & Waters, D. B. (1984). Family therapy as a right of passage: The play's the thing. *Family Process, 23,* 89–100.

Koestler, A. (1978). *Janus: A summing up.* New York: Vintage.

Kohlberg, L. (1963). Moral development and identification. In H. Stevenson (Ed.), *Child psychology: 62nd yearbook of the National Society for the Study of Education.* Chicago: University of Chicago Press.

Kohlberg, L. (1964). Development of moral character and moral ideology. In M. L. Hoffman, & L. W. Hoffman (Eds.), *Review of child development research* (vol. 1). New York: Sage.

Kohlberg, L. (1966). A cognitive developmental analysis of childrens' sex role concepts and attitudes. In E. E. Maccoby (Ed.), *The development of sex differences.* Stanford, CA: Stanford University Press.

Kohlberg, L. (1969). Stage and sequence: The cognitive developmental approach to socialization. In D. Goslin (Ed.), *Handbook of socialization theory and research.* Chicago: Rand McNally.

Kohut, H. (1965). Autonomy and integration. *Journal of the American Psychoanalytic Association, 13,* 851–856.

Kohut, H. (1966). Forms and tranformations of narcissism. *Journal of the American Psychoanalytic Association, 14,* 243–272.

Kohut, H. (1968). The psychoanalytic treatment of narcissistic personality disorders. *The Psychoanalytic Study of the Child, 23,* 86–113.

Kohut, H. (1969). Panel on narcissistic resistance. *Journal of the American Psychoanalytic Association, 17,* 941–954.
Kohut, H. (1971). *The analysis of the self.* New York: International Universities Press.
Kohut, H. (1977). *The restoration of the self.* New York: International Universities Press.
Kolodny, R. C., Masters, W. H., & Johnson, V. (1979). *Textbook of sexual medicine.* Boston: Little, Brown.
L'Abate, L., & Milan, M. (Eds.). (1985). *Handbook of social skills training and research.* New York: Wiley.
Lankton, S. R., & Lankton, C. H. (1983). *The answer within: A clinical framework of Ericksonian hypnotherapy.* New York: Brunner/Mazel.
Lapierre, K. (1979). Family therapy training at the Ackerman Institute: Thoughts of form and substance. *Journal of Marital and Family Therapy, 5,* 53–58.
Lewis, R. (1972). A developmental framework for the analysis of premarital dyadic formation. *Family Process, 11,* 17–48.
Lewis, R. A., & Spanier, G. B. (1979). Theorizing about the quality and stability of marriage. In W. R. Burr, R. Hill, F. I. Nye, & I. L. Reiss (Eds.), *Contemporary Theories About the Family, Vol. I.* London: Free Press.
Lidz, T., Cornelison, A. R., Fleck, S., & Terry, D. (1957). Schism and skew in families of schizophrenics. *American Journal of Psychiatry, 64,* 241–248.
Liddle, H. A., Breunlin, D. C., Schwartz, R. C., & Constantine, D. C. (1984). Training family therapy supervisors: Issues of content, form and context. *Journal of Marital and Family Therapy, 10,* 139–150.
Lorion, R. P. (1978). Research on psychotherapy and behavior change with the poor. In S. L. Garfield & A. E. Bergin (Eds.), *Handbook of psychotherapy and behavior change: An empirical analysis.* New York: Wiley.
Luckey, E. (1960a). Marital satisfaction and congruent self-spouse concepts. *Social Forces, 39,* 153–157.
Luckey, E. (1960b). Marital satisfaction and its association with congruency of perception. *Marriage and Family Living, 22,* 49–54.
Mahler, M. S. (1963). Thoughts about development and individuation. *The Psychoanalytic Study of the Child, 18,* 307–324.
Mahler, M. S. (1965). On the significance of the normal separation-individuation phase. In M. Schur (Ed.), *Drives, affects and behavior,* (vol. 2). New York: International Universities Press.
Mahler, M. S., & Kaplan, L. (1977). Developmental aspects in the assessment of narcissistic and so-called borderline personalities. In P. Hartocollis (Ed.), *Borderline personality disorders: The concept, the syndrome, the patient.* New York: International Universities Press.
Mahler, M. S., & La Perriere, K. (1965). Mother-child interaction during separation-individuation. *Psychoanalytic Quarterly, 34,* 483–498.
Mahler, M. S., & McDevitt, J. (1968). Observations on adaptation and defense in statu nascendi. *Psychoanalytic Quarterly, 37,* 1–21.
Mahler, M. S., Pine, F., & Bergman, A. (1970). The mother's reaction to her toddler's drive for individuation. In E. J. Anthony & T. Benedek (Eds.), *Parenthood: Its psychology and psychopathology.* Boston: Little, Brown.
Mahoney, M. (1974). *Cognition and behavior modification.* Cambridge, MA: Ballinger Publishing Co.
Maslow, A. (1954). *Motivation and personality.* New York: Harper & Row.
Maslow, A. (1962). *Toward a psychology of being.* New York: Van Nostrand.
Masters, V. & Johnson, W. (1970). *Human sexual inadequacy.* New York: Bantam Books.
Masterson, J. F. (1972). *Treatment of the borderline adolescent: A developmental approach.* New York: John Wiley.
Masterson, J. F. (1975). The splitting defense mechanism of the borderline adolescent: Developmental and clinical aspects. In J. Mack (Ed.), *Borderline states.* New York: Grune & Stratton.

Masterson, J. F. (1981). *The narcissistic and borderline disorders: An integrated approach*. New York: Brunner/Mazel.

Masterson, J. F. (1985). *The real self: A developmental, self and object relations approach*. New York: Brunner/Mazel.

Masterson, J. F., & Costello, J. (1980). *From borderline adolescent to functioning adult: The test of time*. New York: Brunner/Mazel.

McGoldrick, M., & Gerson, R. (1985). *Genograms in family assessment*. New York: Norton.

Meichenbaum, D. (1977). *Cognitive-Behavior Modification*. New York: Plenum Press.

Mezydlo, L., Wauck, L., & Foley, J. (1973). The clergy as marriage counselors: A service revisited. *Journal of Religion and Health, 22,* 278–288.

Miller, J. G. (1971a). Living systems: The group. *Behavioral Science, 16,* 302–398.

Miller, J. G. (1971b). The nature of living systems. *Behavioral Science, 16,* 277–291.

Minuchin, S. (1974). *Families and family therapy*. Cambridge, MA: Harvard University Press.

Moos, R., & Moos, B. (1981). *Family environment scale manual*. Palo Alto, CA: Counseling Psychologist Press.

Murray, H. A. (1938). *Explorations in personality*. New York: Oxford University Press.

Napier, A. Y., & Whitaker, C. A. (1978). *The family crucible*. New York: Harper & Row.

Neumann, E. (1954a). *The origins and history of consciousness* (vol. 1). New York: Harper & Row.

Neumann, E. (1954b). *The origins and history of consciousness: The psychological stages and the evolution of consciousness* (vol. 2). New York: Harper & Row.

Olson, D. H., & Killorin, E. (1985). *Clinical rating scale for the circumplex model*. St. Paul, MN: Family Social Science, University of Minnesota.

Olson, D. H., Portner, J., & Lavee, Y. (1985). *FACES III*. St. Paul, MN: Family Social Science, University of Minnesota.

Olson, D. H., Russell, C. S., & Sprenkle, D. H. (1983). Circumplex model of marital and family systems: VI theoretical update. *Family Process, 22,* 69–83.

Olson, D. H., Sprenkle, D. H., & Russell, C. S. (1979). Circumplex model of marital and family systems I: Cohesion and adaptability dimensions, family types and clinical applications. *Family Process, 18,* 3–28.

Papp, P. (1983). *The process of change*. New York: Guilford.

Patterson, G. R., & Hops, H. (1972). Coercion, a game for two: Intervention techniques for marital conflict. In R. C. Ulrich & P. Mountjoy (Eds.), *Behavior modification in clinical psychology*. New York: Appleton-Century-Crofts.

Pattison, E. M. (1976). The fatal myth of death in the family. *American Journal of Psychiatry, 133,* 674–678.

Perry, J. W. (1966). *The lord of the four quarters*. New York: George Braziller.

Piaget, J. (1926). *The language and thought of the child*. New York: Harcourt, Brace and World.

Piaget, J. (1928). *Judgement and reasoning in the child*. New York: Harcourt, Brace and World.

Piaget, J. (1929). *The child's conception of the world*. New York: Harcourt, Brace and World.

Piaget, J. (1930). *The child's conception of physical causality*. New York: Harcourt, Brace and World.

Piaget, J. (1932). *The moral judgement of the child*. New York: Harcourt, Brace and World.

Piaget, J. (1952). *The origins of intelligence in children*. New York: International Universities Press.

Piaget, J. (1954). *The construction of reality in the child*. New York: Basic Books.

Piaget, J. (1969). *The mechanisms of perception* (G. N. Seagrim, trans.). London: Routledge and Kegan Paul.

Piaget, J. (1977). *The development of thought: Equilibrium of cognitive structures*. (A. Rosin, Trans.). New York: Viking Press.

Piercy, F. P., Laird, R. A., & Mohammed, Z. (1983). A family therapist rating scale. *Journal of Marital and Family Therapy, 9,* 45–59.

Pincus, L., & Dare, C. (1978). *Secrets in the family.* New York: Pantheon Books.

Pinsof, W. M., & Catherall, D. R. (1986). The integrative psychotherapy alliance: Family, couple and individual therapy scales. *Journal of Marital and Family Therapy, 12,* 137–151.

Pleck, J. H. (1984). *The myth of masculinity.* Cambridge, MA: MIT Press.

Rappaport, A., & Harrell, J. (1972). A behavioral exchange model for marital counseling. *The Family Coordinator, 21,* 203–212.

Reiss, D. (1971). Varieties of consensual experience I: A theory for relating family interaction to individual thinking. *Family Process, 10,* 1–28.

Roberts, J. (1989). Mythmaking in the land of imperfect specialness: Lions, laundry baskets and cognitive deficits. *Journal of Psychotherapy and the Family, 4,* 81–110.

Rogers, C. (1951). *Client centered therapy.* Boston: Houghton Mifflin.

Rogers, C. (1957). The necessary and sufficient conditions of therapeutic personality change. *Journal of Consulting Psychology, 21,* 95–103.

Rogers, C. (1961). *On becoming a person.* Boston: Houghton Mifflin.

Rogers, L. E. (1972). Dyadic systems and transactional communication in a family context. Unpublished doctoral dissertation, Michigan State University.

Rogers, L. E., & Bagarozzi, D. A. (1983). An overview of relational communication and implications for therapy. In D. Bagarozzi, A. P. Jurich & R. Jackson (Eds.), *Marital and family therapy: New perspectives in theory, research and practice.* New York: Human Sciences Press.

Rosen, S. (1982). *My voice will go with you: The teaching tales of Milton H. Erickson.* New York: Norton.

Rossi, E. (Ed.) (1980). *Collected papers of Milton H. Erickson on hypnosis.* New York: Irvington.

Russell, C. S., Atilano, R. B., Anderson, S. A., Jurich, A. P., & Paff-Bergen, L. (1984). Intervention strategies: Predicting family therapy outcome. *Journal of Marital and Family Therapy, 10,* 241–251.

Ryder, R. R. (1987). The common dance. *Journal of Family Psychology, 1,* 66–76.

Sabatelli, R. M. (1984). The Marital Comparison Level Index: A measure for assessing outcomes relative to expectations. *Journal of Marriage and the Family, 46,* 651–662.

Sager, C. J. (1976). *Marriage contracts and couple therapy: Hidden forces in intimate relationships.* New York: Brunner/Mazel.

Satir, V. (1967). *Conjoint family therapy.* Palo Alto, CA: Science and Behavior Books.

Sattler, J. M. (1978). The effects of therapist-client racial similarity. In A. S. Gurman & A. M. Razin (Eds.), *Effective psychotherapy: A handbook of research.* New York: Pergamon.

Schmid, K. D., Rosenthal, S. L., & Brown, E. D. (1988). A comparison of self-report measures of two family dimensions: Control and cohesion. *American Journal of Family Therapy, 16,* 73–77.

Schulman, M. L. (1974). Idealization in engaged couples. *Journal of Marriage and the Family, 36,* 139–147.

Schumm, W. R., Figley, C. R., & Jurich, A. P. (1979). Dimensionality of the Marital Communication Inventory: A preliminary factor analytic study. *Psychological Reports, 45,* 123–128.

Seltzer, W. (1989). Myths of destruction: A cultural approach to families in therapy. *Journal of Psychotherapy and the Family, 4,* 17–34.

Seltzer, W. J., & Seltzer, M. R. (1983). Material, myth and magic: A cultural approach to family therapy. *Family Process, 22,* 3–14.

Selvini Palazzoli, M. (1986). Toward a general model of psychotic family games. *Journal of Marital and Family Therapy, 12,* 339–349.

Selvini Palazzoli, M., Boscolo, L., Cecchin, G., & Prata, G. (1977). Family rituals: A powerful tool in family therapy. *Family Process, 16,* 445–453.

Selvini Palazzoli, M., Boscolo, L., Cecchin, G., & Prata, G. (1978). A ritualized prescription in family therapy: Odd days and even days. *Journal of Marriage and Family Counseling, 4,* 3–9.

Selvini Palazzoli, M., Cirillo, S., Selvini, M., & Sorrentino, A. M. (1989). *Family games.* New York: Norton.

Shapiro, R. (1974). Therapist attitudes and premature termination in family and individual therapy. *Journal of Nervous and Mental Disease, 159,* 101–107.

Shapiro, R., & Budman, S. (1973). Defection, termination and continuation in family and individual therapy. *Family Process, 12,* 55–67.

Shaw, J., & Bagarozzi, D. A. (1986, April). The treatment of adult incest victims: Combining individual and marital therapy. Paper presented at the annual meeting of the American Association of Sex Educators, Counselors and Therapists, San Francisco.

Speer, D. C. (1971). Family systems: Morphostasis and morphogenesis, or is homeostasis enough? *Family Process, 9,* 259–278.

Stanton, M. D. (1981). An integrated structural/strategic approach to family therapy. *Journal of Marital and Family Therapy, 7,* 427–439.

Stevens, A. (1982). *Archetypes: A natural history of the self.* New York: William Morrow.

Stierlin, H. (1981). *Separating parents and adolescents.* New York: Jason Aronson.

Stone, M. H. (1980). *The borderline syndrome: Constitution, personality and adaptation.* New York: McGraw-Hill.

Strayhorn, J. M. (1978). Social exchange theory: Cognitive restructuring in marital therapy. *Family Process, 17,* 437–448.

Sullivan, H. S. (1953). *The interpersonal theory of psychiatry.* New York: Norton.

Sullivan, H. S. (1954). *The psychiatric interview.* New York: Norton.

Tharp, R. G. (1963). Psychological patterning in marriage. *Psychological Bulletin, 60,* 97–117.

Thomlinson, R. A. (1974). A behavioral model for social work intervention with the marital dyad. *Dissertation Abstracts International, 35,* 1227A.

Urban, H. B., & Ford, D. H. (1971). Some historical and conceptual perspectives on psychotherapy and behavior change. In A. E. Bergin & S. L. Garfield (Eds.), *Handbook of psychotherapy and behavior change.* New York: John Wiley.

Uyeshiba, K. (1958). *Aikido.* Tokyo: Kowado.

Vander Mey, B. J., & Neff, R. L. (1984). Adult-child incest: A sample of substantiated cases. *Family Relations, 33,* 549–557.

Waller, W., & Hill, R. (1951). *The family: A dynamic interpretation.* New York: Dryden.

Wamboldt, F. S., & Wolin, S. J. (1989). Reality and myth in family life. *Journal of Psychotherapy and the Family, 4,* 141–166.

Watts, A. (1954). *Myth and ritual in Christianity.* New York: Macmillan.

Watzlawick, P. (1978). *The language of change.* New York: Basic Books.

Watzlawick, P., Beavin, J. H., & Jackson, D. D. (1967). *Pragmatics of human communication.* New York: Norton.

Watzlawick, P., Weakland, J., & Fisch, R. (1974). *Change: Principles of problem formation and problem resolution.* New York: Norton.

Waxenberg, B. (1973). Therapists' empathy, regard and genuineness as factors in staying in or dropping out of short-term, time-limited family therapy. *Dissertation Abstracts International, 34,* 1288B.

Wheelwright, P. (1962). *Metaphor and reality.* Bloomington: Indiana University Press.

Williamson, D. (1981). Personal authority via termination of the intergenerational boundary: A "new" stage in the family life cycle. *Journal of Marital and Family Therapy, 7,* 441–452.

Williamson, D. (1982a). Personal authority via termination of the hierarchical boundary: Part II—the consultation process and the therapeutic method. *Journal of Marital and Family Therapy, 8,* 23–37.

Williamson, D. (1982b). Personal authority in family experience via termination of the intergenerational hierarchical boundary: Part III—Personal authority defined and the power of play in the change process. *Journal of Marital and Family Therapy, 8,* 309–323.

Winnicott, D. (1965). *The maturational process and the facilitating environment*. New York: International Universities Press.
Wolin, S. J., & Bennett, L. A. (1984). Family rituals. *Family Process, 23*, 401–420.
Wynne, L. C., Ryckoff, I. M., Day, J., & Hirsch, S. I. (1958). Pseudomutuality in the family relations of schizophrenics. *Psychiatry, 21*, 205–220.
Zeig, J. (1980). *A teaching seminar with Milton H. Erickson*. New York: Brunner/Mazel.
Zetzel, E. R. (1970). *The capacity for emotional growth*. New York: International Universities Press.

Index

abandonment, themes of, 26, 35, 48, 56–57, 80, 82, 134, 207, 294–97
"accommodation capacity" of myth, 25, 198
adaptability of family:
  definition of, 36
  see also Family Adaptability and Cohesion Scales III
Adler, A., 28
Aikido, 199
Alcoholics Anonymous, 200
alcoholism, 27, 29, 200–1, 291
Alexander, F., 50
Alexander, J. F., 275–76, 278
ambivalence:
  about intimacy, 56, 68, 70, 197, 279
  conflict and, 132–33
  of therapist, 295
  toward a child, 210, 272
analogies, in therapy, 62–63, 284
analytic psychology, 16
Anderson, C., 18
Anderson, S. A., 1, 15, 22, 28, 36, 57, 63, 86, 94, 100, 102, 206, 274, 276, 278, 286
anger avoidance, 289
anima archetype, 268
anxiety, 23, 26, 107, 134, 163, 247–48, 265
Asbury, F. R., 278
Ashby, R. W., 6
Atilano, R. B., 96, 278
autonomy, 63, 134–36, 170
  of child, 210, 240, 271
  of couple, 164–67

Bagarozzi, D. A., 1, 14, 15, 17, 22, 28, 35, 42, 43, 57, 63, 78–79, 82, 94, 96, 98, 99–102, 106, 114, 139, 150, 152, 156, 249, 277, 282

Bagarozzi, J. I., 28
Balzer, F. J., 278
Bambrick, A., 276, 278
Bandura, A., 45
barriers to divorce and separation:
  external, 97, 110–11, 140, 195, 239
  internal, 97, 110–11, 140, 195
Barton, C., 275–76, 278
basic needs, concept of, 72
Bateson, G., 96, 198, 201, 211
Beavers, W. R., 36
Beavin, J. H., 6, 96, 98, 162, 278
Beck, A. T., 16, 22–24, 50, 275
behavioral contracting, 246
behavioral exchanges, 150–52
behavioral indicators, 51, 137, 157
behavioral management techniques, 246
behavioral strategies, 66–68, 100, 101
Bennett, L. A., 14
Berenson, D., 198, 201
Bergin, A. E., *Handbook of Psychotherapy and Behavior Change: An Empirical Analysis*, 7
Bergman, A., 8
Bettelheim, B., 10, 22, 199
Bienvenu, M. J., 97
"binding centripetal force", 81
biofeedback, 100
Birdwhistell, Ray, 18
Bishop, D. S., 36
"bisociation", 198
Blos, P., 86
borderline personality disorder, 8, 26–27, 39, 50, 176, 256
Boscolo, L., 252
Boszormenyi-Nagy, I., 86
Bowen, M., 3, 56, 81, 84, 86
brain hemispheric functioning, 20–22

311